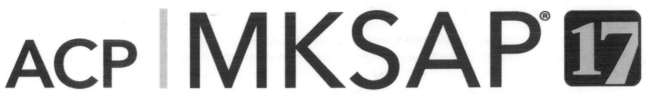

ACP | MKSAP® 17
Medical Knowledge Self Assessment Program®

Pulmonary and Critical Care Medicine

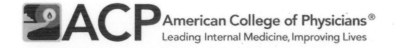
ACP American College of Physicians®
Leading Internal Medicine, Improving Lives

Welcome to the Pulmonary and Critical Care Medicine Section of MKSAP 17!

In these pages, you will find updated information on pulmonary diagnostic testing; airways disease; diffuse parenchymal lung disease; occupational lung disease; pleural disease; pulmonary vascular disease; lung tumors; sleep medicine; high-altitude–related illnesses; principles of ventilation in critical care; common ICU conditions, such as upper airway emergencies, respiratory failure, sepsis, anaphylaxis, and toxicologic emergencies; and other clinical challenges. All of these topics are uniquely focused on the needs of generalists and subspecialists *outside* of pulmonary and critical care medicine.

The publication of the 17th edition of Medical Knowledge Self-Assessment Program (MKSAP) represents nearly a half-century of serving as the gold-standard resource for internal medicine education. It also marks its evolution into an innovative learning system to better meet the changing educational needs and learning styles of all internists.

The core content of MKSAP has been developed as in previous editions—newly generated, essential information in 11 topic areas of internal medicine created by dozens of leading generalists and subspecialists and guided by certification and recertification requirements, emerging knowledge in the field, and user feedback. MKSAP 17 also contains 1200 all-new, psychometrically validated, and peer-reviewed multiple-choice questions (MCQs) for self-assessment and study, including 103 in Pulmonary and Critical Care Medicine. MKSAP 17 continues to include *High Value Care* (HVC) recommendations, based on the concept of balancing clinical benefit with costs and harms, with links to MCQs that illustrate these principles. In addition, HVC Key Points are highlighted in the text. Also highlighted, with blue text, are *Hospitalist*-focused content and MCQs that directly address the learning needs of internists who work in the hospital setting.

MKSAP 17 Digital provides access to additional tools allowing you to customize your learning experience, including regular text updates with practice-changing, new information and 200 new self-assessment questions; a board-style pretest to help direct your learning; and enhanced custom-quiz options. And, with MKSAP Complete, learners can access 1200 electronic flashcards for quick review of important concepts or review the updated and enhanced version of Virtual Dx, an image-based self-assessment tool.

As before, MKSAP 17 is optimized for use on your mobile devices, with iOS- and Android-based apps allowing you to sync your work between your apps and online account and submit for CME credits and MOC points online.

Please visit us at the MKSAP Resource Site (mksap.acponline.org) to find out how we can help you study, earn CME credit and MOC points, and stay up to date.

Whether you prefer to use the traditional print version or take advantage of the features available through the digital version, we hope you enjoy MKSAP 17 and that it meets and exceeds your personal learning needs.

On behalf of the many internists who have offered their time and expertise to create the content for MKSAP 17 and the editorial staff who work to bring this material to you in the best possible way, we are honored that you have chosen to use MKSAP 17 and appreciate any feedback about the program you may have. Please feel free to send us any comments to mksap_editors@acponline.org.

Sincerely,

Philip A. Masters, MD, FACP
Editor-in-Chief
Senior Physician Educator
Director, Clinical Content Development
Medical Education Division
American College of Physicians

Pulmonary and Critical Care Medicine

Committee

Craig E. Daniels, MD, Section Editor[2]
Assistant Professor of Medicine
Division of Pulmonary and Critical Care Medicine
Mayo Clinic College of Medicine
Rochester, Minnesota

Richard S. Eisenstaedt, MD, MACP, Associate Editor[1]
Clinical Professor of Medicine
Temple University School of Medicine
Chair, Department of Medicine
Abington Memorial Hospital
Abington, Pennsylvania

Rendell W. Ashton, MD, FACP[1]
Staff Physician, Cleveland Clinic Respiratory Institute
Associate Director, Medical ICU
Program Director, Pulmonary and Critical Care Fellowship
Respiratory Institute, Cleveland Clinic
Cleveland, Ohio

Sean M. Caples, DO, MS[2]
Assistant Professor of Medicine
Division of Pulmonary and Critical Care Medicine
Mayo Clinic College of Medicine
Rochester, Minnesota

C. Jessica Dine, MD, FACP[2]
Assistant Professor of Medicine
Perelman School of Medicine at the University of
    Pennsylvania
Penn Lung Center
Perelman Center for Advanced Medicine
Philadelphia, Pennsylvania

Stanley Fiel, MD, FACP[2]
Professor of Medicine
Sidney Kimmel Medical College at Thomas Jefferson
    University
Regional Chairman
Department of Medicine
Morristown Medical Center/Atlantic Health System
Morristown, New Jersey

Robert Kempainen, MD[2]
Associate Professor, Department of Medicine
University of Minnesota School of Medicine
Hennepin County Medical Center
Minneapolis, Minnesota

Sumita B. Khatri, MD, MS[2]
Co-Director, Asthma Center
Respiratory Institute, Cleveland Clinic
Associate Professor of Medicine
CCLCM/CWRU School of Medicine
Cleveland, Ohio

Timothy Whelan, MD[2]
Associate Professor of Medicine
Medical Director of Lung Transplantation
Medical University of South Carolina
Charleston, South Carolina

Margaret Wojnar, MD[1]
Professor of Medicine
Division of Pulmonary, Allergy and Critical Care Medicine
Department of Medicine
Penn State Milton S. Hershey Medical Center
Penn State College of Medicine
Hershey, Pennsylvania

Consultant

Darlene Nelson, MD[1]
Assistant Professor
Division of Pulmonary and Critical Care Medicine
Mayo Clinic College of Medicine
Rochester, Minnesota

Editor-in-Chief

Philip A. Masters, MD, FACP[1]
Senior Physician Educator
Director, Clinical Content Development
American College of Physicians
Philadelphia, Pennsylvania

Director, Clinical Program Development

Cynthia D. Smith, MD, FACP[2]
American College of Physicians
Philadelphia, Pennsylvania

Pulmonary and Critical Care Medicine Reviewers

Frantz Duffoo, MD, FACP[1]
Rabeh Elzuway, MD, MSc[1]
Gloria T. Fioravanti, DO, FACP[1]
Lois J. Geist, MD[1]
Jason M. Golbin, DO, MS, FACP[1]
Kristen Kipps, MD[2]
Mark E. Pasanen, MD, FACP[1]
Michael W. Peterson, MD, FACP[1]
Jerry L. Spivak, MD, FACP[2]
Angel O. Coz Yataco, MD[1]

Pulmonary and Critical Care Medicine ACP Editorial Staff

Katie Idell[1], Manager, Clinical Skills Program and Digital Products
Susan Galeone[1], Staff Editor
Margaret Wells[1], Director, Self-Assessment and Educational Programs
Becky Krumm[1], Managing Editor

ACP Principal Staff

Patrick C. Alguire, MD, FACP[2]
Senior Vice President, Medical Education

Sean McKinney[1]
Vice President, Medical Education

Margaret Wells[1]
Director, Self-Assessment and Educational Programs

Becky Krumm[1]
Managing Editor

Katie Idell[1]
Manager, Clinical Skills Program and Digital Products

Valerie A. Dangovetsky[1]
Administrator

Ellen McDonald, PhD[1]
Senior Staff Editor

Megan Zborowski[1]
Senior Staff Editor

Randy Hendrickson[1]
Production Administrator/Editor

Linnea Donnarumma[1]
Staff Editor

Susan Galeone[1]
Staff Editor

Jackie Twomey[1]
Staff Editor

Julia Nawrocki[1]
Staff Editor

Kimberly Kerns[1]
Administrative Coordinator

Rosemarie Houton[1]
Administrative Representative

---

1. Has no relationships with any entity producing, marketing, reselling, or distributing health care goods or services consumed by, or used on, patients.

2. Has disclosed relationship(s) with any entity producing, marketing, reselling, or distributing health care goods or services consumed by, or used on, patients.

Disclosure of Relationships with any entity producing, marketing, reselling, or distributing health care goods or services consumed by, or used on, patients.

Patrick C. Alguire, MD, FACP
Consultantship
National Board of Medical Examiners
Royalties
UpToDate
Stock Options/Holdings
Amgen, Bristol-Myers Squibb, GlaxoSmithKline, Stryker Corporation, Zimmer, Teva Pharmaceutical Industries, Medtronic, Covidien, Express Scripts

Sean M. Caples, DO, MS
Consultantship
Zephyr Labs
Research Grants/Contracts
ResMed Foundation, Ventus Medical

Craig E. Daniels, MD
Patent Holder
Sanovas (bronchoscopy equipment manufacturer)
Research Grants/Contracts
Boehringer Ingelheim, Genentech/Roche

C. Jessica Dine, MD, FACP
Board Member
Sink or Swim
Consultantship
National Board of Medical Examiners

Stanley Fiel, MD, FACP
Advisory Board
Vertex Pharmaceuticals, Boehringer Ingelheim, Gilead Sciences, Novartis, Pfizer
Other
PTC Therapeutics—Data Safety Management Board Chair
Research Grants/Contracts
Cystic Fibrosis Foundation, Gilead Sciences, Vertex Pharmaceuticals, Novartis
Speakers Bureau
Novartis, Sunovion Pharmaceuticals, Mylan, Gilead, Boehringer Ingelheim
Consultantship
Vertex Pharmaceuticals

Robert Kempainen, MD
Consultantship
Association of Pulmonary and Critical Care Medicine
 Program Directors

Sumita B. Khatri, MD, MS
Board Member
American Lung Association of Midland States and National
Employment
Cleveland Clinic
Research Grants/Contracts
Boston Scientific, GlaxoSmithKline, Johnson and Johnson
 (Centocor), Teva Pharmaceuticals, Pfizer
Advisory Board
Asthma and Allergy Foundation of America, Medscape
Consultantship
Boehringer Ingelheim

Kristen Kipps, MD
Employment
UCLA

Cynthia D. Smith, MD, FACP
Stock Options/Holdings
Merck and Co.; spousal employment at Merck

Jerry L. Spivak, MD, FACP
Consultantship
Incyte Corporation, Celgene, Novartis, Merck

Timothy Whelan, MD
Board Member
LifePoint, Inc
Consultantship
InterMune, LifePoint, Inc., Genentech, Boehringer Ingelheim
Research Grants/Contracts
InterMune, Celgene, Sanofi, Boehringer Ingelheim, Gilead,
 Pulmonary Fibrosis Foundation, Actelion, Centocor,
 Genzyme, MedImmune
Advisory Board
Genentech, Boehringer Ingelheim

Acknowledgments

The American College of Physicians (ACP) gratefully acknowledges the special contributions to the development and production of the 17th edition of the Medical Knowledge Self-Assessment Program® (MKSAP® 17) made by the following people:

Graphic Design: Michael Ripca (Graphics Technical Administrator) and WFGD Studio (Graphic Designers).

Production/Systems: Dan Hoffmann (Director, Web Services & Systems Development), Neil Kohl (Senior Architect), Chris Patterson (Senior Architect), and Scott Hurd (Manager, Web Projects & CMS Services).

MKSAP 17 Digital: Under the direction of Steven Spadt, Vice President, Digital Products & Services, the digital version of MKSAP 17 was developed within the ACP's Digital Product Development Department, led by Brian Sweigard (Director). Other members of the team included Dan Barron (Senior Web Application Developer/Architect), Chris Forrest (Senior Software Developer/Design Lead), Kara Kronenwetter (Senior Web Developer), Brad Lord (Senior Web Application Developer), John McKnight (Senior Web Developer), and Nate Pershall (Senior Web Developer).

The College also wishes to acknowledge that many other persons, too numerous to mention, have contributed to the production of this program. Without their dedicated efforts, this program would not have been possible.

MKSAP Resource Site (mksap.acponline.org)

The MKSAP Resource Site (mksap.acponline.org) is a continually updated site that provides links to MKSAP 17 online answer sheets for print subscribers; the latest details on Continuing Medical Education (CME) and Maintenance of Certification (MOC) in the United States, Canada, and Australia; errata; and other new information.

ABIM Maintenance of Certification

Check the MKSAP Resource Site (mksap.acponline.org) for the latest information on how MKSAP tests can be used to apply to the American Board of Internal Medicine for Maintenance of Certification (MOC) points.

Royal College Maintenance of Certification

In Canada, MKSAP 17 is an Accredited Self-Assessment Program (Section 3) as defined by the Maintenance of Certification (MOC) Program of The Royal College of Physicians and Surgeons of Canada and approved by the Canadian Society of Internal Medicine on December 9, 2014. Approval extends from July 31, 2015 until July 31, 2018 for the Part A sections. Approval extends from December 31, 2015 to December 31, 2018 for the Part B sections.

Fellows of the Royal College may earn three credits per hour for participating in MKSAP 17 under Section 3. MKSAP 17 also meets multiple CanMEDS Roles, including that of Medical Expert, Communicator, Collaborator, Manager, Health Advocate, Scholar, and Professional. For information on how to apply MKSAP 17 Continuing Medical Education (CME) credits to the Royal College MOC Program, visit the MKSAP Resource Site at mksap.acponline.org.

The Royal Australasian College of Physicians CPD Program

In Australia, MKSAP 17 is a Category 3 program that may be used by Fellows of The Royal Australasian College of Physicians (RACP) to meet mandatory Continuing Professional Development (CPD) points. Two CPD credits are awarded for each of the 200 *AMA PRA Category 1 Credits*™ available in MKSAP 17. More information about using MKSAP 17 for this purpose is available at the MKSAP Resource Site at mksap.acponline.org and at www.racp.edu.au. CPD credits earned through MKSAP 17 should be reported at the MyCPD site at www.racp.edu.au/mycpd.

Continuing Medical Education

The American College of Physicians (ACP) is accredited by the Accreditation Council for Continuing Medical Education (ACCME) to provide continuing medical education for physicians.

The ACP designates this enduring material, MKSAP 17, for a maximum of 200 *AMA PRA Category 1 Credits*™. Physicians should claim only the credit commensurate with the extent of their participation in the activity.

Up to 19 *AMA PRA Category 1 Credits*™ are available from December 31, 2015, to December 31, 2018, for the MKSAP 17 Pulmonary and Critical Care Medicine section.

Learning Objectives

The learning objectives of MKSAP 17 are to:
- Close gaps between actual care in your practice and preferred standards of care, based on best evidence
- Diagnose disease states that are less common and sometimes overlooked or confusing
- Improve management of comorbid conditions that can complicate patient care
- Determine when to refer patients for surgery or care by subspecialists
- Pass the ABIM Certification Examination
- Pass the ABIM Maintenance of Certification Examination

Target Audience

- General internists and primary care physicians
- Subspecialists who need to remain up-to-date in internal medicine and in areas outside of their own subspecialty area
- Residents preparing for the certification examination in internal medicine
- Physicians preparing for maintenance of certification in internal medicine (recertification)

Earn "Instantaneous" CME Credits Online

Print subscribers can enter their answers online to earn instantaneous Continuing Medical Education (CME) credits. You can submit your answers using online answer sheets that are provided at mksap.acponline.org, where a record of your MKSAP 17 credits will be available. To earn CME credits, you need to answer all of the questions in a test and earn a score of at least 50% correct (number of correct answers divided by the total number of questions). Take any of the following approaches:

1. Use the printed answer sheet at the back of this book to record your answers. Go to mksap.acponline.org, access the appropriate online answer sheet, transcribe your answers, and submit your test for instantaneous CME credits. There is no additional fee for this service.

2. Go to mksap.acponline.org, access the appropriate online answer sheet, directly enter your answers, and submit your test for instantaneous CME credits. There is no additional fee for this service.

3. Pay a $15 processing fee per answer sheet and submit the printed answer sheet at the back of this book by mail or fax, as instructed on the answer sheet. Make sure you calculate your score and fax the answer sheet to 215-351-2799 or mail the answer sheet to Member and Customer Service, American College of Physicians, 190 N. Independence Mall West, Philadelphia, PA 19106-1572, using the courtesy envelope provided in your MKSAP 17 slipcase. You will need your 10-digit order number and 8-digit ACP ID number, which are printed on your packing slip. Please allow 4 to 6 weeks for your score report to be emailed back to you. Be sure to include your email address for a response.

If you do not have a 10-digit order number and 8-digit ACP ID number or if you need help creating a user name and password to access the MKSAP 17 online answer sheets, go to mksap.acponline.org or email custserv@acponline.org.

Disclosure Policy

It is the policy of the American College of Physicians (ACP) to ensure balance, independence, objectivity, and scientific rigor in all of its educational activities. To this end, and consistent with the policies of the ACP and the Accreditation Council for Continuing Medical Education (ACCME), contributors to all ACP continuing medical education activities are required to disclose all relevant financial relationships with any entity producing, marketing, re-selling, or distributing health care goods or services consumed by, or used on, patients. Contributors are required to use generic names in the discussion of therapeutic options and are required to identify any unapproved, off-label, or investigative use of commercial products or devices. Where a trade name is used, all available trade names for the same product type are also included. If trade-name products manufactured by companies with whom contributors have relationships are discussed, contributors are asked to provide evidence-based citations in support of the discussion. The information is reviewed by the committee responsible for producing this text. If necessary, adjustments to topics or contributors' roles in content development are made to balance the discussion. Further, all readers of this text are asked to evaluate the content for evidence of commercial bias and send any relevant comments to mksap_editors@acponline.org so that future decisions about content and contributors can be made in light of this information.

Resolution of Conflicts

To resolve all conflicts of interest and influences of vested interests, the American College of Physicians (ACP) precluded members of the content-creation committee from deciding on any content issues that involved generic or trade-name products associated with proprietary entities with which these committee members had relationships. In addition, content was based on best evidence and updated clinical care guidelines, when such evidence and guidelines were available. Contributors' disclosure information can be found with the list of contributors' names and those of ACP principal staff listed in the beginning of this book.

Hospital-Based Medicine

For the convenience of subscribers who provide care in hospital settings, content that is specific to the hospital setting has been highlighted in blue. Hospital icons (H) highlight where the hospital-based content begins, continues over more than one page, and ends.

High Value Care Key Points

Key Points in the text that relate to High Value Care concepts (that is, concepts that discuss balancing clinical benefit with costs and harms) are designated by the HVC icon (HVC).

Educational Disclaimer

The editors and publisher of MKSAP 17 recognize that the development of new material offers many opportunities for error. Despite our best efforts, some errors may persist in print. Drug dosage schedules are, we believe, accurate and in accordance with current standards.

Readers are advised, however, to ensure that the recommended dosages in MKSAP 17 concur with the information provided in the product information material. This is especially important in cases of new, infrequently used, or highly toxic drugs. Application of the information in MKSAP 17 remains the professional responsibility of the practitioner.

The primary purpose of MKSAP 17 is educational. Information presented, as well as publications, technologies, products, and/or services discussed, is intended to inform subscribers about the knowledge, techniques, and experiences of the contributors. A diversity of professional opinion exists, and the views of the contributors are their own and not those of the American College of Physicians (ACP). Inclusion of any material in the program does not constitute endorsement or recommendation by the ACP. The ACP does not warrant the safety, reliability, accuracy, completeness, or usefulness of and disclaims any and all liability for damages and claims that may result from the use of information, publications, technologies, products, and/or services discussed in this program.

Publisher's Information

Unauthorized Use of This Book Is Against the Law

MKSAP 17 ISBN: 978-1-938245-18-3
(Pulmonary and Critical Care Medicine)
ISBN: 978-1-938245-29-9

Printed in the United States of America.

For order information in the United States or Canada call 800-523-1546, extension 2600. All other countries call 215-351-2600, (M-F, 9 AM – 5 PM ET). Fax inquiries to 215-351-2799 or email to custserv@acponline.org.

Errata

Errata for MKSAP 17 will be available through the MKSAP Resource Site at mksap.acponline.org as new information becomes known to the editors.

Table of Contents

Pulmonary and Critical Care Medicine High Value Care Recommendations

The American College of Physicians, in collaboration with multiple other organizations, is engaged in a worldwide initiative to promote the practice of High Value Care (HVC). The goals of the HVC initiative are to improve health care outcomes by providing care of proven benefit and reducing costs by avoiding unnecessary and even harmful interventions. The initiative comprises several programs that integrate the important concept of health care value (balancing clinical benefit with costs and harms) for a given intervention into a broad range of educational materials to address the needs of trainees, practicing physicians, and patients.

HVC content has been integrated into MKSAP 17 in several important ways. MKSAP 17 now includes HVC-identified key points in the text, HVC-focused multiple choice questions, and, for subscribers to MKSAP Digital, an HVC custom quiz. From the text and questions, we have generated the following list of HVC recommendations that meet the definition below of high value care and bring us closer to our goal of improving patient outcomes while conserving finite resources.

High Value Care Recommendation: A recommendation to choose diagnostic and management strategies for patients in specific clinical situations that balance clinical benefit with cost and harms with the goal of improving patient outcomes.

Below are the High Value Care Recommendations for the Pulmonary and Critical Care Medicine section of MKSAP 17.

- Low-dose chest CT utilizes a lower total radiation dose than standard chest CT and remains as effective for lung cancer screening and for imaging lung nodules and lung parenchyma.
- Vocal cord dysfunction, characterized by (1) mid-chest tightness with exposure to triggers, (2) difficulty breathing in, and (3) partial response to asthma medications, is often misdiagnosed as severe asthma resulting in unnecessary intubations and high health care utilization.
- Although expensive, omalizumab has been shown to reduce emergency department visits and is cost effective in moderate to severe persistent asthma with: (1) symptoms inadequately controlled with inhaled glucocorticoids, (2) allergies to perennial aeroallergens, and (3) serum IgE levels between 30 and 700 U/mL (30-700 kU/L).
- Smoking cessation is the single most clinically efficacious and cost-effective way to prevent COPD, to slow progression of established disease, and to improve survival.

- Screening for COPD with spirometry should not be performed in asymptomatic patients.
- Because inhaled medications are a mainstay of COPD management, good inhaler technique should be ensured (particularly in patients with suboptimal symptom control) before making changes to the drug regimen.
- Long-acting bronchodilators in COPD improve FEV_1, improve health status, and significantly reduce the frequency of exacerbations, but have not been shown to affect mortality.
- The use of inhaled glucocorticoids is not effective as primary therapy or monotherapy in COPD and should only be used in combination with other proven therapies.
- Roflumilast is an oral selective phosphodiestarase-4 (PDE-4) inhibitor and its use should be limited to add-on therapy in severe COPD associated with chronic bronchitis and a history of recurrent exacerbations; it is not a bronchodilator, is expensive, and has not been shown to be effective in other groups of patients with COPD.
- Home treatment of a COPD exacerbation is reasonable in patients with less severe lung disease who do not have significant accompanying illnesses and who are experiencing mild to moderate exacerbations.
- Glucocorticoids for acute exacerbations of COPD have been shown to reduce recovery time, improve lung function and arterial hypoxemia, decrease risk of early relapse, decrease treatment failure, and decrease length of hospital stay; a frequently used regimen is oral prednisone 40 mg/d for 5 days and intravenous glucocorticoids should be reserved for patients unable to tolerate oral therapy.
- Antibiotic use in acute exacerbations of COPD should be limited to patients with increased dyspnea and purulent sputum or those who require mechanical ventilation (invasive or noninvasive).
- Patients with COPD should receive inactivated influenza vaccination annually, and the 23-valent polysaccharide pneumococcal vaccine (PPSV23) should be given to all patients aged 19 to 64 years with COPD, with revaccination at age 65 years or older if 5 years have elapsed since the previous pneumococcal immunization; the 13-valent pneumococcal conjugate vaccine should also be administered at age 65 years or older if 1 year has elapsed since the last PPSV23 immunization (see Item 98).
- There are no data to support the routine use of short- or long-acting bronchodilators or the long term use of systemic glucocorticoids in patients with bronchiectasis.

- Pulmonary rehabilitation programs are effective in patients with bronchiectasis and are associated with significant improvements in exercise capacity and fewer outpatient and emergency department visits.
- High-resolution CT is the diagnostic tool of choice for evaluation of diffuse parenchymal lung disease; there is little role for plain chest radiography or conventional CT imaging (5-mm slice thickness) given the limits of their resolution (see Item 11).
- Cessation of smoking is the primary management for smoking-related diffuse parenchymal lung disease.
- The most recent evidence-based consensus statement recommends against mechanical ventilation for individuals with acute respiratory failure due to either progression or an acute exacerbation of idiopathic pulmonary fibrosis.
- The American Thoracic Society recommends palliation of symptoms rather than intubation and mechanical ventilation for patients with respiratory failure due to progressive idiopathic pulmonary fibrosis (see Item 44).
- In patients with COPD, parameters that portend a poor prognosis and trigger more extensive discussions regarding end-of-life care include an FEV_1 of less than 30% of predicted, oxygen dependence, multiple hospital admissions for COPD exacerbations, significant comorbidities, weight loss and cachexia, decreased functional status, and increasing dependence on others (see Item 69).
- The first step in management of shift work sleep disorder is to address sleep-related behaviors and the sleep environment, referred to as sleep hygiene (see Item 90).
- The overriding principle in management of occupational lung disease is prevention, consisting of interventions in the workplace to avoid exposures as well as early identification of coworkers who may also be at risk.
- Spirometry before and after rechallenge with workplace exposures is a cost-effective way to confirm the diagnosis of occupational asthma (see Item 29).
- Chest radiograph and thoracic ultrasound are important tests in the evaluation of pleural effusion; ultrasound has a higher sensitivity for pleural fluid and no associated radiation exposure.
- Bedside ultrasound is recommended for thoracentesis as it enhances procedural accuracy and safety.
- Observation alone has been shown to be safe for small pneumothoraces in patients with minimal symptoms.
- Advanced therapy for pulmonary hypertension with vasodilators should be reserved for patients with pulmonary arterial hypertension (group 1) as they have not been shown to be efficacious and may be harmful in this group.
- Ventilation-perfusion scanning is a sensitive indicator of chronic thromboembolic pulmonary hypertension and is generally the preferred first imaging modality.
- If prior imaging of the chest is available, it should be reviewed as a low-risk and inexpensive way to assess the stability or growth of the solitary pulmonary nodule.

- In patients with a subcentimeter pulmonary nodule, any previous imaging of the chest should be obtained to establish whether the nodule has remained stable or has grown over time (see Item 3).
- If imaging demonstrates stability of a solitary pulmonary nodule (and no other new findings) for 24 months, no further imaging is required (see Item 65).
- Smoking prevention and cessation are the most important steps in preventing lung cancer.
- The United States Preventive Services Task Force recommends low-dose CT screening for lung cancer in patients between the ages of 55 and 79 years who have a 30-pack-year or more history of smoking and who are currently smoking or quit within the last 15 years.
- Overnight pulse oximetry alone has a high rate of false-positive and false-negative results and has not been validated as a screening tool for obstructive sleep apnea; its use should be limited to patients with low pretest probability, few symptoms, or in patients who prefer to avoid treatment.
- A cost-effective approach to a patient with an inadequate response to obstructive sleep apnea treatment with continuous positive airway pressure (CPAP) therapy is to first check the level of adherence to therapy by downloading and reviewing data from the CPAP device (see Item 49).
- Noninvasive ventilation is associated with decreased ICU mortality, intubation rate, and ICU length of stay in immunocompromised patients and should be considered as an alternative to endotracheal intubation in patients who are appropriate candidates.
- In patients with hypoxemic respiratory failure due to heart failure, noninvasive positive pressure ventilation decreases the need for mechanical ventilation, improves respiratory parameters, and may decrease mortality (see Item 15).
- Bedside ultrasound to assess vena caval dimensions induced by positive-pressure ventilation appears to be highly predictive of volume responsiveness and is a non-invasive alternative to a pulmonary artery catheter.
- Ultrasound-guided central line insertion is associated with a reduction in failure of catheter placement and vessel injury, as well as prevention of pneumothorax.
- When compared with deep sedation, light sedation (a drowsy and cooperative patient) reduces ICU-related posttraumatic stress disorder, time on the ventilator, and mortality.
- Do not routinely transfuse erythrocytes in nonbleeding, hemodynamically stable patients in the ICU with a hemoglobin concentration greater than 7 g/dL (70 g/L) (see Item 93).
- Large-caliber peripheral intravenous access is the preferred route of infusion when large volumes of crystalloid fluid and blood are needed quickly (see Item 8).
- The association between opioid analgesics and central sleep apnea (CSA) is increasingly recognized; reduction or withdrawal of opioids improves CSA (see Item 41).

Pulmonary and Critical Care Medicine

Pulmonary Diagnostic Tests

Pulmonary Function Testing

Pulmonary function testing is essential to the diagnosis and management of respiratory symptoms and pulmonary diseases. Pulmonary function tests are also used in the evaluation and screening of patients who are at risk for lung disease, such as those with occupational exposures or drug toxicity.

Spirometry

Spirometry, the measurement of pulmonary airflow, is a readily available and essential initial test. Spirometry may be performed in the office setting or more formally in a pulmonary function testing laboratory. The results of spirometry are highly dependent on technique and patient effort; therefore, patients should be carefully instructed in the proper technique prior to testing. Proper technique consists of the patient sitting upright with the head erect and the mouthpiece held tightly between the lips. Measurements should be repeated to ensure reproducibility; the two largest values within 150 mL of each other should be used. Normal reference values for spirometry are dependent on age, gender, height, and race.

Measures of interest are the forced expiratory volume exhaled in 1 second (FEV_1) and forced expiratory volume until full exhalation, or forced vital capacity (FVC). The FEV_1/FVC ratio is used to assess for airway obstruction; a value less than 70% (the lower limit of normal) is consistent with airflow obstruction. With evidence of obstruction, the degree of reduction in FEV_1 is used to characterize the degree of obstruction. An FEV_1 of 50% to 80% of predicted is classified as moderately reduced, 34% to 49% of predicted is severely reduced, and less than 34% of predicted is very severely reduced. In patients with evidence of obstruction, a bronchodilator challenge (2 to 4 puffs of a short-acting β_2-agonist) is often given to determine the reversibility of obstruction (which may be helpful in differentiating between asthma and COPD); an increase in FEV_1 of 12% or 200 mL is considered a positive bronchodilator response.

A normal FEV_1/FVC ratio may reflect normal lung function or may indicate a restrictive lung defect. However, if the FEV_1 and the FVC are reduced proportionately with each other and are below the predicted normal values, the spirometry results are consistent with a restrictive defect, which may be confirmed by further testing demonstrating low lung volumes (see Lung Volumes).

Flow-volume loops graphically plot pulmonary airflow during exhalation and inspiration, with characteristic patterns associated with specific clinical conditions (**Figure 1**).

KEY POINT

- An FEV_1/FVC ratio of less than 70% on spirometry is consistent with airflow obstruction.

Bronchial Challenge Testing

In patients with clinical symptoms suggestive of bronchospastic disease (such as cough or unexplained dyspnea) but with normal spirometry, bronchial challenge testing may be diagnostically helpful. Bronchial challenge testing uses a controlled inhaled stimulus to induce bronchospasm in association with spirometry; a positive test is indicated by a drop in the measured FEV_1. Because bronchial challenge testing may induce severe bronchospasm, it should only be performed in a controlled environment such as a pulmonary function testing laboratory.

Methacholine is a commonly used agent that induces cholinergic bronchospasm at low concentrations in patients with asthma. The provocative dose 20% (PD20) is the dose of methacholine that causes a significant drop in the FEV_1 of 20% or greater. The ability to achieve a PD20 at low concentrations of methacholine indicates more easily induced obstruction and is sensitive for detecting asthma.

Similar principles apply to other forms of bronchial challenge testing, such as after exposure to cold air or exercise, in which case a 10% drop in FEV_1 from baseline in the context of a supporting clinical picture is diagnostic.

KEY POINT

- Bronchial challenge testing with a controlled stimulus is helpful in patients with dyspnea or cough of uncertain cause when spirometry results are normal.

Lung Volumes

Lung volume testing directly and indirectly measures the static amount of air in the lungs and can be helpful in the diagnostic evaluation of dyspnea and abnormal spirometry results. Key measures include the total lung capacity (TLC), or the amount of air in the lungs after maximal inhalation, and residual volume (RV), the volume of air remaining in the lungs after a maximal exhalation. Lung volume tests are performed most commonly using body plethysmography. The components that are directly measurable by plethysmography are the functional residual capacity (air in the lungs after a

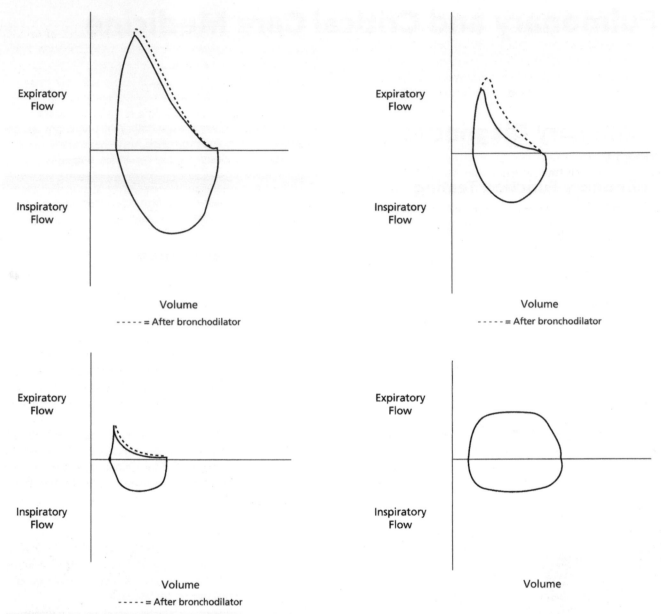

FIGURE 1. *Top left panel*: Flow-volume loop demonstrating normal spirometry, with similar maximum inspiratory and expiratory flows; no significant change is seen after bronchodilator administration. *Top right panel*: Flow-volume loop demonstrating asthma, with a reduction in peak expiratory flow and concave curvature for the expiratory limb while the inspiratory limb remains normal; improvement is seen in expiratory flows (particularly the increase in peak flow) after bronchodilator administration. *Bottom left panel*: Flow-volume loop demonstrating COPD, with a significant reduction in peak expiratory flow and concave appearance of the expiratory limb; no significant change is seen after bronchodilator administration. *Bottom right panel*: Flow-volume loop demonstrating fixed obstruction/tracheal stenosis, with flattening of the peak inspiratory and expiratory flows.

normal expiration), expiratory reserve volume (air in the lungs that is still able to be exhaled after normal expiration), and slow vital capacity (the volume of air maximally exhaled during expiration with a slow exhalation). These measures are then used to calculate the RV and TLC. In the setting of restrictive lung patterns on spirometry, TLC measurement can determine whether restriction is due to a primary parenchymal process or chest cage restriction from factors such as obesity, muscle weakness, or scoliosis. In obstructive lung diseases, an increased TLC is suggestive of hyperinflation and

high compliance, and an increased RV is suggestive of air trapping.

Diffusing Capacity for Carbon Monoxide

The diffusing capacity for carbon monoxide (DLCO) is performed by having the patient take a single, deep breath containing a very low percentage of carbon monoxide and measuring the amount of subsequently exhaled carbon monoxide following a short period of breath holding. Carbon monoxide is rapidly and efficiently taken up by hemoglobin, and the amount absorbed is determined by the amount of blood recruited to the pulmonary alveolar capillary bed and the surface area available for diffusion. DLCO is therefore useful as a measure of the capacity for gas transfer through the alveolar-capillary membrane. Clinical disorders that recruit blood to the alveoli (cardiac shunt, asthma, erythrocytosis, alveolar hemorrhage) can elevate DLCO levels. In contrast, conditions that decrease the surface area available for diffusion, decrease permeability across the alveolar-capillary membrane, or otherwise interfere with gas transfer can reduce DLCO. For example, a reduced DLCO in a patient with a low TLC or restriction on spirometry is suggestive of a parenchymal or interstitial process. The DLCO may also be diminished in COPD (from parenchymal destruction) or in conditions that affect the pulmonary vasculature such as pulmonary hypertension or chronic pulmonary thromboembolic disease.

6-Minute Walk Test

Lung function during exertion using the 6-minute walk test (6MWT) is helpful to assess disability and prognosis in chronic lung conditions. Simple pulse oximetry and oxygen desaturation studies performed at rest and with exertion assess the need for oxygen supplementation. During a 6MWT, oxygen saturation, heart rate, dyspnea and fatigue level, and distance walked at a normal pace in 6 minutes are recorded. This relatively simple maneuver quantifies exercise tolerance, determines effective interventions, and helps predict morbidity and mortality. The 6MWT is routinely used before, during, and after pulmonary rehabilitation programs.

Pulse Oximetry

Pulse oximetry is a noninvasive measurement of arterial hemoglobin saturation. Pulse oximeters have two light-emitting diodes and a photodetector that measures the pulsatile fraction of hemoglobin and algorithmically estimates the arterial hemoglobin saturation. In general, resting oxygen saturation less than or equal to 95% or a desaturation with exercise greater than or equal to 5% is considered abnormal.

Pulse oximetry cannot distinguish between oxygen saturation of hemoglobin and similar abnormal hemoglobins such as carboxyhemoglobin. In patients with high levels of carboxyhemoglobin, as seen in carbon monoxide poisoning, pulse oximetry will provide false-negative results. If the presence of carboxyhemoglobin is suspected, co-oximetry is the preferred test to measure oxyhemoglobin.

Imaging and Bronchoscopy

Imaging

Chest Radiography

A plain chest radiograph allows visualization of the bony structures and contents of the thoracic cavity, including the airways, lungs, heart, pleura, and great vessels (**Figure 2**). It is therefore often the first diagnostic test performed when evaluating any symptoms potentially explained by pathology to any of these structures. The cost and risks to the patient, such as subsequent consequences of radiation exposure (**Table 1**), are lower compared with other chest imaging studies. However, because of the low sensitivity of plain chest radiography in diagnosing

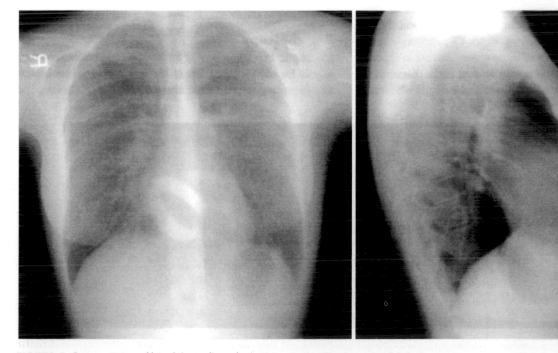

FIGURE 2. Posteroanterior and lateral chest radiographs showing normal cardiopulmonary and skeletal structures.

TABLE 1. Comparison of Radiation Exposure of Chest Imaging Techniques

Imaging Modality	Equivalent Daytime Radiation	Equivalent Number of Chest Radiographs
PA/lateral radiograph	10 days	N/A
Routine CT	3 years	400
HRCT	89 days	43
CTPA	4.3 years	750
Low-dose CT	68 days	33
FDG-PET/CT	5.4 years	809

CTPA = CT pulmonary angiogram; FDG = fluorodeoxyglucose; HRCT = high-resolution CT; N/A = not applicable; PA = posteroanterior.

several cardiopulmonary conditions, CT of the chest is often obtained if the chest radiograph is normal or if clarification of an abnormal chest radiograph finding is needed.

Computed Tomography

The choice of unenhanced CT, contrast-enhanced CT, high-resolution CT (HRCT), or CT pulmonary angiography is dependent on the information being sought based on the differential diagnosis. Contrast may be added to the study to better evaluate the mediastinal structures (for example, to assess for lymphadenopathy) whereas HRCT is indicated if diffuse parenchymal lung disease is suspected. HRCT can help narrow the differential diagnosis based on the distribution of the lung parenchymal abnormalities and the presence or absence of associated findings. Because the HRCT protocol employs thin sections obtained at wide intervals (typically 1 cm between imaged cross sections), this type of CT should not be performed to evaluate suspected lung disease with a focal abnormality or to evaluate pulmonary nodules. CT pulmonary angiography uses a timed bolus of intravenous contrast to opacify the pulmonary arteries and is mainly used in the diagnosis of pulmonary embolism or aortic dissection. Patients who meet

criteria for lung cancer screening should undergo imaging with low-dose chest CT to minimize radiation exposure (see Table 1). Low-dose chest CT images utilize a lower total radiation dose than standard CT chest protocols. The lower dose of radiation decreases the radiation to patients and is as effective in imaging lung nodules and lung parenchyma owing to the high inherent contrast between lung tissue and air.

> **KEY POINT**
> - Low-dose chest CT utilizes a lower total radiation dose than standard chest CT and remains as effective for lung cancer screening and for imaging lung nodules and lung parenchyma.

HVC

Positron Emission Tomography

Patients with a pulmonary nodule or other findings suggestive of malignancy may require PET/CT. This test most commonly uses fluorodeoxyglucose (FDG) as a metabolic marker to identify rapidly dividing cells such as tumor cells and, to a lesser degree, any inflammatory lesion (**Figure 3**). For example, if a pulmonary nodule is identified but no previous imaging is available, PET/CT can help determine the activity of the nodule, as long as the nodule is approximately 1 cm or larger. At smaller sizes, PET/CT imaging may be falsely negative. A nodule that demonstrates no FDG uptake is unlikely to be malignant. Any disease with metabolic activity, including infection, inflammation, and malignancy, can cause an FDG-avid nodule. PET/CT imaging can also be used in the management of known cancer. It can be used for staging the cancer (by determining the presence or absence of metastatic disease), monitoring response to treatments (not only by assessing for a decrease in size but also for a decrease in metabolic activity), and surveillance for recurrence.

Bronchoscopy

H

Fiberoptic bronchoscopy is an endoscopic technique that allows for the visualization of the tracheobronchial lumen and sampling of suspected areas of disease, including the

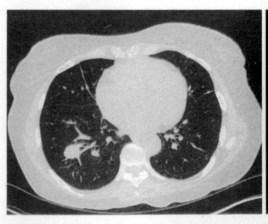 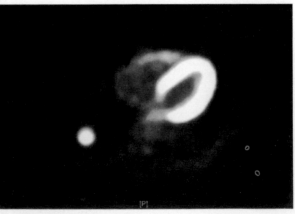

FIGURE 3. A right lower lobe lobulated nodule was identified on an unenhanced chest CT (*left panel*). A high metabolic rate was confirmed on PET/CT (*right panel*) and the patient was subsequently diagnosed with adenocarcinoma of the lung.

CONT.

endobronchial mucosa, lung parenchyma, and accessible lymph nodes. For diagnostic purposes, a flexible broncho-scope is used more commonly than a rigid bronchoscope. A rigid bronchoscope requires general anesthesia, but its larger lumen may be necessary for some therapeutic bronchoscopies such as attempted retrieval of a foreign body. Flexible bronchoscopy can be performed under light to moderate sedation, and, although the flexible bronchoscope's lumen is smaller than that of a rigid bronchoscope, it does allow instruments to be used to help increase its diagnostic yield. Bronchoscopic diagnostic procedures are described in **Table 2**.

The most common indications for a bronchoscopy are (1) evaluation of new respiratory symptoms associated with airway pathology (for example, hemoptysis, stridor); (2) pulmonary infections, especially if they are progressive despite appropriate empiric therapy or occur in immunocompromised patients; (3) diagnosis or staging of primary or metastatic cancer of the lung; (4) diagnosis of an abnormal imaging finding such as a pulmonary nodule, persistent infiltrate, or atelectasis; and (5) diffuse parenchymal lung disease of unknown cause (**Table 3**). A flexible or rigid bronchoscope may also be used therapeutically, such as in instances of airway stenosis (placement of stents or dilation), foreign-body aspiration, or mucus plugging, or to treat a lesion locally with electrocoagulation, laser therapy, or cryotherapy.

Major complications of bronchoscopy are rare and depend on the intervention undertaken; complications include pneumothorax (1%-4%) and significant bleeding (1%) with the use of transbronchial lung biopsy. Patients may also have adverse effects from topical anesthetics and systemic sedatives. Bronchoscopy should be avoided in patients who cannot tolerate possible adverse events, which include hypotension, tachycardia, severe hypoxemia, and bronchospasm. For example, bronchoscopy should be postponed in a patient with a recent myocardial infarction or who requires high amounts of supplemental oxygen. Although hypoxemia, even when severe, is not an absolute contraindication, patients who require high concentrations of supplemental oxygen may require mechanical ventilation to safely perform the bronchoscopy; patients should be informed about this concern in advance of the procedure.

TABLE 2. Bronchoscopic Diagnostic Procedures

Technique	Description	Examples of Indications
Airway inspection	Visualization of the tracheobronchial tree to the level of segmental airways	Hemoptysis
		Localized wheeze
		Persistent atelectasis
		Diagnosis of tracheobronchomalacia
Bronchial washings	Samples from large airways	Diagnosis of infections
		Cell counts in diagnosis of parenchymal lung disease
Bronchoalveolar lavage	Samples from small bronchi and alveoli	Diagnosis of infections
		Cell counts in diagnosis of parenchymal lung disease
Bronchial brushings	Brushings of the endobronchial mucosa for cells	Endobronchial lesions
Endobronchial biopsy	Biopsy of the lumen of the airway	Endobronchial mass or nodules
Transbronchial lung biopsy	Biopsy of the parenchyma	Diffuse lung disease
		Persistent infiltrates
		Posttransplant rejection
Transbronchial needle aspiration	Aspiration of a lymph node or mass adjacent to the airway	Lymphadenopathy
		Pulmonary mass
		Mediastinal mass
Endobronchial ultrasound	Use of an ultrasound probe at the distal end of the bronchoscope	Lymphadenopathy
		Pulmonary mass
Electromagnetic navigation	Images from a recent CT are used to create a 3D model of the patient's airways. During the bronchoscopy, the patient's airways are "linked" with the 3D model whenever the bronchoscope reaches a locatable anatomic landmark. An electromagnetic guidance system at the bronchoscope is then used to create a map of the airways and guide the physician to the area of interest.	Pulmonary mass or nodule

3D = three-dimensional.

TABLE 3. Common Indications for Diagnostic Bronchoscopy

Indication	Comments
Hemoptysis	Patients with active hemoptysis without an obvious explanation warrant an airway inspection via bronchoscopy and chest imaging. Bronchoscopy may be useful in localizing an active bleeding source as well as for treatment of endobronchial abnormalities causing bleeding. However, bronchoscopy is not indicated for all patients presenting with hemoptysis from known causes, including respiratory infection or heart failure exacerbation.
Stridor or localized wheeze	Bronchoscopy can identify the location of airway obstruction and may also treat the underlying cause (for example, removal of a foreign body or balloon dilation of a stricture).
Pulmonary infections	Bronchoscopy can provide microbiologic data in patients who have respiratory infections of diverse causes. Most pulmonary infections do not require bronchoscopy for diagnosis, especially if the patient is otherwise healthy and is improving with therapy. However, bronchoscopy should be considered for all patients with a pulmonary infection who are immunocompromised and do not respond to empiric treatment. These patients commonly have opportunistic infections including *Pneumocystis jivorecii* pneumonia and fungal infections.
Diagnosis and/or staging of bronchogenic carcinoma	Bronchoscopic biopsy of lung nodules and masses coupled with lymph node aspiration can help diagnose and stage lung cancers.
Diagnosis of pulmonary metastases	Diagnosis of metastatic disease may be made by bronchoscopy and biopsy in patients presenting with new pulmonary nodules in the setting of a known primary cancer.
Evaluation of a pulmonary nodule	Diagnostic specimens can be obtained via bronchoscopic biopsy for tissue diagnosis.
Persistent pulmonary infiltrate	Patients with a persistent pulmonary infiltrate may benefit from bronchoscopy to diagnose or exclude noninfectious causes of pulmonary infiltrates, such as eosinophilic lung disease, cryptogenic organizing pneumonia, and cancer.
Mucus plugging	When mucus plugging is severe enough to cause atelectasis and interfere with oxygenation or ventilation, bronchoscopy may evacuate the mucus plug.
Foreign-body aspiration	Bronchoscopy is the intervention of choice to extract foreign bodies wedged in airways.
Diffuse parenchymal lung disease	Surgical lung biopsy is the diagnostic method of choice for most patients with diffuse parenchymal/interstitial lung diseases. However, selected diseases, including sarcoidosis, are diagnosed with a high degree of accuracy via bronchoscopic techniques, which may obviate the need for a more invasive surgical biopsy.

KEY POINT

- Fiberoptic bronchoscopy is an endoscopic technique that allows for the visualization of the tracheobronchial lumen and sampling of suspected areas of disease, including the endobronchial mucosa, lung parenchyma, and accessible lymph nodes.

Endobronchial Ultrasound

Endobronchial ultrasound is a bronchoscopic technique that involves the use of an ultrasound probe at the distal end of the bronchoscope. The ultrasound-tipped bronchoscope can identify mediastinal lymph nodes and increase the yield of a transbronchial needle aspiration by allowing direct visualization of the needle entering the lymph node. This can be used to visualize and biopsy structures adjacent to an airway. For example, endobronchial ultrasound has been particularly useful in the staging of lung cancer, given its high specificity and sensitivity in identifying and staging lymph node involvement of the mediastinum and hila. Peripheral bronchoscopic ultrasound techniques can also aid in the successful biopsy of any lesion adjacent to an airway, including pulmonary nodules.

Airways Disease
Asthma

Asthma is a common chronic respiratory condition characterized by reversible airway obstruction that is caused by airway inflammation and bronchial hyperresponsiveness.

The current view of asthma is that it is a heterogeneous disorder with various phenotypes rather than one condition. Differentiation of asthma subtypes may allow therapeutic approaches to be tailored for the individual patient, resulting in maximal treatment efficacy with minimal adverse effects. Commonly observed clinical syndromes of asthma as well as confounding factors that worsen underlying asthma will be discussed in this chapter.

Epidemiology and Natural History

Asthma affects approximately 8% of the population in the United States. Allergic asthma is strongly associated with a personal or family history of allergies or atopy (maternal asthma in particular), maternal smoking while pregnant, and exposure to environmental tobacco smoke in childhood. Children with allergic asthma are commonly diagnosed during preschool years, and many have mild symptoms that resolve. However, some individuals with childhood allergic asthma progress to chronic airflow obstruction with increasingly severe symptoms that persist into adulthood. Although the cause is unclear, this worsening of asthma into adulthood is likely related to environmental stimuli such as viral infections, workplace exposures, or exposure to tobacco smoke (first-hand or second-hand) as well as individual predisposition (for example, family history, antioxidant activity in the lung). Importantly, adult-onset asthma can occur with or without a history of childhood asthma and may be underrecognized in older adults. Therefore, an initial clinical suspicion should be followed by diagnostic testing, particularly in those without a previous history of asthma. Asthma can present in a variety of ways, from early-onset childhood asthma with allergies, to very late-onset adult nonallergic asthma associated with obesity or chronic sinus infections.

There is a higher prevalence and severity of asthma in people with lower income, children, and black populations. This difference is likely related to multiple factors, including limited access to primary and specialty care, delayed disease recognition and suboptimal management, expectations about disease control, unhealthy dietary patterns, and ongoing exposure to triggers and environmental elements.

KEY POINT

- Asthma affects approximately 8% of the population in the United States.

Pathogenesis

The underlying pathophysiology in asthma is airway inflammation. Chronic airway inflammation results in the production and release of multiple mediators that may result in epithelial damage, smooth muscle hypertrophy, airway fibrosis, and remodeling in some patients (**Figure 4**).

Airway inflammation is usually triggered at the epithelial level. In allergic asthma, exposure of the airway to allergens following sensitization causes mast cell degranulation and initiation

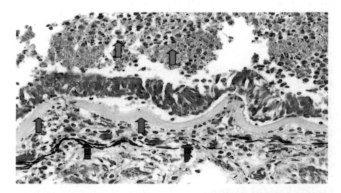

FIGURE 4. Airway tissue in a patient with severe asthma demonstrating subbasement membrane thickening (*red arrows*), disruption of elastic fibers (*blue arrows*), and infiltration with inflammatory cells and filling of the airway lumen with mucus and inflammatory cells (*green arrows*).

of an inflammatory cascade. In nonallergic asthma, epithelial stimulation and initiation of inflammation can occur with viral or bacterial infections or exposure to noxious chemicals.

In allergic asthma, allergen exposure triggers mast cell activation and a robust response from the T-helper 2 (Th2) subset of lymphocytes. Immediate release of histamine and interleukins recruits other cell types, and the activation of Th2 lymphocytes further potentiates airway inflammation. The Th2 response appears to be modulated by Treg cells, a newly discovered, seemingly protective lymphocyte subset. Some patients also experience a late-phase asthmatic response, which manifests as a secondary decrease in FEV_1 4 to 8 hours after immediate exposure.

Bronchial biopsies in patients with allergic and even nonallergic asthma demonstrate accumulation of eosinophils, mast cells, and CD4+ T lymphocytes. When chronic, this results in airway remodeling with structural changes such as mucus cell hyperplasia, subepithelial thickening of basement membrane, smooth muscle hypertrophy, connective tissue deposition, and airway fibrosis.

Risk Factors

The degree to which individual predisposition and environmental factors play a role in asthma is unclear. Genetic susceptibility may be modulated through DNA methylation, which can be altered by environmental factors such as diet and in utero exposures. Genetic studies have identified gene clusters, some of which have been associated with childhood but not adult asthma. However, no single gene or gene cluster accounts for all types of asthma.

Exposures to indoor environmental allergens, environmental tobacco smoke, and viruses can predispose individuals to asthma. Common allergens are indoor mold, house dust, domestic animals, and cockroaches. Maternal smoking during pregnancy and after delivery increases immune responsiveness and the risk for asthma in the infant. Rhinovirus infections in early childhood may also play a role in increasing airway inflammation.

The hygiene hypothesis suggests that exposure to microbial diversity appears to protect against asthma by shifting Th cells to a Th1 instead of a predominantly Th2 phenotype. Breast feeding, exposure to microbial diversity, and avoidance of environmental tobacco smoke have been associated with reduced incidences of asthma; however, a definitive strategy to prevent the development of asthma has not been established.

KEY POINT

- Exposures to indoor environmental allergens, environmental tobacco smoke, and viruses can predispose individuals to asthma.

Symptoms and Clinical Evaluation

Patients with asthma classically present with a history of episodes of coughing, chest tightness, shortness of breath, and wheezing. The cough may be spastic and dry or may be productive of mucus. Some patients have only cough or shortness of breath, as asthma presents differently in different patients. For example, some patients may have an unremitting cough after exposure to cold air or after respiratory tract infections, and other patients with asthma may have significant breathlessness even without cough that is worse with any activity. Patients may identify the onset of symptoms with specific triggers, such as known allergen exposure, inhaled irritants, respiratory tract infections, and exercise. Other conditions that mimic asthma should be considered (**Table 4**).

In patients with suspected asthma, the first step in evaluation is usually spirometry to assess for the presence and severity of airway obstruction (as indicated by a reduced FEV_1/FVC ratio) and its reversibility (with a 12% or greater improvement in FEV_1 after administration of a bronchodilator).

TABLE 4. Differential Diagnosis of Asthma	
Condition	**Characteristics**
COPD	Airway obstruction is less reversible; typically seen in older patients with smoking history
Vocal cord dysfunction	Abrupt onset and end of symptoms; monophonic wheeze; more common in younger patients; confirm with laryngoscopy or flow-volume loop
Heart failure	Dyspnea and often wheezing; crackles on auscultation; limited response to asthma therapy; cardiomegaly; edema; elevated BNP; other features of heart failure
Bronchiectasis	Cough productive of large amount of purulent sputum; rhonchi and crackles are common; may have wheezing and clubbing; confirmed by CT imaging
Allergic bronchopulmonary aspergillosis	Recurrent infiltrates on chest radiograph; eosinophilia; positive skin testing to *Aspergillus* antigens, high IgE levels, positive to *Aspergillus*; frequent need for glucocorticoid treatment
Cystic fibrosis	Cough productive of large amount of purulent sputum; rhonchi and crackles are common; prominent clubbing; may have wheezing. GI symptoms due to pancreatic insufficiency with possible sinus diseases are common, but recurrent respiratory tract infections may be present without GI or other systemic involvement.
Mechanical obstruction	More localized wheezing; if central in location, flow-volume loop may provide a clue
Eosinophilic granulomatosis with polyangiitis (formerly known as Churg-Strauss syndrome)	Autoimmune small-vessel vasculitis presents with peripheral eosinophilia, lung symptoms similar to asthma; skin changes such as purpura and sensory or motor neuropathy are other systemic symptoms; + ANCA in 40%-60% patients, mostly p-ANCA

ANCA = antineutrophil cytoplasmic antibodies; BNP = B-type natriuretic peptide; GI = gastrointestinal; p-ANCA = perinuclear antineutrophil cytoplasmic antibodies.

Although not routinely tested, some patients with asthma may have lung volumes evaluated for dyspnea or cough; patients with air trapping associated with asthma-related airway obstruction may demonstrate an increase in residual volume. Between attacks and exacerbations, spirometry can be normal in patients with suspected asthma. Therefore, a bronchial challenge test may be helpful for diagnosis if positive or make the diagnosis less likely if negative (see Pulmonary Diagnostic Tests).

Chest radiographs are often normal or may demonstrate widened rib spaces and a flattened diaphragm, resulting from air trapping due to chronic airflow obstruction. Eosinophils can be found in sputum, and allergy evaluation with skin testing or blood testing for specific IgE antibodies may aid in the assessment of risk and management of asthma. For individuals in whom allergies may be a trigger or contributing factor, referral to an allergist for allergen skin testing or blood tests for common inhaled allergens may enable patients to avoid exposures. Exhaled nitric oxide testing is a newer noninvasive breath test. Nitric oxide is normally present in airways but is increased in certain types of airway inflammation (asthma, eosinophilic airway inflammation). When elevated, it supports the diagnosis of asthma in the appropriate clinical context.

KEY POINTS

- Patients with asthma classically present with episodic symptoms of cough, chest tightness, shortness of breath, and wheezing.

- In patients with suspected asthma, the first step in evaluation is usually spirometry to assess for the presence and severity of airway obstruction (as indicated by a reduced FEV_1/FVC ratio) and its reversibility (with a 12% or greater improvement in FEV_1 after administration of a bronchodilator).

Asthma Syndromes

Allergic Asthma

Allergic asthma is the most common form of asthma in adults. Patients with atopy may present with allergic asthma early in life, experience a period of stability, and then may have recurrence later. However, allergic asthma can also manifest initially during adulthood. Family history is often positive for allergies and asthma. Symptoms may be seasonal, requiring trigger avoidance and stepping up of asthma therapy during times of known exacerbations. Individuals with perennial allergies may need more sustained controller therapy, with modification (stepping up or stepping down) of treatment based upon sequential monitoring and assessment. Additionally, superimposed viral infections or other nonallergic triggers (such as sinus diseases) may exacerbate underlying allergic asthma.

Cough-Variant Asthma

Asthma can present with a persistent or episodic cough in the absence of other common symptoms usually associated with asthma. Extrinsic triggers such as cold air or irritants can stimulate or make the cough worse. Spirometry and bronchial challenge testing can be helpful to establish the diagnosis and distinguish asthma from other causes of cough, such as upper airway cough syndrome (rhinosinusitis, postnasal drip) and gastroesophageal reflux. Treatment of cough-variant asthma is similar to usual guideline-based therapy for asthma.

See MKSAP 17 General Internal Medicine for a discussion of chronic cough.

Exercise-Induced Bronchospasm

In exercise-induced bronchospasm (EIB), symptoms occur in patients with asthma with exercise that requires increased respiratory ventilation. Increased ventilation, particularly of cool, dry air, causes drying of airway surfaces, which triggers bronchoconstriction via several mechanisms. When the airway-drying phenomenon is reversed, a rebound effect (with recruitment and infiltration of inflammatory cells) causes asthma symptoms. In patients with dyspnea with exercise but normal spirometry, methacholine challenge testing can be useful to assess the degree to which symptoms are related to hyperreactivity of the lungs.

If symptoms occur only a few times per week, EIB can be managed with inhaled short-acting β_2-agonists (such as albuterol) given 5 to 20 minutes prior to exercise; this therapy can be protective for 2 to 4 hours. Inhaled glucocorticoids are useful in minimizing the number and severity of exercise-induced asthma episodes. Antileukotriene therapy is also effective for the chronic management of patients with EIB.

Nonpharmacologic management includes warming and humidifying inhaled air with nasal breathing, as well as covering the nose and mouth during exercise in colder environments. A 10-minute pre-exercise warmup (to achieve a 60% to 80% of maximum heart rate) may decrease the occurrence of exercise-related bronchospasm for up to 4 hours.

KEY POINT

- If symptoms occur only a few times per week, exercise-induced bronchospasm can be managed with inhaled short-acting β_2-agonists (such as albuterol) given 5 to 20 minutes prior to exercise; this therapy can be protective for 2 to 4 hours.

Occupational Asthma

Occupational asthma, related to workplace exposures to agents associated with airway hyperreactivity, should be suspected in all adults with asthma because it may be preventable in most cases. Approximately 10% of workers exposed to known sensitizing agents develop asthma; farmers, factory workers, and hairdressers, among others, are at risk. Exposure to animal allergens, plants, grains, wood dust, and chemicals (diisocyanates from spray paint, persulfates), even at low levels, can act as sensitizers through responses similar to other forms of asthma (T lymphocytes, eosinophils, interleukins, mast cells, histamine). Early recognition of an association of asthma symptoms with potential workplace exposure, and testing if

indicated, is important for diagnosis and to guide therapy. Serial monitoring of peak flows throughout the workday, with comparison to a baseline time period away from exposures, can be helpful to support the diagnosis. Similarly, spirometry before and after rechallenge with workplace exposures is helpful to confirm the diagnosis. Treatment of occupational asthma should follow guidelines for typical asthma, and allergen exposure should be controlled or eliminated if possible.

KEY POINT

- Approximately 10% of workers exposed to known sensitizing agents have asthma; farmers, factory workers, and hairdressers, among others, are at risk.

Aspirin-Sensitive Asthma

Also known as aspirin-exacerbated respiratory disease or Samter triad, aspirin-sensitive asthma includes severe persistent asthma, aspirin sensitivity, and hyperplastic eosinophilic sinusitis with nasal polyposis. Asthma is worsened by exposure to aspirin or other NSAIDs, likely because of the inhibition of cyclooxygenase and the resulting increase in leukotriene synthesis. Treatment consists of avoidance of aspirin or NSAIDs along with typical asthma management. For patients who require aspirin use (such as those with coronary artery disease), an aspirin desensitization procedure can be performed. Successful desensitization down-regulates leukotriene receptors and modifies interleukin sensitivity, which may improve asthma symptoms in some patients.

Reactive Airways Dysfunction Syndrome

Reactive airways dysfunction syndrome (RADS) is the development of respiratory symptoms in the minutes or hours after a single inhalation of a high concentration of irritant; airway hyperresponsiveness then persists for an extended period of time. RADS is not a form of typical asthma; it may be a temporary phenomenon that occurs after a short-lived and/or high-dose exposure to an irritant in a patient without asthma. Examples of exposures include inhalation of strong fumes, particulate matter (such as wood smoke), or chemical irritants (such as cleaning supplies). Spirometry may reveal evidence of bronchoconstriction that is reversible. Initial treatment is similar to that of asthma. The clinical course and recovery may allow reduction of medications relatively quickly; however, initial symptoms may also be early manifestations of new-onset asthma that will require chronic management.

Virus-Induced Bronchospasm

A viral respiratory infection can lead to airway hyperresponsiveness and obstruction through nonallergic mechanisms in patients without a history of asthma, and the associated bronchospasm may be limited only to the duration of the infection. Virus-induced bronchospasm in patients without asthma typically resolves 6 to 8 weeks after a respiratory infection. Viral respiratory infections may also exacerbate disease in patients with allergic asthma, with up to half of asthma exacerbations being related to human rhinovirus infection. Patients with asthma often exhibit more severe symptoms from influenza infections (especially the recent H1N1 strain), possibly owing to differential responses of airway epithelial cells in nonasthmatic versus asthmatic airways. Because of this, annual influenza vaccinations are a key part of the management of patients with asthma.

Allergic Bronchopulmonary Aspergillosis

Allergic bronchopulmonary aspergillosis (ABPA) is a chronic hypersensitivity reaction that occurs in response to colonization of the lower airways with *Aspergillus* species. The resulting inflammation causes impaired mucociliary clearance with expectoration of mucus plugs, destruction of pulmonary parenchyma with bronchiectasis, difficult-to-control asthma, and weight loss. Diagnosis is determined by clinical history, testing (positive skin testing to *Aspergillus* antigens, high IgE titers to *Aspergillus*, peripheral eosinophilia), and radiographic findings (proximal bronchiectasis, pleural thickening, transient infiltrates, or atelectasis). Treatment includes systemic glucocorticoids; inhaled glucocorticoids may reduce the need for higher doses of systemic glucocorticoids. Antifungal therapy (such as fluconazole) may be helpful in conjunction with glucocorticoid therapy, and anti-IgE therapy (such as omalizumab) may be used as adjunctive treatment in selected patients.

Common Contributing Factors

Gastroesophageal Reflux Disease

Gastroesophageal reflux disease (GERD) can make underlying asthma worse through direct reflux of acidic gastric contents into the respiratory system, resulting in upper airway inflammation or direct airway injury. The reflux of gastric contents into the lower part of the esophagus can also cause a reflex bronchoconstriction. There is evidence that treating GERD in patients with asthma improves asthma control. In most patients with asthma and suboptimal control of symptoms, a history consistent with GERD is adequate to justify a trial of empiric antacid therapy without further testing for evidence of reflux. Management of GERD in patients with asthma is an important component of therapy; see MKSAP 17 Gastroenterology and Hepatology for a discussion of the diagnosis and management of GERD.

Sinus Disease

Because disorders affecting the upper respiratory tract may affect the lower tract (unified airway concept), sinus disorders may be associated with worsening control of asthma. Patients with frequent asthma exacerbations should be evaluated for occult sinus disease, as untreated upper airway inflammation may contribute to poor asthma control. Treatment of bacterial sinusitis or allergic sinusitis with nasal glucocorticoids can reduce bronchial hyperresponsiveness, shortness of breath, and wheezing.

Obstructive Sleep Apnea

Asthma has been associated with obstructive sleep apnea (OSA), and the relationship appears to be bidirectional. OSA appears to affect asthma control, and continuous positive airway pressure treatment for comorbid OSA improves asthma symptoms, frequency of rescue inhaler use, and quality-of-life scores. In difficult-to-control asthma, OSA is a significant risk factor for frequent exacerbations. Treatment of OSA affects both daytime and nighttime asthma symptoms, suggesting that local and systemic inflammatory pathways are implicated in the association. See Sleep Medicine for a discussion of the diagnosis and management of OSA.

Vocal Cord Dysfunction

The clinical suspicion of paradoxical vocal fold motion (PVFM) disorder, also known as vocal cord dysfunction, should be high when patients describe (1) mid-chest tightness with exposure to particular triggers such as strong irritants or emotions, (2) difficulty breathing in, and (3) symptoms that only partially respond to asthma medications. Symptoms include mid-chest tightness, dyspnea, and lack of symptom relief with asthma treatment. Patients may also note cough and dysphonia, and stridor may be present that may be detected on examination as inspiratory monophonic wheezing. PVFM disorder can occur suddenly; although it can be present with asthma, it is often misdiagnosed as asthma, resulting in high health care utilization and multiple intubations. Adduction of vocal cords during inspiration as seen on laryngoscopy is the gold standard for diagnosis (**Figure 5**); however, the diagnosis is often made clinically based on history. It may also be diagnosed if spirometry happens to capture a flat inspiratory limb on the flow-volume loop. Speech therapy training exercises (to control the laryngeal area and maintain airflow) and treatment of GERD can result in dramatic improvement in PVFM disorder symptoms.

> **KEY POINT**
> - Vocal cord dysfunction, characterized by (1) mid-chest tightness with exposure to triggers, (2) difficulty breathing in, and (3) partial response to asthma medications, is often misdiagnosed as severe asthma resulting in unnecessary intubations and high health care utilization.

HVC

Obesity

Obesity is one of the strongest risk factors for developing asthma, may have a causal role, and affects prognosis and outcomes in asthma. Obese patients with asthma experience more severe asthma with increased symptoms, worse quality of life, and increased health care utilization. Obesity can worsen childhood-onset allergic asthma. Mechanical strain (breathing against the pressure of added chest or abdominal girth) and obesity-related cytokines, called adipokines, can also affect late-onset nonallergic asthma. Dramatic weight loss

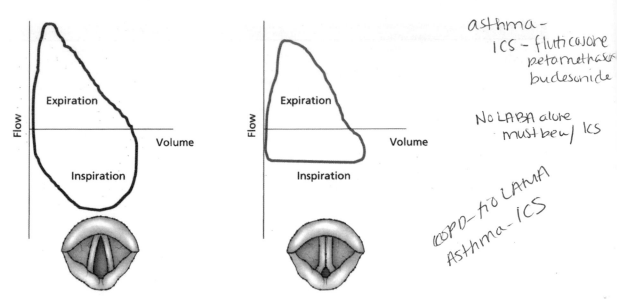

[handwritten notes: asthma- ICS - fluticasone betamethasone budesonide; No LABA alone must be w/ ICS; COPD - to LAMA Asthma- ICS]

FIGURE 5. Flow-volume loops showing maximum inspiratory and expiratory flow-volume relationships in a patient with vocal cord dysfunction during asymptomatic (*left*) and symptomatic (*right*) periods. Note also the marked adduction of the vocal cords with severe reduction of the glottic aperture during a symptomatic period of airway obstruction (*right*).

has proved to be successful in controlling the disease, particularly in a subgroup of middle-aged obese women with non-allergic asthma.

Chronic Management

Goals for the management of asthma outlined by the National Heart, Lung, and Blood Institute include assessment and monitoring, control of factors contributing to symptom exacerbation, pharmacotherapy, and education for partnership in care.

On initial diagnosis of asthma, severity of disease should be determined based on the level of impairment and risk of future exacerbations using the frequency of symptoms, need for quick-relief medications, and degree of obstruction on spirometry (**Table 5**). Appropriate treatment should be initiated based on this assessment (**Figure 6**). Symptoms should be monitored after treatment is initiated; therapy may need to be adjusted as symptom patterns may change over time. If changes in symptoms occur, it is reasonable to reevaluate lung function with spirometry. During times of symptom stability, spirometry should be performed yearly.

Depression is significantly associated with asthma and is present more commonly in patients with asthma than in those with other chronic diseases. A high index of suspicion for and treatment of depression can reduce impairment from asthma. Depression in patients with asthma is underrecognized and has been associated with increased emergency department visits and hospitalizations, decreased lung function, higher medication nonadherence, and increased asthma-related deaths.

Medications

Inhaled glucocorticoids are the mainstay of therapy because of the inflammatory mechanisms underlying asthma. β_2-Agonists are used for symptom relief, and additional medications such as systemic glucocorticoids and anticholinergic agents may be useful in managing asthma in specific situations. Owing to the dynamic nature of asthma, pharmacologic management may require step-wise modification based on periodic assessment of asthma severity.

Quick-Relief Medications

β_2-Agonists are sympathomimetic agents that act on airway β receptors that activate adenylate cyclase, increasing cyclic adenosine monophosphate levels. These activate protein kinase A, which phosphorylates regulatory proteins that mediate bronchodilation. Short-acting β_2-agonists (for example, albuterol, salbutamol) help relieve the acute symptoms of chest tightness, wheeze, shortness of breath, and cough but do not treat or improve the underlying problem of airway inflammation. Long-acting β_2-agonists (LABAs) (for example, salmeterol) are available and should be used in conjunction with inhaled glucocorticoids to avoid potential tolerance to bronchodilators.

Anticholinergic agents dilate bronchial smooth muscle by decreasing the constrictive cholinergic tone in the airways. Although it is less effective than β_2-agonists, the short-acting agent ipratropium can be used as adjunctive quick-relief therapy during asthma exacerbations.

KEY POINT

- In patients with asthma, short-acting β_2-agonists (albuterol, salbutamol) help relieve the acute symptoms of chest tightness, wheeze, shortness of breath, and cough but do not treat or improve the underlying problem of airway inflammation.

[handwritten notes at bottom: ICS- beclomethasone budesonide fluticasone mometasone; ICS - to B2 agonist albut.; ACH →; Ipratropium = Anti ACh; tiotropium = Anti ACh (spiriva)]

TABLE 5. Classification of Asthma Severity

Components of Severity	Intermittent	Persistent		
		Mild	Moderate	Severe
Impairment[a]				
Symptoms	≤2 days/week	>2 days/week but not daily	Daily	Throughout the day
Nighttime awakenings	≤2 ×/month	3-4 ×/month	>1 ×/week but not nightly	Often 7 ×/week
SABA use for symptom control (not prevention of EIB)	≤2 days/week	>2 days/week but not more than 1 ×/d	Daily	Several times a day
Interference with normal activity	None	Minor limitation	Some limitation	Extremely limited
Lung function	Normal FEV_1 between exacerbations FEV_1 ≥80% of predicted FEV_1/FVC normal	FEV_1 ≥80% of predicted FEV_1/FVC normal	FEV_1 ≥60% but <80% of predicted FEV_1/FVC reduced ≤5%	FEV_1 <60% of predicted FEV_1/FVC reduced >5%
Risk				
Exacerbations (consider frequency and severity)[b,c]	0-1/year	>2/year	>2/year	>2/year
Recommended step for initiating treatment (see Figure 6 for treatment steps)[d]	Step 1	Step 2	Step 3; consider short courses of systemic glucocorticoids	Step 4 or 5; consider short courses of systemic glucocorticoids

EIB = exercise-induced bronchospasm; SABA = short-acting β_2-agonist.

[a]Normal FEV_1/FVC ratio: 8-19 years old, 85%; 20-39 years old, 80%; 40-59 years old, 75%; 60-80 years old, 70%.

[b]Frequency and severity may fluctuate over time for patients in any severity category.

[c]Relative annual risk for exacerbations may be related to FEV_1.

[d]In 2 to 6 weeks, evaluate the level of asthma control that is achieved and adjust therapy accordingly.

Source: National Heart, Lung, and Blood Institute; National Institutes of Health; U.S. Department of Health and Human Services. National Asthma Education and Prevention Program. Expert Panel Report 3 (EPR-3): Guidelines for the Diagnosis and Management of Asthma. http://www.nhlbi.nih.gov/files/docs/guidelines/asthsumm.pdf. Published 2007. Accessed June 15, 2015.

Controller Medications

When symptoms related to asthma occur more than twice per week or one night per week, asthma is considered persistent. At this stage, it is appropriate to start controller therapy to reduce airway inflammation from asthma. Inhaled glucocorticoids are the mainstay of controller asthma treatment. They have been shown to improve and control symptoms, reduce exacerbations, and improve lung function. These agents treat the underlying inflammatory disease process, and the inhaled formulation allows drug delivery with minimal systemic absorption and limited side effects. Newer formulations require twice-daily dosing, and varying potency allows careful titration of treatment to minimize potential side effects. Differences in delivery devices (traditional inhaler versus dry powder inhalation formulations) can accommodate patient preferences and capabilities. Traditional inhalers use a pump, and aerosolized medication is delivered. With inhalers, proper (slow and steady) inhalation technique, inhalation chambers (known as spacers), and a breath hold can improve drug deliv- ery and avoid side effects such as thrush. Dry powder inhalers deliver a fine powder to the lungs; they require less coordination but require more forceful inhalation than with a traditional inhaler.

When inhaled glucocorticoids alone do not achieve asthma control, the addition of a LABA has proved to be effective as step-up therapy. Combination preparations that contain an inhaled glucocorticoid and a LABA are available. In addition to bronchodilation, LABAs appear to potentiate anti-inflammatory effects of inhaled glucocorticoids when taken together. However, the LABA portion of the combination preparation can cause side effects (for example, anxiety, tremor, and headache); therefore, stepping down LABA therapy should be considered after a period of sustained asthma control.

In conjunction with inhaled glucocorticoids, long-acting anticholinergic agents (such as tiotropium) may have an anti-inflammatory effect, which has been shown to increase time to severe exacerbation and result in modest

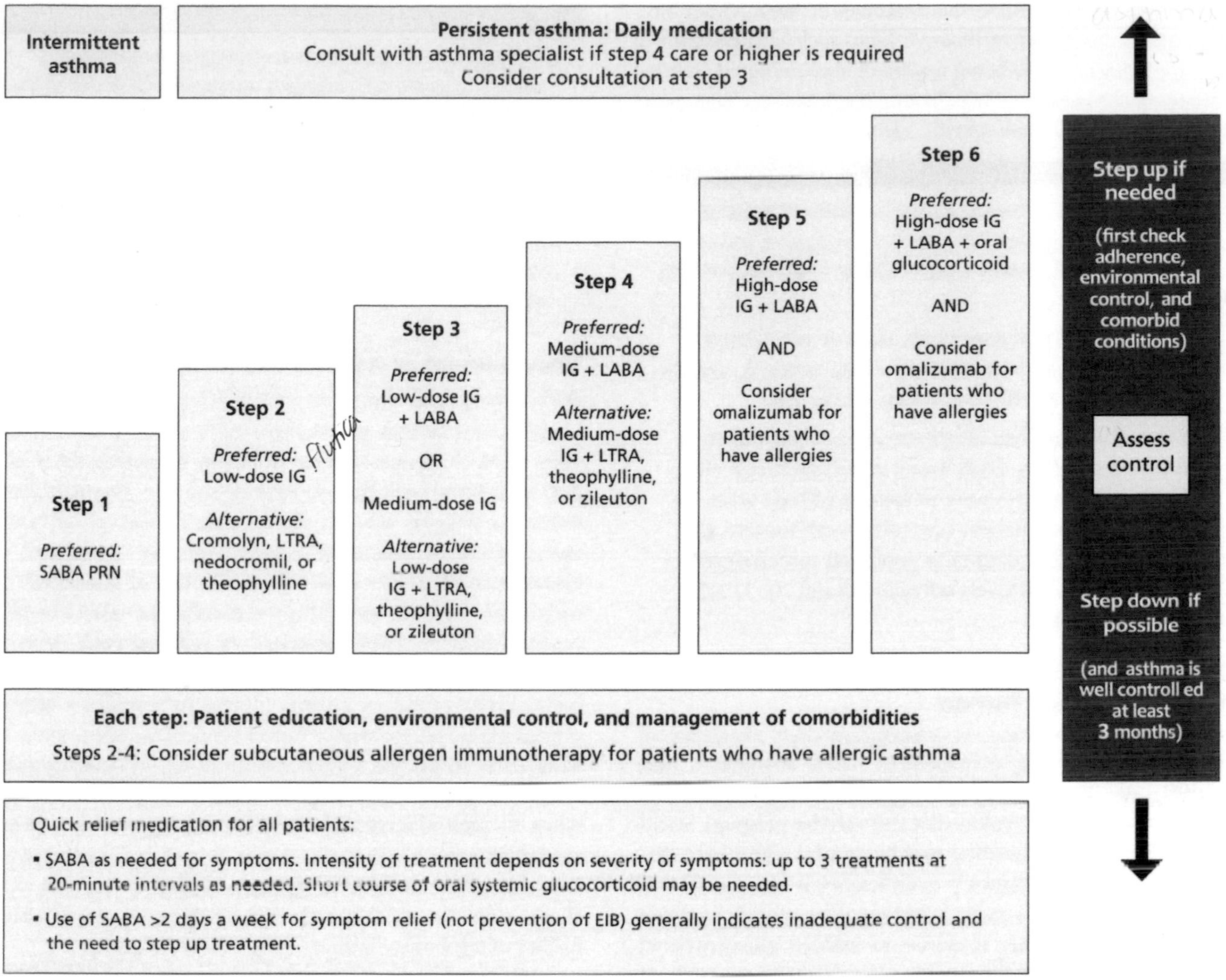

FIGURE 6. Stepwise approach to asthma therapy. EIB = exercise-induced bronchospasm; IG = inhaled glucocorticoids; LABA = long-acting β_2-agonist; LTRA = leukotriene receptor antagonist; PRN = as needed; SABA = short-acting β_2-agonist.

Source: National Heart, Lung, and Blood Institute; National Institutes of Health; U.S. Department of Health and Human Services. National Asthma Education and Prevention Program. Expert Panel Report 3 (EPR-3): Guidelines for the Diagnosis and Management of Asthma. www.nhlbi.nih.gov/files/docs/guidelines/asthsumm.pdf. Published 2007. Accessed June 15, 2015.

sustained bronchodilation. These agents should be considered when inhaled glucocorticoids, LABAs, and leukotriene receptor antagonists (LTRAs) do not provide sufficient control.

LTRAs are not considered first-line controller therapy in any asthma population but can be used as an add-on to inhaled glucocorticoid therapy. LTRAs have a particular role in EIB and aspirin-sensitive asthma, and they can be helpful in sinus disease because they target a different area of the inflammatory cascade.

Theophylline is an older drug from the methylxanthine drug class. Methylxanthines inhibit phosphodiesterase, which is normally responsible for degradation of cyclic adenosine monophosphate, and therefore may have effects on bronchodilation, with potential for some anti-inflammatory capability. Owing to drug toxicity and side effects and improved availability of inhaled glucocorticoids, methylxanthines (such as theophylline) are not commonly used.

Some patients experience severe asthma such that even the optimal inhaled glucocorticoid therapies may not provide sufficient control, and in those situations chronic oral glucocorticoids may be necessary.

Omalizumab, a humanized monoclonal antibody directed at IgE, is the first biologic agent approved by the FDA for use in asthma. Administered subcutaneously every 2 to 4 weeks, omalizumab is indicated in patients with moderate to severe persistent asthma with the following characteristics: (1) symptoms inadequately controlled with inhaled glucocorticoids, (2) evidence of allergies to perennial aeroallergens, and (3) serum IgE levels between 30 and 700 U/mL (30-700 kU/L) (normal range, 0-90 U/mL [0-90 kU/L]). Although it is expensive, omalizumab has been shown to reduce emergency department visits and appears to be cost effective in appropriately selected patients; it is not indicated for use in patients other than those meeting these treatment parameters. This agent can also be useful in the treatment of ABPA. Other biologic agents that target various cytokines such as interleukin-5 and interleukin-13 are being explored, and emerging characterization of biomarkers in individual patients may help guide appropriate use of these specific agents.

KEY POINTS

- Inhaled glucocorticoids are the mainstay of asthma treatment; they have been shown to improve and control symptoms, reduce exacerbations, and improve lung function.

- When inhaled glucocorticoids alone do not achieve asthma control, the addition of a long-acting β_2-agonist has proved to be effective as step-up therapy.

HVC
- Although expensive, omalizumab has been shown to reduce emergency department visits and is cost effective in moderate to severe persistent asthma with: (1) symptoms inadequately controlled with inhaled glucocorticoids, (2) allergies to perennial aeroallergens, and (3) serum IgE levels between 30 and 700 U/mL (30-700 kU/L).

Nonpharmacologic Therapy

Comprehensive asthma care strategies include avoidance of triggers with allergen management (mold abatement, pest control, air filters), reduced exposure to environmental tobacco smoke, and a healthy diet and exercise program. Stress management and counseling may be helpful adjuncts to disease management. Vitamin D insufficiency is associated with a lower level of asthma control, and supplementation has been associated with greater response to inhaled glucocorticoid therapy. Yearly influenza vaccination reduces the risk of asthma exacerbations from influenza.

It is important to address potential barriers to optimal asthma management. For example, prescription of complex treatment regimens may impair adherence, and financial issues associated with acquiring medications may pose a challenge in some patients.

Bronchial thermoplasty (BT) was recently approved by the FDA as an adjunctive therapy for patients with asthma who remain symptomatic despite optimization of medications. A bronchoscopically-introduced catheter is used to apply thermal energy to conducting airways 3 mm or greater in diameter with the goal of reducing smooth muscle thickening in the airway walls. Three bronchoscopic sessions, spaced at least 3 weeks apart, are performed to treat different sections of the lung. After treatment, measures of lung function remain unchanged, but notable outcomes from BT include improved asthma-related symptoms, reduced emergency department visits, and improvement in severity of exacerbations. Adverse effects include a temporary worsening of asthma after the procedure is performed. As experience increases, it is likely that careful patient selection will play an important role in BT outcomes.

KEY POINTS

- Comprehensive asthma care strategies include avoidance of triggers with allergen management (mold abatement, pest control, air filters), reduced exposure to environmental tobacco smoke, and a healthy diet and exercise program.

- Bronchial thermoplasty was recently approved by the FDA as an adjunctive therapy for patients with asthma who remain symptomatic despite optimization of medications.

Management of Asthma Exacerbations

With appropriate education and development of a patient-implemented asthma action plan, many patients can manage early signs of an exacerbation at home. Measurement of airflow with serial peak flow measurements may be particularly helpful in patients who are appropriate candidates for home management by providing a more objective assessment of disease status than the subjective perception of symptoms. At early signs of asthma instability (increased shortness of breath, cough, wheezing, chest tightness, or reduced peak flows to less than 50% of baseline), starting a course of systemic glucocorticoids may improve asthma control. In most cases, antibiotic agents are not necessary unless bronchitis, pneumonia, or sinusitis is suspected. Patients attempting self-management should be given individualized, clear parameters regarding when to seek emergency treatment when treating asthma exacerbations at home (for example, lack of resolution despite three nebulized albuterol treatments, failure to improve with systemic glucocorticoids, early self-referral for patients with a history of respiratory failure or need for intubation).

When evaluating patients with an acute exacerbation, it is important to consider factors that increase the risk of poorer outcomes, which include a history of frequent emergency department visits for asthma, the need for endotracheal intubation and mechanical ventilation to treat previous exacerbations, and poor perception of the presence of reduced lung function. Patients who are not responding to initial treatment and have persistently high work of breathing, particularly high-risk patients (those with lack of improvement with outpatient management, poor access to care, or a history of intubation or near-fatal asthma), should be admitted to the hospital and considered for intensive care management (see Critical Care Medicine). Management should include close monitoring of dyspnea, work of breathing, and vital signs; frequent bronchodilator treatment; and systemic glucocorticoids. Pulse oximetry may be falsely reassuring because patients maintain normal oxygen levels despite high work of breathing, and hypoxia is a late sign of pending respiratory failure. In patients who are at high risk or have lack of symptom resolution with initial therapies, arterial blood gas assessment is vital and may initially reveal hyperventilation with a low arterial P_{CO_2}. Normalization of the P_{CO_2} could be an early indicator of airway muscle fatigue and impending respiratory arrest.

CONT.

Severe Refractory Asthma

Although most patients with asthma achieve symptom control, approximately 10% of patients have severe refractory asthma. Patients are considered to have severe refractory asthma if they have multiple exacerbations per year, a need for high-dose inhaled or oral glucocorticoids, an inability to step down therapy without compromising asthma control, or a history of multiple hospitalizations or intubations. The cause of severe asthma is heterogeneous, and appropriate therapy should be tailored to the specific characteristics of a patient's asthma syndrome. These patients usually require multidisciplinary and specialist care to manage their disease; this may consist of a team of social workers, pulmonary rehabilitation specialists/respiratory therapists, allergists, otolaryngologists, gastroenterologists, and pulmonary specialists. **H**

> **KEY POINT**
>
> - Patients are considered to have severe refractory asthma if they have multiple exacerbations per year, a need for high-dose inhaled or oral glucocorticoids, an inability to step down therapy without compromising asthma control, or a history of multiple hospitalizations or intubations.

Asthma in Pregnancy

Approximately one third of pregnant women with asthma experience worsening asthma symptoms, one third have no change in symptoms, and another third have improvement in symptoms. Lack of asthma control increases the risk for preeclampsia and preterm labor for mothers and low birth weight, small gestational size, and preterm delivery for the infant. Asthma management during pregnancy should consist of optimization of anti-inflammatory therapy, management of gastroesophageal reflux, and smoking cessation. Inhaled glucocorticoids are considered safe in pregnancy, and abundant long-term safety evidence exists for budesonide. Most LTRAs are also considered safe in pregnancy.

> **KEY POINT**
>
> - Inhaled glucocorticoids are considered safe for asthma therapy during pregnancy, and abundant long-term safety evidence exists for budesonide.

Chronic Obstructive Pulmonary Disease

Definition

COPD is characterized by persistent, progressive airflow limitation, which arises from structural lung changes due to chronic inflammation as a result of inhaling noxious particles or gases. Chronic inflammation causes narrowing of the small airways and decreased elastic recoil of the lung, which diminishes the capacity of the airways to remain open during expiration. The resulting increase in air trapping and hyperinflation contributes to progressive airflow limitation. The characteristic symptoms of COPD are chronic dyspnea, cough, and sputum production.

Epidemiology

COPD is the third most common cause of death worldwide and a major cause of chronic morbidity, resulting in an increasingly substantial economic and social burden.

Evidence suggests that up to 50% of the total population with COPD remain undiagnosed. In populations with diagnosed COPD, studies indicate that patients frequently are undertreated, with an estimated 30% to 70% receiving no therapy or suboptimal treatment.

Pathophysiology

The underlying pathophysiology in COPD is chronic inflammation triggered and maintained by inhalation of toxic particles and gases, most commonly from tobacco smoke. Inflammation disrupts normal repair mechanisms and results in thickening and narrowing of the small airways (obstructive bronchiolitis). The inflammatory response also causes release of proteases that dissolve a portion of the adjacent lung tissue, including elastin, the major component of the connective tissue in the lung parenchyma that tethers the small airways open. The loss of elastin causes a decrease in the elastic recoil of the lungs that normally keeps airways open during exhalation. Proteases also damage the airspaces distal to the terminal bronchioles, resulting in permanent enlargement of airspaces with loss of diffusing surface (emphysema). Multiple factors influence the severity of the inflammatory process, including genetics, the level of oxidative stress, and a reduced presence of endogenous antioxidants. However, the degree of inflammation intensifies as disease progresses and the risk of exacerbations increases.

The decreased elasticity of the lung parenchyma causes both static and dynamic hyperinflation. Static hyperinflation occurs because of the loss of the recoil properties of the lung resulting in the inability to fully exhale, leading to permanent increases in end-expiratory lung volumes. In contrast, dynamic hyperinflation occurs when patients begin to inhale before full exhalation of the previous breath has been completed, such that inspiratory air volume exceeds expiratory volume, trapping air within the lungs with each successive breath. The ability to fully exhale is dependent on the degree of airflow obstruction (associated with the degree of structural changes, inflammation, increases in cholinergic tone, and mucus plugging) and rate of breathing. Both can vary and cause greater hyperinflation during periods of exertion and exacerbation. When the demand for greater minute ventilation occurs, increases in tidal volume and respiration rate ensue, and the available time for exhalation can become insufficient, creating a cycle of air trapping and progressive dynamic hyperinflation. Progressive hyperinflation expands the lungs, flattening and reducing the mechanical effectiveness of the diaphragm, making use of accessory muscles of breathing more crucial, and markedly increasing the work of breathing as chest wall compliance decreases. Because of these changes, the ability to increase minute ventilation is severely compromised in patients with COPD. As disease progresses, dynamic hyperinflation occurs even during quiet breathing, causing worsening dyspnea and significant impairment of exercise and activity intolerance.

Gas diffusion by the lung is also impaired in COPD. The ability to exchange CO_2 and oxygen correlates with the degree of functional impairment of gas exchange and reduction of the available capillary bed for gas diffusion owing to a loss of lung parenchyma.

Risk Factors

Essentially all risk for development and progression of COPD results from an interaction between patient and environmental factors.

It is estimated that up to 20% or more of COPD occurs in non- and never-smokers. However, smoking cessation is the single most clinically efficacious and cost-effective way to prevent COPD. Discontinuation of smoking in patients with established COPD slows disease progression and improves survival. The age at which patients start to smoke, total pack-years smoked, and current smoking status are cumulative predictors of COPD morbidity and mortality.

Relatives of patients with COPD have a higher prevalence of the disease, which cannot be attributed to personal or environmental risk factors. Additionally, there is a higher prevalence of reduced lung function among the children of patients with COPD than in their spouses; this is not well understood but is thought to be related to genetic predisposition. COPD is affected by multiple genes and genetic predisposition, but nongenetic factors (for example, childhood viral respiratory infections, childhood asthma, environmental and occupational pollution, and worldwide use of biomass fuels) likely contribute to increased susceptibility in this subset of patients.

KEY POINT

HVC
- Smoking cessation is the single most clinically efficacious and cost-effective way to prevent COPD, to slow progression of established disease, and to improve survival.

Heterogeneity of COPD

Patients with COPD have traditionally been categorized by the predominant manifestation of their disease; this is typically the degree of irreversible airway obstruction present (emphysema) or the presence of significant inflammation (chronic bronchitis), with or without a component of reversible airways disease (asthma). However, the clinical manifestations of COPD vary significantly between patients, suggesting that COPD is a conglomerate of several different disease processes.

Patients with COPD also typically demonstrate different clinical patterns, or phenotypes, of disease, with variations in severity of symptoms, response to treatment, and outcomes that may occur independent of genetic background. For example, some patients experience more rapid disease progression and more frequent exacerbations despite similar history, monitoring, and treatment. In addition to the "exacerbator" phenotype, the Global Initiative for Chronic Obstructive Lung Disease (GOLD) 2015 guidelines has added a phenotype called asthma COPD overlap syndrome (ACOS), as these patients have features of both asthma and COPD.

Role of Comorbid Conditions

Patients with COPD have a high frequency of comorbid conditions that adversely affect prognosis and significantly contribute to morbidity and mortality. It has been shown that the lung disease is frequently not appropriately treated in patients with COPD and significant comorbid conditions.

Cardiovascular disease is one of the most common comorbid conditions of COPD, and it is the leading cause of mortality in patients with mild to moderate COPD. The risk of cardiovascular injury is also significantly increased in patients with COPD who experience frequent exacerbations. During and immediately following an acute exacerbation of COPD, patients are particularly vulnerable to ischemic heart disease and acute myocardial infarction. Weight loss, muscle wasting, muscle weakness, and osteopenia are also common in patients with severe COPD. The rates of early hospital readmission for COPD exacerbation increase as the number of comorbidities increases.

KEY POINT

- Patients with COPD have a high frequency of comorbid conditions (such as cardiovascular disease, weight loss, muscle wasting, weakness, and osteopenia) that adversely affect prognosis and significantly contribute to morbidity and mortality.

Diagnosis

Spirometric evaluation is required for the clinical diagnosis of COPD. Spirometry is warranted in any patient presenting with dyspnea, chronic cough, or sputum production. Screening for COPD with spirometry should not be performed in asymptomatic patients.

For diagnosis of COPD, spirometry should be performed both before and after administration of an inhaled bronchodilator. A postbronchodilator fixed FEV_1/FVC ratio less than 70% is diagnostic for COPD in a consistent clinical context and differentiates COPD from asthma, which shows reversible airflow obstruction.

Patients with an FEV_1 of less than 35% of predicted should be assessed for adequacy of oxygenation with either arterial blood gas studies or measurement of oxyhemoglobin saturation with pulse oximetry.

Patients who develop symptoms of COPD and have a reduced FEV_1/FVC ratio at a young age (≤40 years of age) should be considered for α_1-antitrypsin deficiency testing. Patients with this disorder are often misdiagnosed with asthma for many years. They may have a modest smoking

$FEV_1/FVC < 70\%$

history and basilar emphysema (although they may present with any pattern of emphysema), and they may have concurrent liver disease. Patients with α_1-antitrypsin deficiency who never smoke may develop symptoms later in life. The pattern of basilar emphysema, liver disease, and family history of emphysema in patients with COPD should prompt consideration of α_1-antitrypsin deficiency in middle age and older patients.

KEY POINTS

HVC
- Screening for COPD with spirometry should not be performed in asymptomatic patients.
- A postbronchodilator fixed FEV₁/FVC ratio less than 70% is diagnostic for COPD in the correct clinical context and differentiates COPD from asthma, which shows reversible airflow obstruction.

Assessment and Monitoring

Initial assessment of patients with COPD includes a comprehensive medical history and physical examination to characterize the degree of impairment of lung function and identify potential comorbidities.

Patient symptoms and their impact on function may be more objectively assessed with either the Modified Medical Research Council (mMRC) Questionnaire or the COPD Assessment Test (CAT). The mMRC (**Table 6**) grades the degree of breathlessness using a 0 to 4 scale, with higher values indicating decreasing exercise tolerance. The CAT provides a numeric scale relating to eight functional parameters (for example, cough, sputum, walking, sleeping, energy level); lower scores indicate fewer symptoms and higher scores indicate more symptoms. The 2015 GOLD classification uses spirometric measures to provide a more objective classification of COPD severity (**Table 7**); a higher GOLD category indicates increased risk.

TABLE 6. Modified Medical Research Council (mMRC) Questionnaire for Assessing Severity of Breathlessness

Score	Description of Dyspnea	Severity
0	I get breathless only with strenuous exercise	None
1	I get short of breath when hurrying on level ground or walking up a slight hill	Mild
2	On level ground, I walk slower than other people my age because of breathlessness, or I have to stop for breath when walking at my own pace	Moderate
3	I stop for breath after walking approximately 100 yards or after a few minutes on level ground	Severe
4	I am too breathless to leave the house, or breathless when dressing	Very severe

TABLE 7. Classification of COPD Severity by Spirometry (In Patients with FEV₁/FVC <70%)

Category	Severity	Spirometry
GOLD 1	Mild	FEV₁ ≥80% of predicted
GOLD 2	Moderate	50% ≤ FEV₁ < 80% of predicted
GOLD 3	Severe	30% ≤ FEV₁ < 50% of predicted
GOLD 4	Very severe	FEV₁ <30% of predicted

The updated GOLD guidelines introduced a new model for classifying the severity of disease using more objective measures. The new classification scheme combines four parameters to categorize the level of risk in an individual patient (**Table 8**):

- Degree of patient symptoms as rated on a numeric scale (the CAT or mMRC questionnaire)
- GOLD classification of airflow obstruction
- Exacerbation risk based on the frequency and severity of previous episodes
- Presence of individual patient comorbidities

Exacerbation risk is determined by assessing exacerbations occurring in the past year; patients are considered high risk if they had any exacerbation leading to hospitalization, or two or more COPD exacerbations that did not require hospitalization.

Although comorbidities are not numerically incorporated into the new model, their presence is important for understanding the effect of COPD in specific patients; this information may be useful in assigning overall risk and in making patient-specific treatment decisions.

These parameters are used to assign a patient to a specific risk group, as outlined in Table 8.

Monitoring of patients with COPD includes ongoing review of symptoms, evaluation for complications of COPD, and assessment of frequency and severity of exacerbations, if present. Patients should be asked about changes in sputum volume, the occurrence of worsening dyspnea, and their psychological wellbeing. In patients on pharmacologic therapy, medication dosage(s) should be confirmed, and therapeutic adherence, side effects of treatment, and level of symptom control should be assessed. Because inhaled medications are a mainstay of COPD management, good inhaler technique should be ensured (particularly in patients with suboptimal symptom control) before making changes to the drug regimen. Follow-up visits should also include periodic reevaluation with spirometry, which is usually performed at least annually in stable patients to document changes in lung function and disease progression. Based on these elements, the efficacy of the therapeutic regimen should be reassessed and adjusted if needed.

TABLE 8. GOLD Model for Classifying Severity of Disease in COPD

Patient Category	Characteristics	Spirometric Classification[a]	Exacerbations Per Year	CAT Score	mMRC Score
A	Low risk, fewer symptoms	GOLD 1-2	≤1	<10	0-1
B	Low risk, more symptoms	GOLD 1-2	≤1	≥10	≥2
C	High risk, fewer symptoms	GOLD 3-4	≥2	<10	0-1
D	High risk, more symptoms	GOLD 3-4	≥2/≥1 with hospital admission	≥10	≥2

CAT = COPD Assessment Test; mMRC = Modified Medical Research Council.

[a]See Table 7 for definitions of spirometric classifications.

Data from the Global Strategy for Diagnosis, Management and Prevention of COPD 2015, © Global Initiative for Chronic Obstructive Lung Disease (GOLD), all rights reserved. Available from http://www.goldcopd.org.

Some patients may experience worsening symptoms and significant declines in lung function over time. **Table 9** provides criteria that can be useful for determining whether and when to refer to a pulmonary specialist.

KEY POINTS

- Monitoring of patients with COPD includes ongoing review of symptoms, evaluation for complications of COPD, and assessment of frequency and severity of exacerbations, if present.

HVC
- Because inhaled medications are a mainstay of COPD management, good inhaler technique should be ensured (particularly in patients with suboptimal symptom control) before making changes to the drug regimen.

TABLE 9. Criteria for Potential Referral of Patients with COPD to a Pulmonary Specialist

Diagnosis of COPD at ≤40 years of age

Frequent exacerbations (≥2/year) despite adequate treatment

Rapid disease course (decline in FEV_1, progressive dyspnea, decreased exercise tolerance, unintentional weight loss)

Severe COPD (FEV_1 <50% of predicted) despite optimal treatment

Need for oxygen therapy

Onset of a comorbid condition (especially cardiovascular disease or event)

Diagnostic uncertainty (for example, coexisting COPD and asthma)

Symptoms disproportionate to severity of airflow obstruction

Confirmed or suspected α_1-antitrypsin deficiency

Patient request for a second opinion

Patient is a potential candidate for lung transplant or lung-volume reduction surgery

Patient has very severe disease and requires elective surgery that may impair respiratory function

Source: Littner MR. In the clinic. Chronic obstructive pulmonary disease. Ann Intern Med. 2011 Apr 5;154(7):ITC4-1-ITC4-15. [PMID: 21464346]

Chronic Management

Therapeutic interventions in COPD have traditionally been guided by the degree of airflow obstruction as determined by spirometry, the subjective assessment of the severity of disease, and consideration of individual patient factors that might affect treatment. However, the new GOLD classification model (see Table 8) allows for risk- and symptom-based, individualized therapy for COPD. This classification scheme is helpful in selecting the level of therapeutic intervention appropriate for the patient's risk and symptom level. Management recommendations for the different categories are outlined in **Table 10**.

The American College of Physicians, American College of Chest Physicians, American Thoracic Society, and European Respiratory Society offer a simple, evidence-based classification and treatment scheme for stable COPD (**Table 11**, on page 20).

Pharmacologic Treatment

No pharmacologic agent is able to reduce the progressive decline in lung function seen in patients with COPD. However, a variety of medical treatments may reduce symptoms, diminish the frequency and severity of exacerbations, reduce the frequency of hospitalization, and improve exercise tolerance and health status. Medications used to treat COPD are summarized in **Table 12** on page 21.

Bronchodilators

Bronchodilators are the mainstay of therapy in COPD; they relax airway smooth muscle, increase airway diameter, and decrease breathlessness, hyperinflation, and air trapping. Bronchodilators may also improve exercise tolerance, quality of sleep, and quality of life.

β_2-Agonists or anticholinergic agents are generally preferred over methylxanthines, which have a more extensive side-effect profile. Additionally, inhaled agents are recommended over oral agents based on efficacy and decreased side effects. However, the predominance of data does not support the superiority of any one inhaled bronchodilator over another. Inhaled bronchodilators are available in both short- and long-acting forms.

TABLE 10. Initial Pharmacologic Management of COPD[a]

Patient Category[b]	Recommended First Choice	Alternative Choice	Other Possible Treatments[c]
A	Short-acting anticholinergic PRN *or* Short-acting β_2-agonist PRN	Long-acting anticholinergic *or* Long-acting β_2-agonist *or* Short-acting β_2-agonist *and* Short-acting anticholinergic	Theophylline
B	Long-acting anticholinergic *or* Long-acting β_2-agonist	Long-acting anticholinergic *and* Long-acting β_2-agonist	Short-acting β_2-agonist *and/or* Short-acting anticholinergic *or* Theophylline
C	Inhaled glucocorticoid + Long-acting β_2-agonist *or* Long-acting anticholinergic	Long-acting anticholinergic *and* Long-acting β_2-agonist *or* Long-acting anticholinergic *and* Phosphodiesterase-4 inhibitor *or* Long-acting β_2-agonist *and* Phosphodiesterase-4 inhibitor	Short-acting β_2-agonist *and/or* Short-acting anticholinergic *or* Theophylline
D	*Inhaled* glucocorticoid + Long-acting β_2-agonist *and/or* Long-acting anticholinergic	Inhaled glucocorticoid + Long-acting β_2-agonist *and* Long-acting anticholinergic *or* Inhaled glucocorticoid + Long-acting β_2-agonist *and* Phosphodiesterase-4 inhibitor *or* Long-acting anticholinergic *and* Long-acting β_2-agonist *or* Long-acting anticholinergic *and* Phosphodiesterase-4 inhibitor	N-acetylcysteine *or* Short-acting β_2-agonist *and/or* Short-acting anticholinergic *or* Theophylline

PRN = as needed.

[a]Medications in each box are listed in alphabetical order, not necessarily in order of preference.

[b]See Table 8 for definitions of patient categories.

[c]Medications in this column can be used alone or in combination with other options in the Recommended First Choice and Alternative Choice columns.

Data from the Global Strategy for Diagnosis, Management and Prevention of COPD 2015, © Global Initiative for Chronic Obstructive Lung Disease (GOLD), all rights reserved. Available from http://www.goldcopd.org.

[handwritten: dce\nebprn]

Short-acting bronchodilators (short-acting β_2-agonists [SABAs]) and short-acting anticholinergics [also known as short-acting muscarinic agents [SAMAs]) provide rapid onset of action (within minutes of administration) and have a duration of action of 3 to 6 hours. They are recommended as initial monotherapy, administered on an as-needed basis, in patients with mild COPD and intermittent and/or exertional symptoms of disease (category A) (see Table 10). Short-acting

[handwritten: AntiMuscarinic AntiACh = Tio.]

bronchodilators also have an important role as add-on therapy, either alone or in combination, with other recommended therapies in higher-risk (categories B, C, and D) disease.

Long-acting bronchodilators consist of long-acting β_2-agonists (LABAs) and long-acting anticholinergics (also known as long-acting muscarinic agents [LAMAs]). These agents have demonstrated efficacy in improving FEV_1,

TABLE 11. ACP, ACCP, ATS, and ERS Treatment Recommendations for Patients with Symptomatic, Stable COPD

Degree of Airflow Obstruction	Recommendation	Strength of Recommendation/ Quality of Evidence
FEV_1 60%-80% of predicted	Inhaled bronchodilators	Weak/Low
FEV_1 <60% of predicted	Monotherapy with either a long-acting inhaled anticholinergic or a long-acting β_2-agonist[a]	Strong/Moderate
	Combination therapy (long-acting inhaled anticholinergics, long-acting β_2-agonists, or inhaled glucocorticoids)	Weak/Moderate
FEV_1 <50%[b] of predicted	Pulmonary rehabilitation[c]	Strong/Moderate

ACP = American College of Physicians; ACCP = American College of Chest Physicians; ATS = American Thoracic Society; ERS = European Respiratory Society.

[a]Choice of specific monotherapy should be based on patient preference, cost, and adverse effect profile.

[b]Clinicians should consider pulmonary rehabilitation for symptomatic or exercise-limited patients with an FEV_1 ≥50% of predicted (weak recommendation/moderate evidence).

[c]In addition to pharmacologic therapy.

Source: Qaseem A, Wilt TJ, Weinberger SE, et al; American College of Physicians; American College of Chest Physicians; American Thoracic Society; European Respiratory Society. Diagnosis and management of stable chronic obstructive pulmonary disease: a clinical practice guideline update from the American College of Physicians, American College of Chest Physicians, American Thoracic Society, and European Respiratory Society. Ann Intern Med. 2011 Aug 2;155(3): 179-91. [PMID: 21810710]

improving health status, and significantly reducing the frequency of exacerbations; however, long-acting bronchodilators have not been shown to affect mortality. Some LABAs have a slower onset of action than SABAs, but the duration of action is greater. Salmeterol and formoterol have a 12-hour duration of action, whereas indacaterol and olodaterol have a 24-hour duration of action and provide significantly greater bronchodilating effects than salmeterol or formoterol. Agents with a duration of action of at least 24 hours are sometimes referred to as ultra-LABAs. LAMAs also have a slower onset of action compared with SAMAs, but they provide a 12- to 24-hour duration of action (aclidinium and glycopyrronium are 12 hours; umeclidinium and tiotropium are 24 hours). Newer 24-hour agents are sometimes referred to as ultra-LAMAs. Long-acting bronchodilators are used in the treatment of COPD when patients remain symptomatic on SABAs or require frequent SABA use to control symptoms, as outlined in Table 10. All patients using long-acting bronchodilators should also have a short-acting bronchodilator (SABA or SAMA) available for rescue use.

- Bronchodilators are the mainstay of therapy in COPD; all patients with COPD using long-acting bronchodilators should also have a short-acting bronchodilator available for rescue use.

- Long-acting bronchodilators in COPD improve FEV_1, **HVC** improve health status, and significantly reduce the frequency of exacerbations, but have not been shown to affect mortality.

Inhaled Glucocorticoids

The use of inhaled glucocorticoids is not considered appropriate as primary therapy or monotherapy in COPD, which differentiates COPD treatment from asthma treatment. However, combination treatment with an inhaled glucocorticoid and LABA or LAMA is recommended for highly symptomatic patients with frequent exacerbations (category C and D disease) (see Table 10).

In older patients with advanced COPD, inhaled glucocorticoids appear to be associated with an increased incidence of pneumonia, but this association has been difficult to confirm in this high-respiratory-risk population and has not been associated with increased mortality. Routine treatment with inhaled glucocorticoids does not improve decline of lung function, and the safety data with long-term use are not definitive. Patients taking inhaled glucocorticoids should be monitored for adverse drug effects, such as osteopenia, hyperglycemia, and cataracts. The potential for harm in treating patients with advanced COPD with inhaled glucocorticoids needs to be balanced against the potential benefit of reducing exacerbations and improving respiratory symptoms and quality of life.

A short-term trial of oral glucocorticoids is not recommended as a means of identifying patients who may respond to inhaled glucocorticoids.

- The use of inhaled glucocorticoids is not considered **HVC** appropriate as primary therapy or monotherapy in COPD.

Systemic Glucocorticoids

Oral glucocorticoids are reserved for limited periodic use in treating exacerbations of COPD and may provide some benefit in decreasing hospital readmission rates after exacerbation. Long-term oral glucocorticoid therapy has limited, if any, benefit in COPD and carries a high risk for other significant side effects (such as muscle weakness and decreased functional status) in addition to those associated with inhaled glucocorticoids. Long-term oral glucocorticoids should not be used to treat COPD. However, select patients with ACOS may benefit from oral glucocorticoids, provided they have a reversible asthma component that predominates their symptomatic disease.

TABLE 12. Drug Treatment for COPD

Agent	Side Effects	Notes
Bronchodilators		
Inhaled short-acting β_2-agonists (albuterol, fenoterol, levalbuterol, metaproterenol, pirbuterol, terbutaline)	Tachycardia and hypokalemia (usually dose dependent), but generally well tolerated by most patients	Generally used as needed for mild disease with few symptoms
Inhaled short-acting anticholinergic agents (ipratropium)	Dry mouth, mydriasis on contact with eye, tachycardia, tremors, rarely acute narrow angle glaucoma; this drug class has been shown to be safe in a wide range of doses and clinical settings	Not to be used with tiotropium; generally used as needed for mild disease with few symptoms; avoid using both short- and long-acting anticholinergics
Inhaled long-acting anticholinergic agents (tiotropium, aclidinium, umeclidinium, glycopyrronium)	Dry mouth, mydriasis on contact with eye, tachycardia, tremors, rarely acute narrow angle glaucoma	Not to be used with ipratropium; use when short-acting bronchodilators provide insufficient control of symptoms for patients with an FEV_1 <60% of predicted
Inhaled long-acting β_2-agonists (salmeterol, formoterol, arformoterol, indacaterol, olodaterol)	Sympathomimetic symptoms such as tremor and tachycardia; overdose can be fatal	Use as maintenance therapy when short-acting bronchodilators provide insufficient control of symptoms for patients with an FEV_1 <60% of predicted; not intended to be used for treatment of exacerbations of COPD or acute bronchospasm
Methylxanthines (theophylline, aminophylline; sustained and short-acting)	Tachycardia, nausea, vomiting, disturbed pulmonary function, and disturbed sleep; narrow therapeutic index; overdose can be fatal with seizures and arrhythmias	Used as maintenance therapy; generally use only after long-acting bronchodilator treatment to provide additional symptomatic relief of exacerbations; may also improve respiratory muscle function
Oral β_2-agonists (albuterol, metaproterenol, terbutaline)	Sympathomimetic symptoms such as tremor and tachycardia	Used as maintenance therapy; rarely used because of side effects but may be beneficial for patients who cannot use inhalers
Oral Phosophodiesterase-4 Inhibitor		
Roflumilast	Diarrhea, nausea, backache, decreased appetite, dizziness	Used to reduce risk for exacerbations in patients with severe COPD (blood levels not required) with chronic bronchitis and history of exacerbations; roflumilast should not be used with methylxanthines owing to potential toxicity; very expensive and should be used only in select patients
Anti-Inflammatory Agents		
Inhaled glucocorticoids (fluticasone, budesonide, mometasone, ciclesonide, beclomethasone)	Dysphonia, skin bruising, oral candidiasis, rarely side effects of oral glucocorticoids (see below)	Most effective in patients with a history of frequent exacerbations and when used in conjunction with long-acting bronchodilators; not approved by the FDA for treatment for COPD
Oral glucocorticoids (prednisone, prednisolone)	Skin bruising, adrenal suppression, glaucoma, osteoporosis, diabetes mellitus, systemic hypertension, pneumonia, cataracts, opportunistic infection, insomnia, mood disturbance	Use for significant exacerbations of COPD with taper; avoid, if possible, in stable COPD to limit glucocorticoid toxicity; consider inhaled glucocorticoids to facilitate weaning of systemic glucocorticoids
Combination Agents		
Combined inhaled long-acting β_2-agonist and inhaled glucocorticoid in a single inhaler (fluticasone/salmeterol, budesonide/formoterol)	Same/combined effects of both drug classes	Fluticasone/salmeterol is approved by the FDA as maintenance therapy and for prevention of exacerbations; budesonide/formoterol metered-dose inhaler is approved by the FDA as maintenance therapy; combinations are not to be used for treatment of acute bronchospasm
Combined short-acting β_2-agonist plus anticholinergic in a single inhaler (fenoterol/ipratropium, salbutamol/ipratropium)	Same/combined effects of both drug classes	Not to be used with tiotropium; generally used as needed for mild disease with few symptoms; avoid using both short- and long-acting anticholinergics; this combination therapy may be used for maintenance therapy only if patients have well-controlled disease on this combination treatment and do not require rescue therapy if/when expense is a determining factor

(Continued on the next page)

TABLE 12. Drug Treatment for COPD *(Continued)*		
Agent	**Side Effects**	**Notes**
Combined inhaled glucocorticoid and ultra-long-acting β₂-agonist in a single inhaler (fluticasone/vilanterol)	Same/combined effects of both drug classes	Not to be used for treatment of acute bronchospasm
Combined anticholinergic plus ultra-long-acting β₂-agonist in a single inhaler (umeclidinium/vilanterol)	Same/combined effects of both drug classes	Not to be used for treatment of acute bronchospasm

Oral or intravenous glucocorticoids may be used in the management of acute exacerbations of COPD that require hospital admission. Although oral therapy has been shown to be noninferior to intravenous therapy, critically ill patients and those with nausea are candidates for intravenous therapy. Patients responding to intravenous glucocorticoids should be switched to oral glucocorticoids, and the dose of oral glucocorticoid should be tapered after discharge. The optimal dose and duration of glucocorticoid therapy in management of an acute exacerbation remains uncertain. Recent clinical trials continue to demonstrate a pattern that supports noninferiority of shortened duration of therapy and low-dose regimens. A recent systematic review found no significant differences in clinical outcomes between short-duration (<7 days) and longer-duration (>7 days) glucocorticoid treatment. Additionally, a recent randomized clinical trial showed that prednisone, 40 mg orally daily for 5 days, was not inferior to prednisone, 40 mg orally daily for 14 days, with regard to re-exacerbation within 6 months. Although the optimal dose and duration is not known, these data demonstrate shortened duration and reduced daily dosing of glucocorticoid therapy can decrease the total glucocorticoid exposure without worsening outcomes. 🄷

Methylxanthines
Methylxanthines have shown modest treatment benefit in COPD, likely due to a bronchodilating effect mediated by nonselective inhibition of phosphodiesterase. However, the potential toxicity of this class of drugs coupled with their reduced efficacy has led to increasingly limited use. Although they may be helpful in any classification of COPD, they tend to be used in selected patients with late-stage disease or for patients in whom other preferred therapies have proved ineffective for symptomatic relief; they may also be used when other medications are not available or affordable. Methylxanthines are available in oral and intravenous formulations. However, they have a narrow therapeutic window, are poorly tolerated in older patients, and have multiple drug interactions.

Phosphodiesterase-4 Inhibitors
Inhibition of phosphodiestarase-4 (PDE-4) decreases inflammation, which may be helpful in a limited number of patients with COPD in whom inflammation is a significant factor.

Roflumilast is an oral selective PDE-4 inhibitor and is currently the only available drug in this class. It is used primarily as add-on therapy in severe COPD (categories C and D) associated with chronic bronchitis and a history of recurrent exacerbations despite other therapies; it has been shown to improve symptoms and reduce risk and frequency of exacerbations in these individuals. However, it is not a bronchodilator, is expensive, and has not been shown to be effective in other groups of patients with COPD; therefore, it is not indicated for acute bronchospasm, rescue, or treatment of primary emphysema. Common side effects include diarrhea, nausea, weight loss, headache, and some psychiatric adverse events (anxiety, depression, insomnia). Roflumilast is contraindicated in patients with liver impairment and has significant drug interactions.

α₁-Antitrypsin Augmentation Therapy
α₁-Antitrypsin replacement therapy has been shown to slow the progression of COPD in select young patients with severe hereditary α₁-antitrypsin deficiency and established emphysema. However, this therapy is not recommended for patients with COPD that is unrelated to this deficiency.

Antibiotics
Use of antibiotics, other than for the treatment of infectious exacerbations, is currently not indicated.

There has been increasing interest in the chronic use of macrolide antibiotics to prevent COPD exacerbations based on their dual antimicrobial and anti-inflammatory effects. Several clinical trials to assess prophylactic use and benefit have demonstrated a reduction in the rate of exacerbation in patients with moderate to severe COPD with one or more exacerbations in the previous year despite optimal maintenance inhaler therapy; further evaluation is needed before routine use can be recommended in this patient population. Benefit and use of prophylactic macrolide therapy for patients with stable COPD has not been demonstrated and is presently not recommended. Macrolide antibiotics have the potential to precipitate growth of macrolide-resistant bacterial organisms and/or development of macrolide-resistant strains of nontuberculous mycobacteria and should be used with caution. In addition, potentially fatal arrhythmias have occurred in association with azithromycin.

Other Agents

Routine use of antitussive agents is not recommended because there is no evidence of their efficacy.

Mucolytic drugs reduce sputum viscosity and are often prescribed in patients with COPD. N-acetylcysteine is an oral mucolytic drug that has been shown to improve mucociliary clearance and modulate the inflammatory response. It has antioxidant properties and may be helpful in preventing exacerbations in patients with moderate to severe COPD. However, further evaluation is needed before routine use of N-acetylcysteine can be recommended for treatment of patients with stable COPD. In other patients, the overall benefit of mucolytic therapy appears to be minimal, and routine use of mucolytics is not recommended.

The use of statins is not recommended in patients with moderate to severe COPD who are at risk for COPD exacerbations; however, some patients with COPD may meet accepted criteria for initiation of statins owing to the presence of cardiovascular risk factors.

Use of oral and parenteral opioids is very effective to treat dyspnea in severe COPD; however, data on nebulized delivery are insufficient. Use of opioids is common in patients in hospice care. Patients with refractory or disabling dyspnea who are not enrolled in hospice also benefit from symptom relief provided by opioids, which are likely underutilized in this population.

Use of pulmonary vasodilators (phosphodiesterase-5 inhibitors, calcium channel blockers, nitric oxide) is not recommended until further safety and efficacy data are available. There is no evidence supporting the use of leukotriene-modifying agents in COPD treatment.

Vaccination

Influenza vaccination has been shown to reduce serious illness (such as lower respiratory tract infections that require hospitalization) and death in patients with COPD. These vaccines should be administered annually in all patients with COPD.

Pneumococcal vaccination with the 23-valent polysaccharide vaccine should be given to all patients aged 19 to 64 years with COPD, with revaccination at age 65 years if 5 years have elapsed since the previous pneumococcal immunization. All patients (with or without COPD) should also receive the 13-valent pneumococcal conjugate vaccine at age 65 years, although the polysaccharide and conjugate vaccines should be given sequentially rather than together for optimal effect (see MKSAP 17 General Internal Medicine).

Nonpharmacologic Therapy
Smoking Cessation

Smoking cessation has been demonstrated to reduce the rate of decline in FEV_1 and risk of exacerbations in COPD. Smoking cessation is the most important goal in the management of COPD in patients who smoke, regardless of the level of disease severity. Counseling and pharmacotherapy can be effective to increase cessation success (see MKSAP 17 General Internal Medicine).

KEY POINTS

- Smoking cessation is the most important goal in the management of COPD in patients who smoke, regardless of the level of disease severity. **HVC**

- The use of antibiotics in COPD should be limited to infectious exacerbations. **HVC**

- Roflumilast is an oral selective phosphodiesterase-4 (PDE-4) inhibitor and its use should be limited to add-on therapy in severe COPD associated with chronic bronchitis and a history of recurrent exacerbations; it is not a bronchodilator, is expensive, and has not been shown to be effective in other groups of patients with COPD. **HVC**

Pulmonary Rehabilitation

All patients with COPD can benefit from exercise maintenance. Pulmonary rehabilitation is recommended for all symptomatic patients with an FEV_1 less than 50% of predicted and specifically for those hospitalized with an acute exacerbation of COPD. Pulmonary rehabilitation may also be considered in symptomatic or exercise-limited patients with an FEV_1 greater than or equal to 50% of predicted. These programs include education, functional assessment, nutrition counseling, and follow-up to reinforce behavioral techniques for change. They also include an exercise training component (≥30 minutes three times weekly for 6 to 8 weeks) that has been shown to improve endurance, flexibility, and upper and lower body strength. Exercise training can provide sustained benefit for post-exacerbation symptoms such as breathlessness following the completion of even a single rehabilitation program. This benefit does not wane after a rehabilitation program ends; however, sustaining benefit requires continuation of routine exercise. When combined with other forms of therapy (medical therapy, smoking cessation, nutrition counseling, and education), pulmonary rehabilitation has been shown to decrease patients' perceived intensity of breathlessness, reduce dyspnea and fatigue, facilitate increased participation in daily activities, and enhance health-related quality of life, including improvements in anxiety and depression.

KEY POINT

- All patients with COPD can benefit from pulmonary rehabilitation and exercise maintenance; pulmonary rehabilitation is recommended for all symptomatic patients with an FEV_1 less than 50% of predicted and specifically for those hospitalized with an acute exacerbation of COPD.

Oxygen Therapy

Long-term oxygen therapy in specific patients with COPD improves survival and has beneficial effects on hemodynamics, hematologic characteristics, exercise capacity, general alertness, mental status, hand grip, and motor speed. When provided during exercise, oxygen therapy can increase duration of endurance and reduce breathlessness at the end of exercise.

The need for oxygen therapy should be evaluated in all stable patients with an FEV_1 less than 35% of predicted or in patients with clinical symptoms or signs suggestive of respiratory failure or right-sided heart failure. A determination of the need for long-term oxygen therapy is initially based on resting arterial Po_2 or oxygen saturation values, which should be repeated and confirmed twice over a 3-week period. If resting oxygen saturation is less than 88%, arterial blood gas studies should be performed and long-term oxygen therapy should be initiated. When starting long-term oxygen therapy, a 6-minute walk test should be performed to assess and titrate oxygen levels with activity. The use of ambulatory oxygen is not supported for patients who do not meet the selection criteria.

Use of long-term oxygen therapy (>15 hours per day) has been shown to prolong life in patients meeting the following criteria: (1) chronic respiratory failure and/or severe resting hypoxemia, defined as an arterial Po_2 less than or equal to 55 mm Hg (7.3 kPa) or oxygen saturation less than or equal to 88% breathing ambient air, with or without hypercapnia; and/or (2) if there is evidence of pulmonary hypertension, peripheral edema suggesting right-sided heart failure, or polycythemia, in combination with an arterial Po_2 less than 60 mm Hg (8.0 kPa) or oxygen saturation less than 88% breathing ambient air.

Noninvasive Mechanical Ventilation

In select patients with COPD, noninvasive positive pressure ventilation may improve breathing pattern, diminish dyspnea, and increase oxygenation, resulting in improved sleep continuity, symptoms of daytime somnolence, exertional dyspnea, and awake arterial Po_2 levels. Candidates for this therapy are patients with stable severe and very severe COPD. The combination of noninvasive ventilation with long-term oxygen therapy is used in a select subset of patients with pronounced daytime hypercapnia. In patients with both COPD and obstructive sleep apnea, continuous positive airway pressure improves both survival and risk of hospital admissions. In addition to performing arterial blood gas studies to assess changes in Pco_2, dyspnea and exercise capacity should also be evaluated.

Noninvasive ventilation also has a significant role in management for patients with very severe COPD during an acute exacerbation and/or acute respiratory infection (for example, chronic bronchitis, pneumonia) and may be helpful to avoid intubation (see Critical Care Medicine).

Lung Volume Reduction Surgery

Lung volume reduction surgery is a palliative procedure that carries a high risk of perioperative mortality, and it is indicated only in a very clearly defined group of patients (**Table 13**). This

TABLE 13. Eligibility Criteria for Lung Volume Reduction Surgery in Patients with COPD

Severe COPD
Remain symptomatic despite maximal pharmacologic therapy
Completed pulmonary rehabilitation
Evidence of bilateral predominant upper-lobe emphysema on CT scan
Postbronchodilator total lung capacity of >100% **and** residual lung volume >150% of predicted
Maximum FEV_1 >20% and ≤45% of predicted and D_{LCO} ≥20% of predicted
Ambient air arterial Pco_2 ≤60 mm Hg (8.0 kPa) **and** arterial Po_2 ≥45 mm Hg (6.0 kPa)

Information from Global Initiative for Chronic Obstructive Lung Disease (GOLD), Global Strategy for the Diagnosis, Management, and Prevention of Chronic Obstructive Lung Disease. http://www.goldcopd.org/guidelines-global-strategy-for-diagnosis-management.html. Updated 2015. Accessed July 1, 2015.

surgery improves the mechanical efficiency of respiratory muscles and increases the elastic recoil of the lungs to improve expiratory flow and reduce exacerbations. Although lung volume reduction surgery may improve exercise capacity, lung function, dyspnea, and health-related quality of life in some patients, it has not been shown to increase survival when compared with pharmacologic therapy alone.

Lung Transplantation

Lung transplantation improves quality of life and functional capacity in select patients with very severe COPD. Patients who may be considered appropriate candidates for lung transplantation should meet the criteria described in **Table 14**.

Common complications of lung transplantation include acute rejection, opportunistic infections (such as cytomegalovirus), fungal infections (such as *Candida, Aspergillus, Cryptococcus, Pneumocystis*), bacterial infections (such as *Pseudomonas, Staphylococcus* species), bronchiolitis obliterans, lymphoproliferative disease, and overall increased postoperative mortality. Double lung transplantation has similar or slightly higher survival rates compared with single lung transplantation.

TABLE 14. Recommended Criteria for Lung Transplantation in Patients with COPD

History of exacerbation associated with acute hypercapnia (arterial Pco_2 >50 mm Hg [6.7 kPa])
Pulmonary hypertension
Cor pulmonale
Pulmonary hypertension and cor pulmonale
FEV_1 <20% of predicted with D_{LCO} <20% of predicted **or** homogeneous distribution of emphysema

Data from the Global Strategy for Diagnosis, Management and Prevention of COPD 2015, © Global Initiative for Chronic Obstructive Lung Disease (GOLD), all rights reserved. Available from http://www.goldcopd.org.

Acute Exacerbations

Definition

An exacerbation of COPD is defined as a sustained worsening of the patient's COPD. Exacerbations are marked by increased breathlessness and are usually accompanied by increased cough and sputum production. The degree of exacerbation is considered mild when a change in the clinical condition is noted but no change in medication is necessary. An exacerbation is considered moderate when medication changes are made. A severe exacerbation results in hospitalization.

KEY POINT

- An exacerbation of COPD is defined as a sustained worsening of the patient's COPD; exacerbations are marked by increased breathlessness and are usually accompanied by increased cough and sputum production.

Prevention

The strongest predictors of exacerbation are: (1) a history of previous exacerbation and (2) the baseline severity of airflow limitation. However, exacerbations of COPD can be prevented by optimizing treatment with appropriate interventions based on risk classification and overall disease management; this includes immunizations and lifestyle changes such as maintaining physical activity and addressing anxiety and depression. Interruption of maintenance therapy for COPD is associated with an increased risk of exacerbation. Smoking cessation has the greatest capacity to influence the natural history of COPD and reduce future exacerbations; therefore, all measures (including counseling and pharmacologic support) should be given to assist patients in stopping smoking. Exacerbations may also commonly be precipitated by respiratory infections (either bacterial or viral), and efforts should be made to minimize exposure to possible sources of infection. Additionally, environmental exposures, such as to pollutants, may trigger exacerbations and should be avoided.

In patients who experience an exacerbation, early outpatient pulmonary rehabilitation is safe and produces clinically significant improvements in health status at 3 months, possibly decreasing the risk of future exacerbations.

KEY POINT

- The strongest predictors of exacerbation of COPD are (1) a history of previous exacerbation and (2) the baseline severity of airflow limitation.

Initial Assessment and Setting of Care

Initial assessment of the severity of an exacerbation is based on the patient's medical history and clinical signs of severity (**Table 15**). Studies helpful in the evaluation may include pulse oximetry to assess oxygenation or guide oxygen therapy; a chest radiograph to rule out an alternative diagnosis; a complete blood count to identify the presence of polycythemia, anemia, or leukocytosis; arterial blood gas studies; a biochemical panel to assess for electrolyte and glycemic abnormalities;

TABLE 15. Criteria for Assessment of COPD Exacerbations

Medical History
Severity of COPD based on degree of airflow limitation
Duration of worsening or new symptoms
Number of previous episodes (exacerbations/hospitalizations)
Comorbidities
Current treatment regimen
Previous requirement for mechanical ventilation
Signs/Degree of Severity
Use of accessory respiratory muscles
Paradoxical chest wall movements
Worsening or new onset of central cyanosis
Development of peripheral edema
Hemodynamic instability
Deteriorated mental status

Data from the Global Strategy for Diagnosis, Management and Prevention of COPD 2015, © Global Initiative for Chronic Obstructive Lung Disease (GOLD), all rights reserved. Available from http://www.goldcopd.org.

and an electrocardiogram to evaluate for a possible cardiac comorbidity.

The decision regarding the appropriate setting of treatment is usually based on the severity of the underlying lung disease, the severity of the exacerbation, and the presence of comorbidities.

Up to 80% of COPD exacerbations may appropriately be treated at home. The risk of dying from an exacerbation is closely related to the development of acidotic respiratory failure and possible need for ventilatory support in addition to the presence of significant comorbid conditions; therefore, treatment at home is reasonable in patients with less severe lung disease who do not have significant accompanying illnesses and who are experiencing mild to moderate exacerbations. Patients with more severe disease (symptom/risk evaluation categories C or D) without evidence of impending respiratory failure may also be candidates for home therapy, particularly if professionally administered home care services are available. However, the exact criteria for this approach (versus hospitalization) are not well defined and vary by health care setting, requiring individualization of setting of care decisions for these patients.

The criteria for hospital admission are described in **Table 16**. If an exacerbation is life-threatening, the patient should be immediately admitted to the ICU (see Critical Care Medicine). Criteria for ICU admission are discussed in **Table 17**.

KEY POINTS

- Home treatment of a COPD exacerbation is reasonable in patients with less severe lung disease who do not have significant accompanying illnesses and who are experiencing mild to moderate exacerbations.

HVC

(Continued)

TABLE 16. Criteria for Hospital Assessment of an Acute Exacerbation of COPD

Marked increase in intensity of symptoms (such as sudden onset of resting dyspnea)

Severe underlying COPD

Onset of new physical signs (such as cyanosis, peripheral edema)

An exacerbation that fails to respond to initial medical management

Presence of high-risk comorbid conditions (such as heart failure or newly occurring arrhythmias)

Frequent exacerbations

Advanced age

Patient inability to care for him- or herself

Inadequate home care available

Data from the Global Strategy for Diagnosis, Management and Prevention of COPD 2015, © Global Initiative for Chronic Obstructive Lung Disease (GOLD), all rights reserved. Available from http://www.goldcopd.org.

TABLE 17. Criteria for ICU Admission for an Acute Exacerbation of COPD

Despite adequate, appropriate treatment (oxygen, noninvasive ventilation), the patient experiences:

Persistent/worsening hypoxemia (arterial P_{O_2} <40 mm Hg [5.3 kPa]), **and/or**

Severe/worsening respiratory acidosis (pH <7.25) and requires endotracheal intubation with mechanical ventilation

Severe dyspnea that responds inadequately to initial emergency therapy

Changes in mental status (such as confusion, lethargy, coma)

Hemodynamic instability with need for vasopressors

Data from the Global Strategy for Diagnosis, Management and Prevention of COPD 2015, © Global Initiative for Chronic Obstructive Lung Disease (GOLD), all rights reserved. Available from http://www.goldcopd.org.

KEY POINTS *(continued)*

- The criteria for hospital admission in patients with a COPD exacerbation include a marked increase in the severity of symptoms, the presence of severe underlying COPD, failure to respond to initial medical treatment or a change in medications, advanced age, and/or lack of sufficient in-home care.

Goals and Therapeutic Management

A primary goal of treatment is to minimize the overall impact of an exacerbation, and a secondary goal is to prevent future episodes. When an exacerbation occurs, components of treatment include both respiratory support and pharmacologic treatments.

Supplemental oxygen therapy should be provided to maintain an arterial P_{O_2} greater than 60 mm Hg (8.0 kPa) or an oxygen saturation of 88% to 92%. In patients with severe underlying lung disease who are at risk for acidotic respiratory failure, arterial blood gases should be checked 30 to 60 minutes after initiating oxygen therapy to assess for carbon dioxide retention and development of acidosis. Patients with severe underlying lung disease or severe exacerbations should be monitored closely for evidence of respiratory decompensation and the need for ventilatory support.

In patients with impending respiratory failure, noninvasive mechanical ventilation may be helpful in avoiding intubation. However, endotracheal intubation and mechanical ventilation are indicated in patients experiencing life-threatening hypoxemia, progressive hypercapnia, and/or severely altered mental status in whom a decision has been made to pursue invasive therapy (see Critical Care Medicine).

Short-acting bronchodilator therapy is a mainstay of therapy for treating COPD exacerbation, and a SABA or SAMA should be administered either alone or as combination therapy. The role of long-acting bronchodilators for treating COPD exacerbations has not been defined.

Glucocorticoids for acute exacerbations of COPD have been shown to reduce recovery time, improve lung function and arterial hypoxemia, decrease risk of early relapse, decrease treatment failure, and decrease length of hospital stay. Guidelines recommend oral glucocorticoids, although intravenous glucocorticoids are frequently administered in hospitalized patients. The optimal dose and duration of glucocorticoid therapy for COPD exacerbation has not been established, but a frequently used regimen is prednisone, 40 mg/d for 5 days. Tapering during the post-discharge period is reasonable.

Although the role of antibiotics in treating COPD exacerbations is not well defined, they appear to be most effective in patients with (1) increased dyspnea, sputum volume, and sputum purulence; (2) two of the preceding symptoms if one of the two symptoms is increased purulence; or (3) a requirement for mechanical ventilation (invasive or noninvasive). Empiric antibiotic therapy should be chosen on the basis of local bacterial resistance patterns. Commonly used regimens include an advanced macrolide, a cephalosporin, or doxycycline. If symptoms do not respond to initial antibiotic therapy, sputum cultures should be obtained, particularly to assess if *Pseudomonas aeruginosa* is present. The length of antibiotic treatment is usually 5 to 10 days.

Palliative Care and Hospice

Progressive respiratory failure, comorbid cardiovascular disease, malignancies, and the presence of other disease continue to be the primary cause of death in patients with COPD hospitalized for an exacerbation. Therefore, palliative and hospice care are important components of care for patients with advanced and complicated COPD.

Palliative care should be made available to all patients with advanced COPD early in their clinical course. Hospice services are focused on patients with very advanced COPD and a limited life expectancy; these services may be provided in either inpatient or home settings.

In patients with COPD, parameters that portend a poor prognosis and should trigger more extensive discussions regarding end-of-life care include an FEV_1 of less than 30% of predicted, oxygen dependence, multiple hospital admissions for COPD exacerbations, significant comorbidities, weight loss and cachexia, decreased functional status, and increasing dependence on care takers.

KEY POINTS

HVC
- Glucocorticoids for acute exacerbations of COPD have been shown to reduce recovery time, improve lung function and arterial hypoxemia, decrease risk of early relapse, decrease treatment failure, and decrease length of hospital stay; a frequently used regimen is oral prednisone 40 mg/d for 5 days.

HVC
- Antibiotic use in acute exacerbations of COPD should be limited to patients with increased dyspnea and purulent sputum or those who require mechanical ventilation (invasive or noninvasive).

Bronchiectasis

Definition

Bronchiectasis is irreversible pathologic dilation of the bronchi or bronchioles resulting from an infectious process occurring in the context of airway obstruction, impaired drainage, or abnormality in antimicrobial defenses. The pattern of lung involvement varies greatly with the underlying cause and may be focal or diffuse. Focal bronchiectasis may occur owing to either extrinsic changes (airway tumor, aspirated foreign body, scarred or stenotic airway) or intrinsic changes (bronchial atresia) to the airway. Diffuse bronchiectasis is more commonly associated with underlying systemic or infectious disease (bacterial infection, nontuberculous mycobacterial [NTM] infection, reactivated tuberculosis, cystic fibrosis [CF]).

Causes

The causes of bronchiectasis are listed in **Table 18**. The affected area of the lung may be helpful in defining the associated underlying disease. For example, CF-related bronchiectasis has more pronounced involvement of the upper lung fields. Upper lobe predominance is also suggestive of allergic bronchopulmonary aspergillosis, congenital causes, and causes associated with autoimmune or connective tissue diseases/syndromes. The mid-lung fields may be preferentially affected with NTM or *Mycobacterium avium* complex (MAC) infection (see MKSAP 17 Infectious Disease). Chronic recurrent aspiration, end-stage fibrotic disease, or recurrent infections associated with immunodeficiency more commonly affect the lower lung fields. Primary ciliary dyskinesia can be either central or diffuse. Bronchiectasis is associated with postradiation fibrosis, which corresponds with the lung tissue included in the radiation port.

Presentation

Symptoms of bronchiectasis include chronic cough with purulent sputum and recurrent pneumonia (in both smokers and nonsmokers). Pulmonary function tests commonly detect mild to moderate airflow obstruction, which may overlap with

TABLE 18. Causes of Bronchiectasis

Categories	Causes
Congenital	Cystic fibrosis
	Primary ciliary dyskinesia
Infections	Typical and atypical mycobacterial infection
	Recurrent infection, postinfectious (viral, bacterial, fungal)
Inhalation	Recurrent aspiration
	Chronic hypersensitivity pneumonitis
	Smoke inhalation
Traction (scarring)	Usual and nonspecific interstitial pneumonias
	Asbestosis
	Radiation therapy
Systemic inflammatory disorders	Collagen vascular disease (rheumatoid arthritis, scleroderma, systemic lupus erythematosus)
	Sarcoidosis
Local immunologic reactions	Allergic bronchopulmonary aspergillosis
	Asthma
	Lung transplant rejection
Autoimmune disease	Rheumatoid arthritis
	Sjögren syndrome
Connective tissue disease	Tracheobronchomegaly (Mounier-Kuhn syndrome)
	Cartilage deficiency (Williams-Campbell syndrome)
	Marfan syndrome
Immune deficiency	Immunoglobulin deficiency
	HIV infection
	Job syndrome (elevated IgE, eczema, and recurrent respiratory infection)
	Agammaglobulinemia
	Common variable immune deficiency
	Secondary immunodeficiency (chronic lymphocytic leukemia, HIV)
Inflammatory bowel disease	Ulcerative colitis
	Crohn disease
Obstruction	Tumor
	Foreign body
	Lymphadenopathy
Other	α_1-Antitrypsin deficiency
	Yellow nail syndrome (nail dystrophy, lymphedema, and pleural effusions)
	Young syndrome (azoospermia and recurrent sino-pulmonary infections due to ciliary dysfunction)

other disease findings (COPD). Physical findings may include crackles and/or wheezing on lung auscultation. Some patients present with digital clubbing.

Diagnosis

High-resolution CT (HRCT) is diagnostically definitive for bronchiectasis. For every diagnosed patient, it should be determined whether there is an underlying cause that can be treated. This may involve testing for chronic bacterial or mycobacterial infections, assessing for the presence of connective tissue disease, and evaluating immune function. In selected patients, testing for CF or α_1-antitrypsin deficiency may be appropriate if suspected. However, even with rigorous evaluation, more than half of all cases are still considered idiopathic.

KEY POINTS

- Symptoms of bronchiectasis include chronic cough with purulent sputum and recurrent pneumonia (in both smokers and nonsmokers).
- High-resolution CT is diagnostically definitive for bronchiectasis.

Treatment

Overall goals of therapy for bronchiectasis are to reduce symptoms, improve quality of life, and prevent acute exacerbations. If a modifiable cause for bronchiectasis is identified, treating the cause is the primary priority.

Inhaled hypertonic saline in conjunction with chest physiotherapy is often used for airway clearance. Mucolytic agents such as acetylcysteine may be used to reduce viscosity and liquefy sputum secretions but are not routinely recommended owing to lack of definitive benefit. Dornase alfa (an enzyme that selectively cleaves DNA in sputum from degenerating neutrophils and reduces sputum viscosity) is beneficial in patients with CF-related bronchiectasis but not in patients with bronchiectasis due to other causes.

Pulmonary rehabilitation programs are effective in patients with bronchiectasis; they are associated with significant improvements in exercise capacity and fewer outpatient and emergency department visits.

Although some patients with bronchiectasis show significant improvement in FEV_1 following administration of a bronchodilator, there are no data to support the routine use of short- or long-acting bronchodilators in bronchiectasis.

Anti-inflammatory therapy with inhaled glucocorticoids may be used in the treatment of bronchiectasis. In patients with non-CF bronchiectasis who also have COPD, inhaled glucocorticoids combined with SABA/LABA have a role for those patients who have two or more exacerbations annually. There is no evidence to support inhaled glucocorticoids alone in treating bronchiectasis. Short-duration systemic glucocorticoids have been used for exacerbations of bronchiectasis. However, because of side effects, long-term systemic glucocorticoids should not be used.

The macrolide antibiotic azithromycin has demonstrated clinical benefit in treatment of bronchiectasis; however, because of the potential to foster significant increases in antibiotic-resistant organisms, chronic NTM infection should be ruled out before initiating chronic macrolide therapy in bronchiectasis.

Oral, inhaled, and/or intravenous antibiotics are increasingly used in the management of bronchiectasis owing to a better understanding of the role of mucus stasis in bacterial colonization of the lung. In patients with bronchiectasis who experience recurrent exacerbations (≥ 3 episodes per year), use of oral or inhaled antibiotics to suppress microbial load and reduce future exacerbations is best supported in patients with CF rather than non-CF bronchiectasis. If *Pseudomonas aeruginosa* and/or methicillin-resistant *Staphylococcus aureus* is detected, consensus-based guidelines suggest treatment to attempt eradication.

KEY POINTS

- If a modifiable cause for bronchiectasis has been identified, treating the cause is the primary priority.
- There are no data to support the routine use of short- or long-acting bronchodilators or the long term use of systemic glucocorticoids in patients with bronchiectasis. **HVC**
- Pulmonary rehabilitation programs are effective in patients with bronchiectasis and are associated with significant improvements in exercise capacity and fewer outpatient and emergency department visits. **HVC**

Treatment of Exacerbations

Exacerbations of bronchiectasis may be difficult to differentiate from baseline symptoms. However, changes in sputum volume, viscosity, or purulence; increased cough; wheezing; shortness of breath; hemoptysis; and/or declines in lung function are considered evidence of exacerbation.

Therapy for an exacerbation is ideally guided by routine sputum and acid-fast bacilli culture results to identify a possible predominant organism for treatment. Empiric therapy should be based on previous respiratory cultures until current culture data are available, as resistant organisms commonly colonize bronchiectatic airways. Once culture and sensitivity data are available, antimicrobial therapy should be tailored to treat known pathogens. Although there is no clear evidence for determining the appropriate length of the therapeutic course, 2 weeks is commonly suggested.

Cystic Fibrosis in Adults

CF results from mutations in the CF transmembrane conductance regulator (*CFTR*) gene. It causes epithelial mucus dehydration and viscous secretions, which then cause occlusion of respiratory airways and contribute to the persistent airway infections and progressive tissue destruction that characterizes CF. However, CF is a multisystem disease that may also involve obstruction of the pancreatic ducts, biliary tree, and vas deferens.

CF is an autosomal recessive disorder that occurs with a frequency of 1 in 2000 to 3000 live births. Approximately 1000 new cases of CF are diagnosed annually, and approximately

70,000 people are affected worldwide. Approximately 7% of patients with CF remain undiagnosed until adulthood (≥18 years of age).

Because of late diagnosis and treatment advances, CF is no longer considered a pediatric disease. By 2012, adults made up nearly 50% of the population with CF, and it is expected that adult patients with CF will very soon outnumber pediatric patients. The mean predicted survival age has increased over the last decade by almost 10 years, to 41.1 years of age as of 2012.

Diagnosis

Diagnosis of CF in adults may be obscured by an atypical and/or delayed presentation. However, the presence of certain conditions in an adult should increase suspicion for CF (**Table 19**).

Diagnosis is based on a combination of CF-compatible clinical findings in conjunction with either biochemical (sweat testing, nasal potential difference) or genetic (*CFTR* mutations) techniques. Use of the sweat test has been the mainstay of laboratory confirmation, although infection with *Burkholderia cepacia* is pathognomonic for CF. Once a CF diagnosis is confirmed, all patients should undergo *CFTR* mutational analysis to determine if *CFTR* modulator therapy may be an option.

Associated comorbidities in adults with CF include diabetes mellitus (present in up to 30% of patients), infertility due to azoospermia (present in 95% of men) and multifactorial causes in women, osteoporosis (present in 23% of patients), and liver disease. Liver disease occurs in 10% of patients with CF. The most common abnormality is fatty infiltration and intrahepatic cholestasis, with up to 5% to 15% of patients developing multilobular cirrhosis and portal hypertension.

Treatment

The pillars of CF management are airway clearance, antibiotic therapy, nutritional support, and psychosocial support. The primary objectives of CF treatment are maintaining lung health and controlling/minimizing the impact of CF-affected organ disease.

The vast majority (95%) of patients with CF die from complications of lung infection. The cardinal feature of CF lung disease is pulmonary exacerbation, which serves as a significant predictor of lung function decline, decreased quality of life, and increased morbidity. The Cystic Fibrosis Foundation (CFF) practice guidelines recommend use of chronic medications to improve lung function and reduce exacerbations. These medications include mucolytics, hydrating agents, inhaled antibiotics, oral macrolide antibiotics, and *CFTR* potentiators. Despite monitoring and management, patients may still experience exacerbations. Treatment for end-stage lung disease is with transplantation.

The goals of antibiotic treatment of CF bacterial infection(s) are to reduce bacterial burden, attempt/achieve early bacterial eradication, and/or prevent bacterial colonization of the lung (such as with *P. aeruginosa*). The CFF practice guidelines recommend that antibiotic treatment be provided for a minimum of 10 days, but a 14- to 21-day course is often necessary. Therapy may be extended even longer in patients with severe disease.

Similarly, additional recommendations are provided by the CFF for managing other CF-affected organ disease (pancreatic insufficiency; need for transplantation; sinus, liver, and bone disease; reproductive issues); these can be found on the CFF website (www.cff.org).

KEY POINTS

- The diagnosis of cystic fibrosis is based on a combination of compatible clinical findings in conjunction with either biochemical (sweat testing, nasal potential difference) or genetic (*CTFR* mutations) techniques.

- The pillars of cystic fibrosis management are airway clearance, antibiotic therapy, nutritional support, and psychosocial support.

Diffuse Parenchymal Lung Disease

Overview

Interstitial lung diseases were initially named because of abnormalities identified in the pulmonary interstitium on histopathology. However, these disorders also typically involve the distal lung parenchyma, smaller airways, vasculature, and pleura. As a result, diffuse parenchymal lung disease (DPLD) is a more accurate and inclusive term for describing these diseases than is interstitial lung disease. DPLD represents a heterogeneous group of disorders that are classified based on similar clinical, radiographic, physiologic, and pathologic criteria. The term DPLD excludes pulmonary hypertension and COPD. In general, DPLDs are not infectious in origin, they most commonly present with dyspnea and cough, and imaging abnormalities are most often diffuse rather than focal.

Classification and Epidemiology

In comparison with the prevalence of either COPD or cardiogenic causes of shortness of breath, the DPLDs are extremely

---

TABLE 19. Conditions Suggesting the Possible Diagnosis of Cystic Fibrosis in Adults

Recurrent pancreatitis
Male infertility
Chronic sinusitis
Severe nasal polyposis
Nontuberculous mycobacterial infection
Allergic bronchopulmonary aspergillosis
Bronchiectasis
Positive sputum culture for *Burkholderia cepacia*

rare. Accurate estimates of the prevalence of DPLD remain elusive. Current estimates place the prevalence of DPLD at approximately 70 per 100,000 persons. Although this is the most widely accepted prevalence, it likely underestimates the true prevalence of the disorder. Approximately 30% to 40% of cases are idiopathic.

There are hundreds of DPLDs, which often leads to confusion on how best to diagnose them. The most useful classification system defines those with a known cause or association versus those that are idiopathic (**Table 20**). Pulmonary pathology specimens are the gold standard for diagnosis of DPLD of both unknown and known causes; however, for the idiopathic

TABLE 20. Classification and Distinguishing Features of Select Forms of Diffuse Parenchymal Lung Disease	
Known Causes	
Drug induced	Examples: amiodarone, methotrexate, nitrofurantoin, chemotherapeutic agents (see www.pneumotox.com for a complete listing)
Smoking related	"Smokers" respiratory bronchiolitis characterized by gradual onset of persistent cough and dyspnea. Radiograph shows ground-glass opacities and thickened interstitium. Smoking cessation improves prognosis.
	Desquamative interstitial pneumonitis and pulmonary Langerhans cell histiocytosis are other histopathologic patterns associated with smoking and DPLD.
Radiation	May occur 6 weeks to months following radiation therapy
Chronic aspiration	Aspiration is often subclinical and may exacerbate other forms of DPLD
Pneumoconioses	Asbestosis, silicosis, berylliosis
Connective tissue diseases	
Rheumatoid arthritis	May affect the pleura (pleuritis and pleural effusion), parenchyma, airways (bronchitis, bronchiectasis), and vasculature. The parenchymal disease can range from nodules to organizing pneumonia to usual interstitial pneumonitis.
Systemic sclerosis	Nonspecific interstitial pneumonia pathology is most common; may be exacerbated by aspiration due to esophageal involvement; antibody to Scl-70 or pulmonary hypertension portends a poor prognosis. Monitoring of diffusing capacity for early involvement is warranted.
Polymyositis/ dermatomyositis	Many different types of histology; poor prognosis.
Other connective tissue diseases	Varying degrees of lung involvement and pathology can be seen in other forms of connective tissue disease.
Hypersensitivity pneumonitis	Immune reaction to an inhaled low-molecular-weight antigen; may be acute, subacute, or chronic. Noncaseating granulomas are seen.
Unknown Causes	
Idiopathic interstitial pneumonias	
Idiopathic pulmonary fibrosis	Chronic, insidious onset of cough and dyspnea, usually in a patient aged >50 y. Usual interstitial pneumonia pathology (honeycombing, bibasilar infiltrates with fibrosis). Diagnosis of exclusion.
Acute interstitial pneumonia	Dense bilateral acute lung injury similar to acute respiratory distress syndrome; 50% mortality rate.
Cryptogenic organizing pneumonia	May be preceded by flu-like illness. Radiograph shows focal areas of consolidation that may migrate from one location to another.
Sarcoidosis	Variable clinical presentation, ranging from asymptomatic to multiorgan involvement. Stage 1: hilar lymphadenopathy. Stage 2: hilar lymphadenopathy plus interstitial lung disease. Stage 3: interstitial lung disease. Stage 4: fibrosis. Noncaseating granulomas are hallmarks.
Rare DPLD with Well-Defined Features	
Lymphangioleiomyomatosis	Affects women in their 30s and 40s. Associated with spontaneous pneumothorax and chylous effusions. Chest CT shows cystic disease.
Chronic eosinophilic pneumonia	Chest radiograph shows "radiographic negative" heart failure, with peripheral alveolar infiltrates predominating. Other findings may include peripheral blood eosinophilia and eosinophilia on bronchoalveolar lavage.
Pulmonary alveolar proteinosis	Median age of 39 years, and males predominate among smokers but not in nonsmokers. Diagnosed via bronchoalveolar lavage, which shows abundant protein in the airspaces. Chest CT shows "crazy paving" pattern.
DPLD = diffuse parenchymal lung disease.	

forms of disease, histopathologic patterns correlate with disease prognosis as well as response to anti-inflammatory treatment (such as glucocorticoids).

Diagnostic Approach and Evaluation

Patients with DPLD most often present with nonspecific symptoms of dyspnea and cough. A careful history with attention to time course is useful in raising the suspicion for DPLD and narrowing the differential diagnosis. For symptoms of shorter duration, lasting days to weeks rather than over months, infection and heart failure remain the most likely cause. If these causes are excluded or empiric treatment in this population is unsuccessful, the acute- or subacute-onset DPLDs should be considered.

Causes of DPLD can be classified into several broad categories, which include connective tissue diseases, occupational or other exposures, drug-induced lung injuries, idiopathic disorders, and primary disorders (**Figure 7**). For each of these categories, the differential diagnoses overlap with the idiopathic interstitial pneumonias. Therefore, in patients with suspected DPLD, a careful history that includes the time

course of symptoms, smoking and exposure history, rheumatologic review of systems, family history of autoimmune and lung disease, and past medication use helps assess potential risk and focus the differential diagnosis.

Plain chest radiography findings may be highly variable in patients with DPLD. Chest films may show increased interstitial reticular or nodular infiltrates in different patterns of distribution, but they may be normal in up to 20% of patients. Therefore, if clinical suspicion for DPLD exists, the evaluation should not stop if the chest radiograph is normal.

Characteristics on high-resolution CT (HRCT) of the chest have pulmonary pathology correlates that can help narrow the differential diagnosis. HRCT provides detailed resolution of the pulmonary parenchymal architecture. Advances in HRCT imaging techniques along with improved understanding of the correlation between HRCT findings and surgical biopsy histopathology findings have made HRCT the diagnostic tool of choice for evaluation of DPLD. There is little role for the use of conventional CT imaging (5-mm slice thickness) for this population given the limits of its resolution. HRCT, clinical presentation (including time course of symptoms), physical findings, and, when necessary, lung biopsy and histopathology allow clinicians to reach selected diagnoses from hundreds of DPLDs.

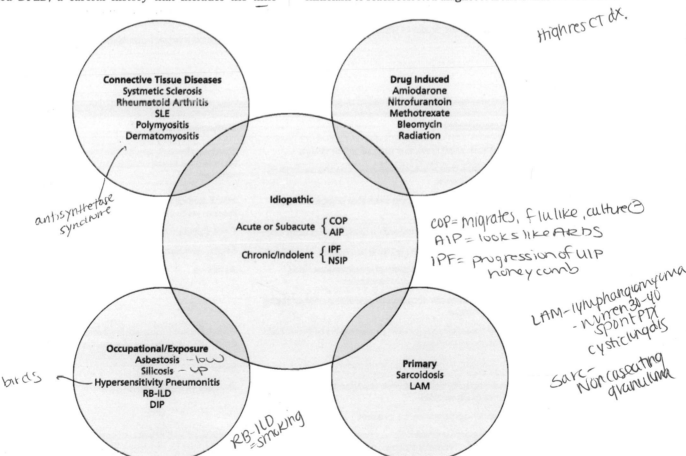

FIGURE 7. Broad categories of diffuse parenchymal lung disease. AIP = acute interstitial pneumonia; COP = cryptogenic organizing pneumonia; DIP = desquamative interstitial pneumonia; IPF = idiopathic pulmonary fibrosis; LAM = lymphangioleiomyomatosis; NSIP = nonspecific interstitial pneumonia; RB-ILD = respiratory bronchiolitis-associated interstitial lung disease; SLE = systemic lupus erythematosus.

For patients with more chronic symptoms, pulmonary function testing is helpful diagnostically to exclude obstructive lung disease as a primary cause of a patient's dyspnea symptoms. When restrictive or combined obstructive/restrictive diseases are identified and the presentation is more insidious (>6 months), DPLD should be considered.

Once there is clinical suspicion of DPLD, pulmonary consultation is appropriate.

KEY POINTS

- Causes of diffuse parenchymal lung disease can be classified into several broad categories, which include connective tissue diseases, occupational or other exposures, drug-induced lung injuries, idiopathic disorders, and primary disorders.

- The diagnosis of diffuse parenchymal lung disease should be considered in patients with insidious onset dyspnea and cough (>6 months) once infection, heart failure, and COPD are ruled out; consistent pulmonary function testing has a restrictive or combined obstructive/restrictive pattern.

- **HVC** High-resolution CT is the diagnostic tool of choice for evaluation of diffuse parenchymal lung disease; there is little role for plain chest radiography or conventional CT imaging (5-mm slice thickness) given the limits of their resolution.

High-Resolution CT Scanning

Patterns and Distribution

Disease patterns on HRCT generally correlate with pathologic findings on open lung biopsy. Specific terminology is used to describe findings noted on HRCT (**Table 21**). This terminology, in conjunction with the distribution of disease, allows the thoracic radiologist to describe patterns of disease associated with specific pathology (**Table 22**). Coexisting patterns of disease are common and can make definitive characterization from the CT scan imaging alone difficult. The combination of history, physical examination, serologic evaluation, and HRCT can obviate the need for diagnostic lung biopsy in 60% or more of patients. For those without a clear diagnosis following this evaluation, surgical lung biopsy may be considered. **H**

Associated Findings

Outside of the lung parenchyma, additional findings may be present in the mediastinum, pleura, and soft tissues that assist in making a diagnosis. For example, mediastinal and hilar lymphadenopathy is a common finding in sarcoidosis, whereas significantly enlarged lymph nodes are a rare finding in patients with idiopathic pulmonary fibrosis (IPF). Similarly, pleural effusions are rare in IPF but can be seen in connective tissue disease–associated DPLD such as systemic lupus erythematosus. Pleural plaques can help identify a history of asbestos

[handwritten note: lady windermere – lingula bronchiect MAC]

TABLE 21. Thoracic Radiology Terminology for Parenchymal Findings in DPLD

Pattern	Characteristics	Pathophysiology
Septal	Peripheral: short lines that extend to the pleura	Disease affecting any component of the septum (connective tissue containing lymphatics and pulmonary venules)
	Central: polygonal arcades that outline the secondary pulmonary lobule	
Reticular	On radiograph: interlacing lines that suggest a net	HRCT further defines the abnormality, whether septal lines or walls of a cyst
Nodular	Spherical lesions (<1 cm) with widespread distribution	Centrilobular: artery and small airway pathology
	Locations: centrilobular, lymphatic (septal), or random	Septal (see above)
Reticulonodular	On radiograph: intersection of innumerable lines producing the effect of micronodules	As above
	HRCT: Discerns the location of nodules as either septal or centrilobular	
Ground glass	Hazy increased opacity with preservation of bronchial and vascular markings	Partial filling of airspaces; interstitial thickening from fluid, cells, and/or fibrosis; partial collapse of alveoli; increased capillary blood volume or a combination of these
Consolidation	Denser opacity that obscures vascular markings, unlike ground-glass opacity	Exudate or other product that replaces alveolar air
	Air bronchograms may be present	
Honeycomb change	Closely approximated ring shadows that resemble a honeycomb; typically subpleural with well-defined walls	Destroyed and fibrotic lung containing cystic airspaces
Mosaic attenuation	Patchy regions of differing attenuation	On expiratory images, decreased areas of attenuation represent bronchial or bronchiolar obstruction

DPLD = diffuse parenchymal lung disease; HRCT = high-resolution CT.

TABLE 22. Patterns of Disease Associated with Diagnosis of DPLD

Lung Disease	Imaging	Comments
Acute interstitial pneumonia	Diffuse ground-glass with consolidation	Indistinguishable from ARDS with a risk factor
Organizing pneumonia	Patchy ground glass, consolidation, peripheral and basal predominance	Connective tissue diseases, infections, vasculitis, lymphoma, adenocarcinoma
Idiopathic pulmonary fibrosis/usual interstitial pneumonia	Basal- and peripheral-predominant septal line thickening with traction bronchiectasis and honeycomb changes	This is the usual interstitial pneumonia pattern and can be seen in connective tissue disease, asbestosis, and chronic hypersensitivity pneumonitis; idiopathic pulmonary fibrosis is a diagnosis of exclusion
Nonspecific interstitial pneumonia	Ground glass, basal predominance	Idiopathic and common finding in connective tissue disease
Respiratory bronchiolitis	Centrilobular nodules and ground-glass opacity in an upper-lung predominant distribution	May be an asymptomatic finding in an active smoker
Desquamative interstitial pneumonia	Basal- and peripheral-predominant ground-glass opacity with occasional cysts	—
Hypersensitivity pneumonitis	Acute: centrilobular micronodules that are upper- and mid-lung predominant Chronic: mid- and upper-lung predominant septal lung thickening with traction bronchiectasis; usual interstitial pneumonia pattern may be seen	Acute: associated with flulike illness Chronic: often cannot identify a causative antigen
Sarcoidosis	Upper-lobe predominant fibrosis; mediastinal and hilar lymphadenopathy; cystic changes including development of aspergilloma; airways-centered changes	Findings for sarcoidosis are often not specific; DPLD with diffuse mediastinal and hilar lymphadenopathy greater than 2 cm in size should raise suspicion

ARDS = acute respiratory distress syndrome; DPLD = diffuse parenchymal lung disease.

Langerhoans small cysts smoking PH (handwritten margin note)

exposure and possible asbestosis. Bone abnormalities are notable in individuals with ankylosing spondylitis.

 ### Surgical Lung Biopsy

Video-assisted thoracoscopic lung biopsy is an option for patients who have disparate findings on history, physical examination, imaging, and laboratory studies. Although generally well tolerated, there are reports of individuals whose disease has worsened after the procedure. Therefore, risk stratification and assessment of potential benefit are necessary when deciding whether to pursue biopsy. **H**

Diffuse Parenchymal Lung Diseases with a Known Cause

Smoking-Related Diffuse Parenchymal Lung Disease

Tobacco smoke is associated with the development of multiple DPLDs, including IPF. There are also several disorders that generally only develop in individuals who have an active smoking history.

Respiratory bronchiolitis–associated interstitial lung disease is used to describe disease in active smokers who have imaging findings of centrilobular micronodules with a pathologic finding of respiratory bronchiolitis on biopsy.

Desquamative interstitial pneumonia is due to extensive, diffuse macrophage filling of alveolar spaces with predominant cough and dyspnea symptoms and bilateral ground-glass opacities on chest imaging. Pulmonary Langerhans cell histiocytosis is characterized by thin-walled cysts with accompanying nodules and is often associated with pulmonary hypertension. All of these diseases are subacute and present in active smokers. Pulmonary function tests usually reveal an obstructive pattern with a severely decreased DLCO in individuals with more severe disease. For those with milder disease, pulmonary function tests can be normal, restrictive, or obstructive. Cessation of smoking is the primary management. Although glucocorticoids are used in individuals with more severe disease, the benefit of their use is uncertain.

KEY POINTS

- Tobacco smoke is associated with the development of multiple diffuse parenchymal lung diseases, including idiopathic pulmonary fibrosis.
- Cessation of smoking is the primary management for smoking-related diffuse parenchymal lung disease.

HVC

Connective Tissue Diseases

The prevalence of pulmonary manifestations in individuals with known connective tissue diseases is extremely high.

Patients with DPLD associated with connective tissue disease typically present with dyspnea.

DPLD is most often identified after an established diagnosis of connective tissue disease, although occasionally DPLD will be the first manifestation of connective tissue disease. As a result, all patients with suspected DPLD should be screened with a careful rheumatologic review of systems and physical examination to assess for the possibility of connective tissue disease. It is important to identify an underlying autoimmune disorder because of its effect on prognosis, drug therapy recommendations, and management of comorbidities that may adversely affect pulmonary outcomes.

For example, progressive pulmonary disease is now the primary cause of mortality in systemic sclerosis. Cyclophosphamide may have some short-term benefit in treating the lung disease, and managing the gastroesophageal dysmotility associated with systemic sclerosis may help avoid aspiration and further lung injury.

Another connective tissue disease commonly associated with DPLD is rheumatoid arthritis. DPLD associated with rheumatoid arthritis is more common in males than females and, as with other autoimmune diseases, may present prior to manifestations of arthritis. Parenchymal lung disease may include pleural disease, rheumatoid nodules, bronchitis, bronchiectasis, organizing pneumonia, and bronchiolitis, as well as a pattern of usual interstitial pneumonia (UIP). Similar to individuals with IPF, a UIP pattern on CT imaging indicates a poor prognosis. Currently, these manifestations of rheumatoid arthritis are often treated with glucocorticoids and disease-modifying agents; however, there are little data to suggest clear efficacy for this strategy.

KEY POINTS

- The prevalence of pulmonary manifestations in individuals with known connective tissue diseases is extremely high, and these patients typically present with dyspnea.

- All patients with diffuse parenchymal lung disease should be clinically assessed for an underlying autoimmune disorder because of its effect on prognosis, drug therapy recommendations, and management of comorbidities.

Hypersensitivity Pneumonitis

Hypersensitivity pneumonitis (HP) is the result of an immunologic response to repetitive inhalation of antigens. The most common sources of antigens are thermophilic actinomyces, fungi, and bird droppings. Antigens, however, are not limited to these origins and can include bacterial, protozoal, animal, or insect proteins, and even small molecular chemical compounds.

The acute form of HP presents within 48 hours of a high-level exposure and will often be associated with fevers, flulike symptoms, cough, and shortness of breath. Radiographic imaging can demonstrate bilateral hazy opacities, while HRCT imaging of the chest shows findings of ground-glass opacities and centrilobular micronodules that are upper- and mid-lung predominant (**Figure 8**). Symptoms typically wane within 24

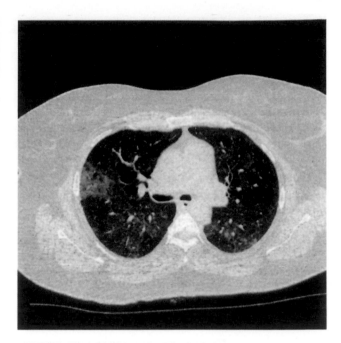

FIGURE 8. Chest CT demonstrating hypersensitivity pneumonitis with patchy, bilateral ground-glass opacities and centrilobular micronodules in this mid-lung section.

to 48 hours after removal from the exposure. Recurrence of symptoms with exposure to the respiratory antigen is the hallmark of this disorder, and careful attention to the history will help identify the cause.

Subacute and chronic forms of the disease also occur and are believed to be associated with more chronic low-level exposures to inhaled antigen. Bird fancier's disease is the classic example of this disorder, in which individuals are chronically exposed to an antigen from a domestic bird within the home. Patients will ultimately present with cough, dyspnea, malaise, and weight loss. HRCT findings include centrilobular micronodules in upper- and mid-lung distribution as well as evidence of septal line thickening and fibrosis.

The primary treatment is to remove the offending antigen. For this reason, it is extremely important to obtain a careful history to identify potential exposures. Glucocorticoids are used for patients with more severe symptoms and for those with evidence of fibrosis.

KEY POINTS

- The most common sources of antigens causing hypersensitivity pneumonitis are thermophilic actinomyces, fungi, and bird droppings; symptoms wane 24 to 48 hours after removal from exposure and recur with re-exposure to respiratory antigens.

- Radiographic imaging in hypersensitivity pneumonitis may demonstrate bilateral hazy opacities, while high-resolution CT imaging of the chest shows findings of ground-glass opacities and centrilobar micronodules that are upper- and mid-lung predominant.

(Continued)

- The primary treatment for hypersensitivity pneumonitis is to remove the offending antigen; glucocorticoids are used for patients with more severe symptoms and for those with evidence of fibrosis.

Drug-Induced Parenchymal Lung Disease

In patients who present with diffuse abnormalities on chest imaging, drug-induced parenchymal lung disease should be considered and investigated. Hundreds of drugs have been described in association with drug-induced lung disease. A few classic drug-induced lung syndromes are described in **Table 23**. Symptoms can develop acutely after drug initiation, but some medications have more subacute symptoms. Therefore, a careful medication history should be taken and should include medications that may have been discontinued after chronic treatment. The primary management of these disorders is removal of the offending agent.

Radiation-Induced Parenchymal Lung Disease

Symptoms of acute radiation pneumonitis typically occur 6 to 12 weeks after exposure. Patients present with cough, dyspnea, and occasionally fever and malaise. Differentiating these symptoms from infection and drug-induced pneumonitis is difficult given the common use of chemotherapy in combination with radiation. HRCT shows hazy ground-glass opacities.

TABLE 23. Select Drug-Induced Parenchymal Lung Diseases

Drug	Clinical Points	Radiographic Findings and Treatment
Amiodarone	More common in: Older patients Increased dosage and higher cumulative dose First year of therapy (but can occur late)	Multiple radiographic presentations possible including ground-glass opacities, subpleural nodules, and reticular abnormalities Very long half-life prevents clearance from the pulmonary parenchyma: Rare improvement with discontinuation of the drug alone High risk of recurrence with tapering of glucocorticoids
Methotrexate	Occurs in less than 5% of patients treated Unpredictable time to presentation No clear correlation between dose and disease severity	Diffuse reticular and ground-glass attenuation Patients generally do well after stopping medication Glucocorticoids are often given and duration is based on response
Nitrofurantoin	Acute (more common): Fevers, chills, cough, shortness of breath, chest pain; rash can occur in 10%-20% of patients Peripheral eosinophils common Chronic: Distinct from the acute form Onset months to years after prolonged exposure	Acute: Faint bilateral lower lobe septal lines; moderate pleural effusions may be present. Treatment: Often will resolve with discontinuation but will recur with repeat exposure. Chronic: Reticular opacities with subpleural lines and thickened peri-bronchovascular areas. Treatment: Possible benefit of glucocorticoids from anecdotal reports.
Busulfan	Occurs in less than 8% of patients treated Used solely as a conditioning regimen for HSCT today; often combined with other agents associated with pulmonary toxicity Injury typically occurs 30 days to 1 year after exposure	Multiple patterns including: ground glass opacities, reticulation, bibasilar septal lines, asymmetric peripheral and peribronchial consolidation, centrilobar nodules, and dependent consolidation Optimal treatment unknown and is often supportive Glucocorticoids may be used for more progressive disease
Bleomycin	Risk significantly increases with cumulative dose Increased age, renal insufficiency, concomitant chemotherapy and/or radiation also increases risk of toxicity Typically subacute presentation 1 to 6 months after exposure; may resemble hypersensitivity pneumonitis but with more rapid onset and progressive course	Imaging patterns suggest the multiple possible pathologic findings seen: Consolidation with ground glass (diffuse alveolar damage) Septal line thickening, traction bronchiectasis, and honey comb change (end-stage fibrosis) Patchy ground glass with subpleural consolidation or peribronchial consolidation (organizing pneumonia) Diffuse ground glass with centrilobar micronodules (hypersensitivity pneumonitis) Glucocorticoids are used for more severe disease and disease may recur with tapering of steroids

HSCT = hematopoietic stem cell transplantation.

CONT.

The factor that is most pathognomonic of radiation pneumonitis is the imaging finding of a nonanatomic straight line demarcating involved versus uninvolved lung parenchyma. Although abnormalities most often occur within the radiation field, it is possible for changes to occur outside of the field as well. Typically, acute changes will resolve within 6 months, but some patients may be left with a well-demarcated area of fibrosis, volume loss, and bronchiectasis.

Treatment of radiation pneumonitis is determined by the severity of symptoms. For patients with evidence of organizing pneumonia, there is likely a benefit to the use of glucocorticoids. Glucocorticoid therapy use is based on animal data suggesting a beneficial effect by suppressing the inflammatory response from acute radiation. For those with milder disease, the inflammation may resolve, obviating the need for glucocorticoids.

KEY POINTS

- In patients who present with diffuse abnormalities on chest imaging, drug-induced lung disease should be considered and investigated.

- Radiation pneumonitis presents with cough, dyspnea, and hazy ground-glass opacities (pathognomonic finding is a nonanatomic straight line between involved and uninvolved lung) on high-resolution CT 6 to 12 weeks after radiation exposure.

Diffuse Parenchymal Lung Diseases with an Unknown Cause

Idiopathic Pulmonary Fibrosis

IPF is the most common idiopathic interstitial pneumonia. It occurs predominantly in older individuals; the diagnosis of IPF is rare in those younger than 60 years of age. Gradual onset of dyspnea and cough over months to years is typical. Physical examination reveals dry inspiratory crackles at the bases. Nearly 50% of patients will have clubbing. More severe disease is associated with secondary pulmonary hypertension and evidence of right-sided heart failure on examination. Initial evaluation findings are often similar to more common conditions such as heart failure (due to crackles on lung examination) or COPD (a smoking history is common). Pulmonary function testing will most often show a restrictive abnormality with a reduced diffusing capacity; however, an isolated reduction in diffusing capacity and normal pulmonary function can also be seen (see Pulmonary Diagnostic Tests). All other identifiable causes of fibrotic lung disease must be excluded before the diagnosis can be made. When select HRCT features are present that establish a definite pattern of UIP (see Table 22) in the appropriate clinical setting, the diagnosis of IPF is established.

Prognosis remains poor, and individuals diagnosed with IPF have an estimated average survival of 3 to 5 years. There is, however, variability in the disease course. Some individuals will have slowly progressive declines in their forced vital capacity, while others can have a rapid decline leading to death. Still others will demonstrate stepwise declines in their pulmonary function tests with acute declines followed by subsequent stabilization.

An acute decline may manifest as an acute exacerbation of IPF. This is a well-defined clinical syndrome that develops in a small portion of patients with IPF. The clinical course of an acute exacerbation is acute to subacute onset (typically <30 days) of worsening dyspnea, and the medical evaluation does not reveal another cause for dyspnea such as infection, heart failure, or pulmonary embolism. HRCT shows new-onset diffuse ground-glass opacities. Patients may develop frank respiratory failure due to an exacerbation or stabilize at a new, worsened baseline.

The most common cause of death in IPF is respiratory failure. For individuals who develop severe respiratory distress for which there is no underlying reversible cause, supportive mechanical ventilation is of little long-term benefit. Therefore, the most recent evidence-based consensus statement recommends against mechanical ventilation for individuals with acute respiratory failure due to either progression or an acute exacerbation of IPF. In these circumstances, the focus should be on palliation of the patient's underlying dyspnea.

Treatment of IPF is primarily supportive, with optimization of fitness and oxygenation, as well as treatment of associated conditions. Recent clinical trials have led to a clearer understanding of the pharmacologic approach to patients with carefully diagnosed IPF. Therapies used in the past focused on anti-inflammatory therapy (for example, prednisone), with or without immune modulators (such as azathioprine). These therapies should be avoided because they were associated with increased mortality when compared with placebo in patients with mild to moderate respiratory impairment due to IPF. Antioxidant therapy with N-acetylcysteine was not found to be beneficial in decreasing the progression of IPF or reducing the frequency of exacerbations of IPF.

The most current models of disease focus on the interplay among alveolar epithelial cells, the extracellular matrix, and myofibroblasts that lead to fibrosis. Knowledge of these pathways has led to the development of two newly approved FDA therapies for the treatment of IPF: nintedanib and pirfenidone. Nintedanib is a tyrosine kinase inhibitor known to block pathways that lead to activation of the fibroblast. Similarly, pirfenidone is a novel therapeutic agent that regulates transforming growth factor β (TGF-β) and tumor necrosis factor α (TNF-α) activity through an unknown mechanism. Although these therapies are an important step forward in the management of IPF, they are not curative.

Lung transplantation remains the only therapy that clearly prolongs life in a select subset of patients with IPF. Early referral to a lung transplant center for suitable individuals interested in transplantation remains an appropriate early intervention for individuals with IPF.

- Treatment of idiopathic pulmonary fibrosis is supportive, with optimization of fitness and oxygenation, as well as treatment of associated conditions; lung transplantation may be appropriate in a select subset of patients.

HVC

- The most recent evidence-based consensus statement recommends against mechanical ventilation for individuals with acute respiratory failure due to either progression or an acute exacerbation of idiopathic pulmonary fibrosis.

Nonspecific Interstitial Pneumonia

Similar to IPF, NSIP is a disease that predominantly affects the lower lobes of the lung. Unlike IPF, NSIP tends to affect a younger patient population and is strongly associated with connective tissue disease. The largest group of patients with NSIP is those with systemic sclerosis; however, many autoimmune disorders have been associated with NSIP, including rheumatoid arthritis, systemic lupus erythematosus, polymyositis/dermatomyositis, and undifferentiated connective tissue disease. Some patients may initially present with only pulmonary manifestations of their underlying autoimmune disorder. For these individuals, the initial diagnosis may be idiopathic NSIP. This cohort of patients should receive continued surveillance for development of connective tissue disease. A careful review of systems is a key component of patient follow-up; new-onset symptoms should prompt further diagnostic assessments. A definitive diagnosis may help to better define the prognosis. The basis for immunosuppressive/immune-modulatory medications in patients with NSIP stems from the treatment response observed in the Scleroderma Lung Study, which was specific for patients with scleroderma and the inflammatory form of NSIP. The generalizability of these data in patients with NSIP due to other causes is less understood. In general, the prognosis for patients with an underlying autoimmune disorder is better than those with IPF; however, more severely affected pulmonary function and more extensive disease on CT imaging portend a worse prognosis.

- Nonspecific interstitial pneumonia predominantly affects the lower lobes of the lung, tends to affect a younger patient population, and is strongly associated with connective tissue disease (most often systemic sclerosis).

Cryptogenic Organizing Pneumonia

Organizing pneumonia is a patchy process that involves proliferation of granulation tissue within alveolar ducts, alveolar spaces, and surrounding areas of chronic inflammation. There are many known causes of this pattern, including acute infections and autoimmune disorders like rheumatoid arthritis. The term cryptogenic organizing pneumonia (COP) is reserved

for individuals who have this pattern but do not have a clear associated cause.

Patients with COP will typically present with symptoms over 6 to 8 weeks that mimic community-acquired pneumonia. The vast majority of individuals will present with symptoms of less than 3 months' duration. Patients typically present with bilateral diffuse alveolar opacities on chest radiograph with normal lung volumes (**Figure 9**). Patients may also present with multiple large nodules or masses that are predominantly peripheral. Although these findings are suggestive of an organizing pneumonia pattern, they are not specific to this disease. Typically, an initial empiric treatment for infection is given but fails; subsequently, noninfectious causes are then considered. Because the imaging findings are not specific, a bronchoscopic or surgical lung biopsy may be necessary to establish the diagnosis.

The prognosis for COP is typically favorable with a good response to glucocorticoids. Similar to idiopathic NSIP, individuals with COP should undergo examination and careful review of systems to ensure that there is not an underlying connective tissue disease. Also similar to idiopathic NSIP, individuals may develop manifestations of an underlying autoimmune disease subsequent to their initial pulmonary presentation.

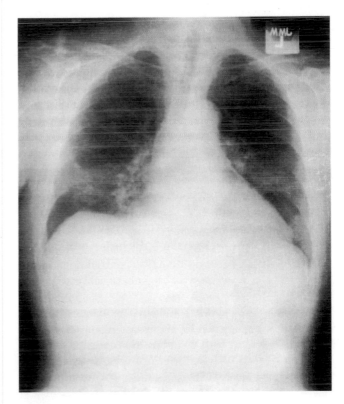

FIGURE 9. Chest radiograph showing cryptogenic organizing pneumonia with multiple patchy bilateral alveolar opacities that are nonspecific and may be difficult to distinguish from more typical infectious pneumonia. Infiltrates may be migratory with resolution of established opacities as new areas appear on serial imaging. Imaging may also be nonspecific, showing interstitial infiltrates and alveolar opacification or showing one or more rounded nodules that may be interpreted as malignancy.

CONT. In COP, recurrence with tapering of the glucocorticoid dosage is common; however, these recurrences most often respond to readministration and tapering of glucocorticoids. For those with multiple recurrences, careful re-examination for an underlying cause (such as an autoimmune disorder or ongoing exposure) is necessary. This group of patients may require long-term immunosuppressive therapy. **H**

KEY POINT

- The prognosis for cryptogenic organizing pneumonia is typically favorable with a good response to glucocorticoids.

Acute Interstitial Pneumonia

Acute interstitial pneumonia develops rapidly over days to weeks and results in progressive hypoxemic respiratory failure. Radiographic examination reveals bilateral alveolar opacities consistent with pulmonary edema; these findings cannot be reliably discerned from acute respiratory distress syndrome. Similarly, open lung biopsy specimens demonstrate diffuse alveolar damage. Unlike acute respiratory distress syndrome, there are no clearly associated risk factors for respiratory failure. Therefore, the history should be carefully reviewed to ensure that there is nothing to suggest aspiration, sepsis, pneumonia, or inhalational injury that might be amenable to treatment. Consensus recommendations advocate treatment with glucocorticoids. Although little evidence-based data exist, anecdotal reports suggest an improved outcome with this therapy. In addition to glucocorticoids, supportive care (with low tidal volume ventilation and careful attention to avoid complications of critical illness) remains the mainstay of therapy. Mortality rates remain extremely high (approximately 50%). Individuals who recover from the initial illness may relapse or develop chronic lung disease. **H**

KEY POINT

- Acute interstitial pneumonia develops rapidly over days to weeks and results in progressive hypoxemic respiratory failure; treatment consists of glucocorticoids and supportive care, but mortality is still high at 50%.

Sarcoidosis

Sarcoidosis is a multisystem granulomatous disease of unclear cause with a predilection for the lung; pulmonary involvement occurs in more than 90% of patients.

Many patients with pulmonary sarcoidosis are asymptomatic, and lung involvement is frequently discovered incidentally on chest imaging (**Figure 10**). Pulmonary sarcoidosis is classified based on the radiographic pattern (**Table 24**), and spontaneous regression of disease is common. For example, greater than 90% of those with stage I findings have radiographic resolution of their findings within 2 years, whereas 20% of those with stage II or III had spontaneous improvement in their imaging findings over this same time interval.

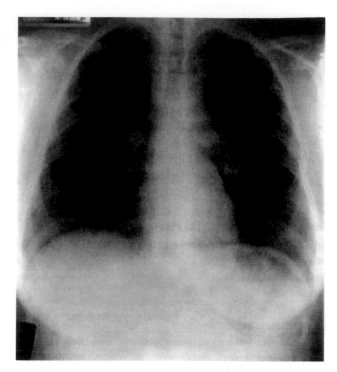

FIGURE 10. Chest radiograph showing stage I pulmonary sarcoidosis with hilar lymphadenopathy and normal lung parenchyma.

TABLE 24. Plain Radiographic Staging of Pulmonary Sarcoidosis

Stage	Radiographic Pattern	Clinical Course and Comments
0	Normal	—
I	Hilar lymphadenopathy with normal lung parenchyma	>90% will have spontaneous resolution without treatment
II	Hilar lymphadenopathy with abnormal lung parenchyma	Approximately 20% rate of spontaneous improvement without treatment
III	No lymphadenopathy with abnormal lung parenchyma	Approximately 20% rate of spontaneous improvement without treatment
IV	Parenchymal changes with fibrosis and architectural distortion	—

Pulmonary function tests will often be abnormal with obstructive, restrictive, or combined physiology on testing. Because sarcoidosis is a diagnosis of exclusion, a careful assessment is warranted in all patients to clarify the diagnosis. Although tissue biopsy (most often via bronchoscopy with transbronchial and lymph node biopsy) is usually required to diagnose sarcoidosis and exclude significant alternative diagnoses, there are several specific clinical situations in which biopsy is not considered necessary (**Table 25**).

[handwritten: Löfgren = transient sarc / hilar full / migratory arthralgia + erythema nod.]

TABLE 25. Clinical Presentations of Sarcoidosis that Do Not Warrant a Biopsy

Syndrome/Sign	Comments
Asymptomatic bilateral hilar lymphadenopathy	No evidence of fevers, malaise, or night sweats to suggest a malignancy
Löfgren syndrome	Bilateral hilar lymphadenopathy, migratory polyarthralgia, erythema nodosum, and fevers
Heerfordt syndrome	Anterior uveitis, parotiditis, fevers (uveoparotid fever), and facial nerve palsy

Glucocorticoids are the mainstay of therapy. Treatment is usually limited to those with evidence of clinical symptoms from organ dysfunction. Because there is a high rate of spontaneous remission and stability, most treatment protocols favor a period of observation without therapy. The decision to initiate glucocorticoid therapy for sarcoidosis should be based on symptoms or physiologic impairment that is attributable to sarcoid disease. There is a paucity of randomized controlled trials to provide guidance regarding whether glucocorticoid therapy will provide definitive benefit. Retrospective data suggest that treatment with glucocorticoids may have short-term symptomatic benefit but does not clearly affect long-term disease outcomes. If glucocorticoids are used for treatment of sarcoidosis, studies suggest that low-dose or alternate-day treatment strategies are as efficacious as higher-dose strategies and appear to have fewer side effects. Studies also show that once glucocorticoid therapy has begun, many patients will remain on this therapy for prolonged periods. Tapering regimens are often prolonged and should be based on clear, attributable symptoms or physiologic metrics in conjunction with careful and frequent follow-up.

Pulmonary hypertension may develop in some individuals with sarcoidosis owing to multiple physiologic reasons, including DPLD, pulmonary vascular disease, pulmonary artery compression from significant lymphadenopathy, left ventricular dysfunction, and pulmonary venous occlusion. For individuals who develop pulmonary hypertension without evidence of left ventricular dysfunction, mortality is significantly higher, with a median survival of approximately 3 years. For this group of patients, as well as individuals with significant limitations due to pulmonary disease, lung transplantation is a viable therapeutic option.

For a discussion of the musculoskeletal manifestations of sarcoidosis, see MKSAP 17 Rheumatology. **H**

KEY POINTS

- Pulmonary involvement occurs in more than 90% of patients with sarcoidosis, but is often asymptomatic.
- Glucocorticoids are the mainstay of therapy for symptomatic pulmonary sarcoidosis.

Lymphangioleiomyomatosis

Lymphangioleiomyomatosis is a rare disorder that occurs sporadically in women or in association with tuberous sclerosis. It manifests as a diffuse cystic lung disease due to infiltration of smooth muscle cells into the pulmonary parenchyma. Genetic mutations within the cells lead to activation of the mammalian target of rapamycin (mTOR) pathway. Diagnosis is based on imaging studies with diffuse thin-walled cysts (**Figure 11**) as well as spontaneous pneumothorax, angiomyolipomas, and elevated vascular endothelial growth factor-D (VEGF-D). Hormonal therapy, which was used in the past, is not effective in altering the disease course. Immunosuppression with sirolimus has demonstrated promise in limiting progression of pulmonary disease in patients with lymphangioleiomyomatosis. *[handwritten: LAM]*

Occupational Lung Disease

When to Suspect an Occupational Lung Disease

Occupational lung diseases affect all aspects of the respiratory tract, from the upper airways to the lower airways and interstitium. Clinical manifestations may include rhinitis, asthma, COPD, constrictive bronchiolitis, and restrictive diseases. Symptom onset following exposure can be acute (reactive airways disease/small airways dysfunction as occurs in acute chlorine gas exposure) as well as prolonged or subacute with a significant latent period (as with asbestosis). Because the clinical presentation of occupational lung disease is highly variable and dependent on the particular exposure, a high index of suspicion is necessary to identify this disorder.

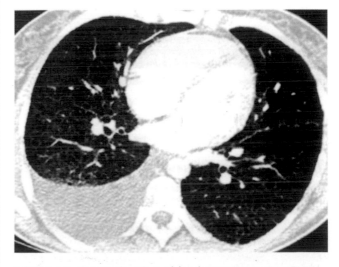

FIGURE 11. CT image of a patient with lymphangioleiomyomatosis showing diffuse thin-walled cysts and a right chylothorax.

Key Elements of the Exposure History

Factors that should raise the index of suspicion for an occupational-associated lung disease are shown in **Table 26**. Careful attention to historical details and a comprehensive occupational history are often crucial to identification of these disorders. In addition to identification of specific exposures, the duration and concentrations of exposures should be elicited. Owing to the variable time of onset of symptoms, the history should include exposures that date back many years. Furthermore, the interviewer should inquire about any potential additional exposures outside the work environment that may affect respiratory health (**Table 27**).

For individuals who work with potentially harmful substances, the U.S. Occupational Safety and Health Administration (OSHA) requires that employers maintain Material Safety Data Sheets (MSDS). These documents outline chemical properties of substances and the known potential health risks. OSHA requires that employers provide the MSDS upon request. These documents may be helpful in determining the risk of lung disease associated with a particular exposure.

When concern for an occupational disease persists but the history is unrevealing, referral to an occupational/environmental lung disease specialist is appropriate.

KEY POINT

- Careful attention to historical details and a comprehensive occupational history are often crucial to identification of occupational lung disease; in addition to identification of specific exposures, the duration and concentrations of exposures should be elicited.

Management

The overriding principle in management of occupational lung disease is prevention. This includes interventions in the work-

TABLE 27. Elements of a Thorough Patient History for Suspected Occupational Lung Disease
Understand the Occupation
What tasks do you perform at your current job?
How long have you been working at your current job?
What other jobs have you had in the past and for how long?
Understand the Type and Extent of Exposure
Are you exposed to vapors, gases, dust, or fumes in your work?
Do you know the amount and type of chemicals used?
Do you have Material Safety Data Sheets (MSDS) from your workplace?
Is your work environment well ventilated?
Does your employer require you to wear protective equipment? Do you wear it for the full duration of your exposure?
Is there visible dust in the air or on surrounding equipment?
Understand the Temporal Relationship of Symptoms to the Work Environment
Were there any changes to your work process prior to the onset of symptoms?
Do symptoms improve when you are away from the work environment? With vacation?
Understand Other Relevant Exposures
What are your hobbies?
Do you have pets in the home?
What is your travel history?

place to avoid exposures as well as early identification of coworkers who may also be at risk. For those who are affected, removal of the offending agent is essential. Symptomatic management often includes pharmacologic interventions.

Workers' compensation issues may require an assessment of the extent to which symptoms and physiologic impairment are directly attributable to a work exposure. These assessments are challenging, and referral to a specialist may be most appropriate.

KEY POINT

- The overriding principle in management of occupational lung disease is prevention, consisting of interventions in the workplace to avoid exposures as well as early identification of coworkers who may also be at risk.

HVC

Surveillance

When primary prevention fails or when a new potential threat is identified, surveillance programs including health screening and serial pulmonary function testing are appropriate. A recent example is the assessment of returning war veterans from Afghanistan and Iraq. Sentinel cases of constrictive

TABLE 26. Conditions that Should Increase Clinical Suspicion of Occupational Lung Disease
The patient raises a concern about possible exposures at work
There is a temporal relationship to clinical symptoms and work:
Symptoms worsen during or after work
Symptoms abate or improve with time off or away from the workplace
Coworkers are affected with similar symptoms
There are known respiratory hazards at work (these can be identified by Material Safety Data Sheets [MSDS] from the workplace)
Failure to respond to initial therapy or symptoms that are further exacerbated upon returning to work
Onset of a respiratory disorder without typical risk factors
Clustering of disease in one geographic area

bronchiolitis have identified multiple potential exposures (open fire pits, diesel exhaust, particulate matter from sand storms, and exposure to rocket fuel) that may result in lung disease. Because of this, a thorough assessment of war veterans for possible evidence of lung disease is recommended and should include symptom review and serial pulmonary function tests for those who are symptomatic. Identification of patients with mild or early disease allows for earlier intervention and counseling.

Asbestos-Related Lung Disease

Asbestos is a silicate mineral fiber previously used as an insulating material that is a major cause of lung disease. Although asbestos use in the United States has been virtually eliminated since its peak in the 1980s, asbestos-related diseases will persist well into this century owing to the long latency period between exposure and disease development (15-35 years). Although developed nations have nearly eliminated its use, asbestos inhalation remains at roughly 2 million metric tons per year worldwide. The result is that asbestos-related diseases will continue to be a major public health concern in the developing world for many years. Currently, approximately 107,000 people die each year owing to asbestos-related mesothelioma, lung cancer, and interstitial lung disease (asbestosis).

Risk Factors

The extent of asbestos exposure correlates with risk for disease, with the most common occupational exposures occurring in the construction, automotive servicing, and shipbuilding industries. Asbestos-related diseases are also commonly found in mining workers and in areas where manufacturing of asbestos has led to contamination of the environment. In this instance, individuals will not have an occupational exposure history.

KEY POINT

- Asbestos exposures are most commonly associated with the construction, automotive servicing, shipbuilding, and mining industries.

Pathophysiology

Asbestos fibers are inhaled and are deposited at the level of airway bifurcations and the alveolus. The lung may clear fibers (typically shorter fibers), whereas others are transported to the interstitium or via the lymphatics to the pleura. Parietal plaques are the most common finding, and the mechanism by which fibers transmigrate and develop plaques remains unclear. Diffuse parenchymal lung disease due to asbestos (asbestosis) is secondary to the extent of the fiber burden. The initial process begins with an alveolitis. If the fiber burden is low, this can resolve spontaneously. With a higher burden, proinflammatory and cytotoxic agents are released by macrophages with resultant recruitment of fibroblasts. If the process is sustained, collagen deposition leads to irreversible chronic fibrosis.

Asbestos-Related Pleural Diseases

Asbestos is associated with multiple forms of pleural disease. Pleural plaques are the most common form of disease and are characterized by smooth, white, raised, irregular lesions affecting predominantly the parietal and, very rarely, the visceral pleura (**Figure 12**). Pleural plaques are asymptomatic in the absence of parenchymal disease and are typically incidentally identified on routine chest radiograph.

Pleural fibrosis is a visceroparietal pleural reaction that may be either localized or diffuse. When the process is diffuse, it can lead to symptomatic restrictive disease. Treatment options for this are limited, and there is little benefit to surgical removal of the pleural layer (decortication) in this cohort. Pleural fibrosis may also lead to the development of rounded atelectasis (**Figure 13**). This is a process in which the lung becomes atelectatic in the region of the pleural fibrosis. The area forms a mass-like lesion that includes bronchi and vessels. These are often asymptomatic but may lead to respiratory impairment if they become large enough. Although these lesions may be concerning for a possible malignancy, they are often distinguished radiographically by a thoracic radiologist as benign.

Benign asbestos pleural effusion may occur either early or late after asbestos exposure. It may be asymptomatic or associated with chest pain. The pleural fluid analysis will be exudative and is often hemorrhagic. Further, eosinophils are present in nearly one third of patients. Benign asbestos pleural effusion is diagnosed only after exclusion of infection, pulmonary

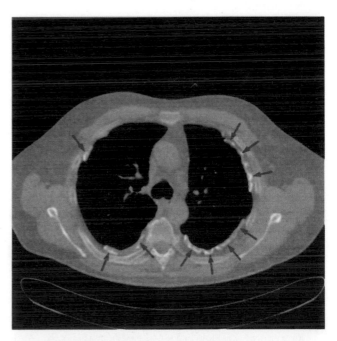

FIGURE 12. Chest CT showing extensive calcified pleural plaques (*arrows*) associated with asbestos exposure.

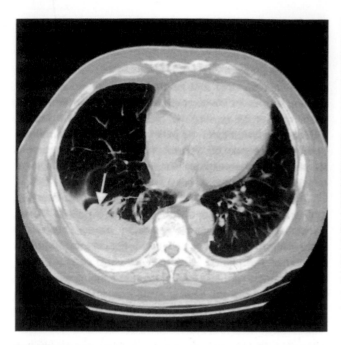

FIGURE 13. Chest CT showing rounded atelectasis (*arrow*) with its typical findings of a round area of lung parenchyma associated with a pleural abnormality and a comet tail that extends into the lung parenchyma.

embolism, and malignancy. Exclusion of mesothelioma is difficult owing to the low sensitivity of cytology and the presence of "reactive" mesothelial cells. Clinicians should have a low threshold to refer for consideration of pleuroscopy for these patients. An experienced thoracic surgeon or interventional pulmonologist can often discern mesothelioma on direct inspection. See Lung Tumors for a discussion of mesothelioma.

Asbestos exposure significantly increases the risk of lung cancer. In a recent report, 19% of patients with extensive asbestos exposure died secondary to lung cancer. For those that were nonsmokers, the risk of lung cancer mortality was 3.6-fold higher than controls. For those with a combined history of smoking and asbestos exposure, the risk of lung cancer mortality was 14.4 times higher than controls. For patients with a history of asbestosis, however, the additional risk of smoking was supra-additive (36.8 times higher than controls). The risk of developing cancer was mitigated by discontinuing smoking at any point. This new information further encourages smoking cessation and highlights the potential importance of lung cancer screening in those with the combined risk factors of smoking and asbestosis.

KEY POINTS

- Asbestos exposure is associated with multiple forms of pleural disease, including pleural plaques, pleural fibrosis, benign asbestos pleural effusion, and mesothelioma.
- Asbestos exposure significantly increases the risk of lung cancer and lung cancer mortality, particularly when combined with smoking.

Silicosis

Silicosis is a spectrum of fibrotic lung diseases related to the inhalation of silica dust. The most common form of silica is quartz, and any occupation that disturbs the earth's crust involves potential risk. Workers in industries that process silica-containing rock or sand are also at risk. Simple silicosis is marked by profusion of small rounded nodules that are upper-lobe predominant. The disease course may be accelerated (3-10 years after exposure) or latent (>10 years after exposure). The lesions may become confluent and lead to progressive massive fibrosis. Although individuals with simple silicosis may be asymptomatic, those with progressive massive fibrosis develop symptomatic shortness of breath.

The incidence of tuberculosis is increased in those with silicosis, and symptoms should prompt an evaluation for possible infection. In addition, altered cellular immunity may account for the increased prevalence of connective tissue disease in those with silicosis. Mine workers are often exposed to multiple dusts and radon, and they have high rates of tobacco use; however, the development of silicosis is also an independent risk factor for the development of lung cancer.

Once fibrotic disease develops, there are no clear therapeutic interventions to alter the disease course. Individuals with continued exposure to silica dust should change to a silica-free environment. Because airways disease and cancer are also associated with silica exposure, smoking cessation is always an appropriate recommendation. Symptomatic treatment includes inhaled bronchodilators, antibiotics for infections, and supplemental oxygen for hypoxemia. For individuals with progressive disease, consideration of lung transplantation referral is appropriate.

KEY POINT

- The incidence of tuberculosis is increased in patients with silicosis, and symptoms should prompt an evaluation for possible infection.

Pleural Disease

There are two main types of abnormalities that affect the pleura: increased fluid (pleural effusion) and air (pneumothorax) in the pleural space.

Pleural Effusion

Pleural effusion is the most common disorder affecting the pleura, with approximately 1.5 million pleural effusions diagnosed each year. These occur as a result of increased fluid formation and/or decreased fluid resorption in the pleural space. There are over 50 known causes and the pathophysiology varies depending on the cause. The vast majority of pleural effusions in the United States are the result of heart failure, pneumonia, or malignancy. A systematic approach to diagnosis is necessary based on the clinical presentation of the patient.

KEY POINT

- The vast majority of pleural effusions in the United States are the result of heart failure, pneumonia, or malignancy.

Evaluation

History and Physical Examination

The history and physical examination guide the initial evaluation of pleural effusion. Signs and symptoms vary depending on the cause but commonly include dyspnea, cough, and pleuritic chest pain. Additional features such as fever, orthopnea, or concurrent arthralgia may provide clues to the underlying cause and can help narrow the differential diagnosis. History of travel, prior and current occupation, medication use, prior surgery (such as coronary artery bypass surgery), malignancy, place of residency, and prior asbestos exposure should also be elicited.

Clinical examination hallmarks include diminished breath sounds, dullness to percussion, and decreased tactile fremitus over the area of the pleural effusion; these findings generally occur only in effusions larger than 300 mL. Other clues on examination include distended neck veins, peripheral edema, right ventricular heave or deep venous thrombosis, stigmata of end-stage liver disease, joint deformities, or synovitis. Each of these findings may help narrow the differential diagnosis and guide additional testing.

Diagnostic Imaging

A chest radiograph is usually the first imaging study obtained when evaluating a pleural effusion. Posteroanterior radiographs will generally show evidence of pleural effusion when there is approximately 200 mL of pleural fluid present, and lateral films will be abnormal when approximately 50 mL of pleural fluid is present.

Thoracic ultrasound also has an increasingly important role in the evaluation of pleural effusion because of its higher sensitivity in the detection of pleural fluid than the clinical examination or chest radiography. Characteristics that can also be seen on ultrasound can help define whether the effusion is simple or complex. A simple effusion can be identified as fluid in the pleural space with homogeneous echotexture as seen in most transudative effusions, whereas a complex effusion is echogenic, frequently with septations (loculations) within the fluid, and is always an exudate. Bedside ultrasound is recommended when performing thoracentesis, as it enhances procedural accuracy and safety.

KEY POINTS

HVC
- Chest radiograph and thoracic ultrasound are important tests in the evaluation of pleural effusion; ultrasound has a higher sensitivity for pleural fluid and no associated radiation exposure.

HVC
- Bedside ultrasound is recommended for thoracentesis, as it enhances procedural accuracy and safety.

Indications for Thoracentesis

A thoracentesis is indicated for any new unexplained pleural effusion. Observation and initiation of therapy without diagnostic thoracentesis are reasonable in the setting of known heart failure or small parapneumonic effusions, or following coronary artery bypass surgery. However, any atypical features (such as fever, pleurisy) or failure to respond to therapy in these patients should prompt consideration of a diagnostic thoracentesis.

Pleural Fluid Analysis

The gross appearance of pleural fluid should be noted while performing a thoracentesis, as it may reveal the diagnosis. Fluid can appear serous, serosanguineous (blood stained), hemorrhagic, or purulent. Bloody fluid is often seen in malignancy, pulmonary embolism with lung infarction, trauma, benign asbestos effusion, or post–cardiac injury syndrome. Purulent fluid can be seen in empyema and lipid effusions. In addition, a putrid odor can point to an anaerobic infection and the smell of ammonia to an urinothorax.

The characterization of pleural fluid as a transudate or exudate helps narrow the differential diagnosis and direct subsequent investigations. The most common criteria used to make this differentiation are the Light criteria (Table 28). Initial testing should include measurement of the pleural fluid total protein and lactate dehydrogenase with concurrent measurement of serum total protein and lactate dehydrogenase to allow assessment of the Light criteria.

Other initial pleural fluid studies include the cell count with differential, pH, and glucose levels. If infection is suspected, Gram stain and microbiologic culture should be performed, and cytology is appropriate in patients with possible malignancy. Additional tests performed in selected patients include amylase, cholesterol, triglycerides, acid-fast bacilli, and *Mycobacterium tuberculosis* culture.

Transudates are usually the result of an imbalance between hydrostatic and oncotic pressures, whereas exudates result primarily from inflammation or impaired lymphatic drainage (such as infections, inflammation, or malignancy) (Table 29). Light criteria can occasionally misclassify transudative effusions as exudates in the setting of ongoing diuresis. In this case it is reasonable to determine the serum albumin to pleural fluid albumin gradient. If it is greater than 1.2 g/dL (12 g/L), the underlying process is likely transudative.

TABLE 28.	Light Criteria
An effusion is considered an exudate if any of the following are met:	
Pleural fluid total protein/serum total protein >0.5	
Pleural fluid LDH/serum LDH >0.6	
Pleural fluid LDH >2/3 the upper limit of normal for serum LDH	
LDH = lactate dehydrogenase.	

TABLE 29. Common Causes of Transudates and Exudates

Transudates	Exudates
Heart failure	Parapneumonic effusions
Hepatic hydrothorax	Malignancy
Nephrotic syndrome	Pulmonary embolism
Hypoalbuminemia	Tuberculosis
Unexpandable (trapped) lung	Autoimmune diseases (RA, SLE)
Urinothorax	Benign asbestos effusion
Atelectasis	Post–coronary artery bypass
Peritoneal dialysis	Pancreatitis
	Post-myocardial infarction
	Yellow nail syndrome (lymphatic disorders)
	Drugs

RA = rheumatoid arthritis; SLE = systemic lupus erythematosus.

TABLE 30. Clinical Significance of Cell Counts in Pleural Fluid

Cell Type	Cell Count	Clinical Significance
Erythrocytes	5000-10,000/µL (5-10 × 10⁹/L)	Bloody appearance, hemothorax if pleural fluid hematocrit >50% peripheral hematocrit; most commonly associated with cancer, pulmonary infarction, asbestos-related effusions, or trauma
Nucleated cells	>50,000/µL (50 × 10⁹/L)	Complicated parapneumonic effusions and empyema
	>10,000/µL (10 × 10⁹/L)	Bacterial pneumonia, acute pancreatitis, and lupus pleuritis
	<5000/µL (5 × 10⁹/L)	Chronic exudates (TB pleurisy and malignancy)
Lymphocytes	>80%	Suggests TB, lymphoma, chronic rheumatoid pleurisy, sarcoidosis, and late post-CABG effusions. Pleural biopsy is indicated if no diagnosis.
Eosinophils	>10%	Suggests air or blood in the pleural space but is nonspecific. Can be seen in parapneumonic effusions, drug-induced pleurisy, eosinophilic granulomatosis with polyangiitis (formerly known as Churg-Strauss syndrome), benign asbestos effusions, malignancy (lymphoma), pulmonary infarction, fungal disease (coccidioidomycosis, cryptococcosis, histoplasmosis), and parasitic disease

CABG = coronary artery bypass graft; TB = tuberculosis.

KEY POINT

- The characterization of pleural fluid as a transudate or exudate helps narrow the differential diagnosis and direct subsequent investigations.

Cell Counts and Differential

Pleural fluid cell counts with differential are helpful in narrowing the diagnosis but are not disease specific (**Table 30**).

Blood Chemistry Studies

Glucose concentration in pleural fluid is equivalent to that of the blood in the absence of pleural pathology. Therefore, a low pleural fluid glucose concentration can be very helpful in the analysis of pleural fluid. A low pleural fluid glucose level results from either increased utilization within the pleural space (bacteria, malignant cells) or decreased transport into the pleural space (rheumatoid pleurisy), and a concentration less than 60 mg/dL (3.3 mmol/L) narrows the differential diagnosis significantly (**Table 31**).

Pleural fluid acidosis (pH <7.30) is seen in complicated parapneumonic effusions, malignancy, tuberculous pleuritis, rheumatoid and lupus pleuritis, and esophageal rupture. By itself it does not distinguish between these entities, but it implies high metabolic activity in the pleural space. In malignancy, a low pH correlates with a poor prognosis and predicts pleurodesis failure. In suspected pleural infection, a pH less than 7.20 should be treated with pleural drainage. Collection and processing of samples for pH must be done carefully. Exposure of the fluid to air in the syringe can increase the pleural fluid pH, and very small amounts of lidocaine can lower pH significantly. It is recommended that pleural fluid pH be tested on a blood gas analyzer within 1 hour of collection.

Pleural fluid amylase is elevated if the pleural fluid to serum amylase ratio is greater than 1.0 and suggests pancreatic

TABLE 31. Pleural Effusions with Glucose Level Less than 60 mg/dL (3.3 mmol/L)

Rheumatoid pleurisy
Complicated parapneumonic effusion or empyema
Malignant effusion
Tuberculous pleurisy
Lupus pleuritis
Esophageal rupture

disease, esophageal rupture, and malignant effusions. It should not be routinely measured but can be useful when an esophageal or pancreatic cause for the effusion is suspected.

A pleural fluid triglyceride level greater than 110 mg/dL (1.24 mmol/L) is characteristic of a chylothorax, and a level less

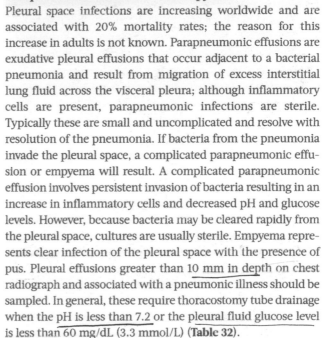

than 50 mg/dL (0.56 mmol/L) reasonably excludes the diagnosis. An intermediate level (between 50-110 mg/dL [0.56-1.24 mmol/L]) should be investigated with a lipoprotein analysis looking for chylomicrons. It is also not a routine pleural fluid study but is appropriate in patients with suspected chylothorax.

Tests for Tuberculous Effusions

Tuberculous pleuritis continues to be a common problem worldwide and should be considered as part of the differential diagnosis in patients with undiagnosed lymphocyte-predominant exudative effusions. Smear and culture of pleural fluid for acid-fast bacilli are very specific but have a low sensitivity (5% and 20%, respectively). Adenosine deaminase is an enzyme present in lymphocytes that is elevated in most tuberculous pleural effusions (sensitivity 95%). In countries with a low incidence of tuberculosis, testing for adenosine deaminase can be useful as a test to rule out tuberculosis. Pleural biopsy is the most likely test to yield a positive mycobacterial culture (>70%).

Adenosine deaminase is pleural effusion in Tb

Tests for Pleural Malignancy

Cytology should be performed on any effusion in which malignancy is suspected. When the suspicion for malignancy is high, it is appropriate to repeat cytology if the first specimen is negative. The overall mean sensitivity is approximately 60%, and the yield from sending more than two samples is very low. One study demonstrated an additional yield of 27% on the second sample and only 5% on the third. The diagnostic rate is higher for adenocarcinoma than mesothelioma and lymphoma. If lymphoma is suspected, flow cytometry should be performed to further characterize the cells present.

Thoracoscopy is the next step in the evaluation of an exudative pleural effusion that is indeterminate and malignancy is suspected. Medical thoracoscopy allows for the direct visualization of the pleural surface and allows for biopsy of pleural sites likely to have a high diagnostic yield. It therefore has a diagnostic sensitivity for malignant disease of greater than

90%. Blind closed pleural biopsy is less sensitive than cytology and should not be performed.

Management

Parapneumonic Effusions and Empyema

Pleural space infections are increasing worldwide and are associated with 20% mortality rates; the reason for this increase in adults is not known. Parapneumonic effusions are exudative pleural effusions that occur adjacent to a bacterial pneumonia and result from migration of excess interstitial lung fluid across the visceral pleura; although inflammatory cells are present, parapneumonic infections are sterile. Typically these are small and uncomplicated and resolve with resolution of the pneumonia. If bacteria from the pneumonia invade the pleural space, a complicated parapneumonic effusion or empyema will result. A complicated parapneumonic effusion involves persistent invasion of bacteria resulting in an increase in inflammatory cells and decreased pH and glucose levels. However, because bacteria may be cleared rapidly from the pleural space, cultures are usually sterile. Empyema represents clear infection of the pleural space with the presence of pus. Pleural effusions greater than 10 mm in depth on chest radiograph and associated with a pneumonic illness should be sampled. In general, these require thoracostomy tube drainage when the pH is less than 7.2 or the pleural fluid glucose level is less than 60 mg/dL (3.3 mmol/L) (Table 32).

A wide range of organisms may cause pleural space infection; the most typical are *Streptococcus pneumoniae*, *Streptococcus milleri*, *Staphylococcus aureus*, and Enterobactcriaceae. Anaerobes have also been cultured in 36% to 72% of empyemas. Consequently, empiric antimicrobial coverage for suspected pleural infection should include anaerobic coverage. The use of intrapleural fibrinolytics has been studied in complicated parapneumonic effusions and has shown limited utility. When combined with a mucolytic agent (deoxyribonuclease), it resulted in a greater decrease in the size of the effusion and lower rate of surgical referral. The size of the drainage tube remains controversial, but several studies have demonstrated equal efficacy

TABLE 32.	Parapneumonic Effusions		
Type	**Pleural Characteristics**	**Pleural Fluid Chemistry**	**Management**
Uncomplicated	Small (<10 mm on lateral decubitus radiographic view), free flowing	pH: unknown Glucose: unknown	Antibiotics and serial follow-up to ensure resolution; if no resolution or ongoing sepsis, consider thoracentesis
	Small to moderate effusion (>10 mm to <1/2 hemithorax), free flowing	pH >7.2 Glucose >60 mg/dL (3.3 mmol/L)	Antibiotics, thoracentesis, and serial follow-up to ensure resolution; if no resolution or ongoing sepsis, consider repeat thoracentesis and need for drainage
Complicated	Loculated or thickened pleura	pH <7.2 **or** glucose <60 mg/dL (3.3 mmol/L)	Antibiotics, thoracostomy tube drainage, serial follow-up; if no resolution, consult thoracic surgeon for possible thorascopic debridement
Empyema	Bacterial organisms seen on Gram stain or aspiration of pus on thoracentesis	pH <7.0	Antibiotics, thoracostomy tube drainage, early consultation with a thoracic surgeon for possible thorascopic debridement

CONT.

and improved patient comfort with the use of smaller, 10 to 14 Fr (3.3 to 4.7 mm) thoracostomy tubes. Effusions refractory to antibiotics and drainage alone require surgical debridement.

KEY POINTS

- Parapneumonic pleural effusion requires thoracostomy tube drainage when the pH is less than 7.2 or the pleural fluid glucose level is less than 60 mg/dL (3.3 mmol/L).

- Anaerobes are cultured in 36% to 72% of empyemas, and empiric antibiotic therapy should include anaerobic coverage.

H **Malignant Pleural Effusion**

The goal of management in malignant pleural effusions is palliation of symptoms. The choice of therapy should be dependent on prognosis, rate of reaccumulation, and the severity of the patient's symptoms. Repeat therapeutic thoracentesis is appropriate for patients with poor prognosis (<3 months) and slow reaccumulation of fluid. In patients with more rapid recurrence of fluid, more definitive measures are warranted. Indwelling pleural catheters with intermittent drainage (managed as an outpatient) is commonly the procedure of choice for management of malignant pleural effusions. Indwelling pleural catheters have been demonstrated to provide significant symptom relief, and 50% to 70% of patients achieve spontaneous obliteration of the pleural space (pleurodesis) after 2 to 6 weeks. Chemical pleurodesis with talc is also very effective, with a success rate of 60% to 90% depending on the degree of lung reexpansion. Pleurectomy and pleuroperitoneal shunt are other management options but are rarely performed.

Pneumothorax

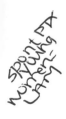

Pneumothorax (air in the pleural space) can occur spontaneously, as a result of trauma, or iatrogenically. Spontaneous pneumothorax is further characterized as a primary spontaneous pneumothorax (PSP) in a person without underlying lung disease or a secondary spontaneous pneumothorax (SSP) in a person with underlying lung disease. Risk factors for PSP are smoking, tall stature, family history, Marfan syndrome, and thoracic endometriosis. SSP is most commonly associated with COPD and presents with increased symptoms and breathlessness due to decreased respiratory reserve.

Physical examination usually reveals reduced lung expansion, hyperresonance to percussion, and diminished breath sounds on the side of the pneumothorax. Tension pneumothorax should be suspected in patients presenting with significant cardiorespiratory distress.

Pneumothorax is diagnosed by detection of a visceral pleural line on a standard chest radiograph (**Figure 14**). The size of the pneumothorax is determined by measuring the distance between the lung margin and the inner chest wall at the level of the hilum. A distance of greater than 2 cm is considered a large pneumothorax.

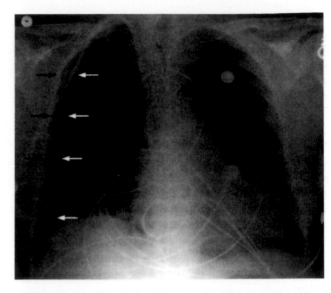

FIGURE 14. This chest radiograph demonstrates a right pneumothorax following the placement of a central venous catheter. The chest wall and parietal pleura are indicated by the black arrows, and the visceral pleura and lung border are indicated by the white arrows. The air in the pleural space is darker than the adjacent lung and also lacks normal lung markings.

Management of a pneumothorax depends on the degree of clinical compromise, size, and whether the pneumothorax is primary or secondary. Breathlessness indicates the need for active intervention as well as supportive treatment (high-flow supplemental oxygen). A large, hemodynamically significant pneumothorax (tension pneumothorax) should be managed with high-flow supplemental oxygen and emergent needle thoracostomy, followed by thoracostomy tube placement and hospitalization. In contrast, observation alone has been shown to be safe for small pneumothoraces in patients with minimal symptoms (**Table 33** and **Table 34**). Patients presenting with SSP are at higher risk for persistent air leak or further expansion of the pneumothorax due to their underlying lung disease. As a result, SSPs are best managed with a small-bore (<14 Fr [4.7 mm]) pleural drain instead of simple aspiration.

TABLE 33. Management of Primary Spontaneous Pneumothorax

Size and Clinical Symptoms	Management
<2 cm on chest radiograph, minimal symptoms	Observation alone; may be managed as an outpatient if easy access to medical care is available if clinical symptoms change
>2 cm on chest radiograph, breathlessness, and chest pain	Needle aspiration; if reaccumulation then insertion of a small-bore (<14 Fr [4.7 mm]) thoracostomy tube
Clinical instability regardless of size	Emergent needle decompression followed by thoracostomy tube insertion[a]

[a]If persistent air leak (>3-5 days), refer to a thoracic surgeon for possible surgical pleurodesis and bleb resection.

TABLE 34. Management of Secondary Spontaneous Pneumothorax

Size and Clinical Symptoms	Management
<2 cm on chest radiograph, minimal symptoms	Admit to hospital for observation and supplemental oxygen
>2 cm on chest radiograph, breathlessness, and chest pain	Insertion of a small-bore (<14 Fr [4.7 mm]) thoracostomy tube
Clinical instability regardless of size	Emergent needle decompression followed by thoracostomy tube insertion[a]

[a]If persistent air leak (>48 hours), refer to a thoracic surgeon for possible surgical bleb resection and pleurodesis; recurrence prevention (pleurodesis) should be offered to all patients after one event of secondary spontaneous pneumothorax.

Recurrence is estimated at 23% to 50% over the first 5 years in PSP and close to 50% in SSP. Intervention to prevent recurrence includes both chemical and mechanical pleurodesis, which is recommended in all SSP and after the second occurrence of a PSP.

All patients should be counseled against air travel until complete resolution of the pneumothorax has been confirmed by chest radiograph. In addition, diving should be discouraged permanently unless a definitive prevention plan (such as surgical pleurectomy) has been performed.

KEY POINTS

- A large, hemodynamically significant pneumothorax (tension pneumothorax) should be managed by high-flow supplemental oxygen and emergent needle thoracostomy followed by thoracostomy tube placement and hospitalization.

- Observation alone has been shown to be safe for small pneumothoraces in patients with minimal symptoms.

Pulmonary Vascular Disease

Pulmonary Hypertension

The pulmonary vasculature is a system of low pressure and high compliance, such that in healthy individuals, pulmonary artery pressures remain relatively unchanged during states of stress and high flow, such as exercise. The normal mean pulmonary artery pressure is approximately 15 mm Hg. Pulmonary hypertension (PH) is defined by a resting mean pulmonary artery pressure of 25 mm Hg or greater. Unabated, PH eventually leads to right ventricular (RV) failure and may directly contribute to death; however, the rate of progression is highly variable and dependent upon the origin of disease and comorbidities.

The current classification system subdivides PH into five groups (Table 35), which are based on similarities in mechanisms,

TABLE 35. Classification of Pulmonary Hypertension

1. PAH
   1.1 Idiopathic PAH
   1.2 Heritable
      1.2.1 *BMPR2*
      1.2.2 *ALK1*, endoglin (with or without hereditary hemorrhagic telangiectasia)
      1.2.3 Unknown
   1.3 Drug- and toxin-induced
   1.4 Associated with
      1.4.1 Connective tissue diseases
      1.4.2 HIV infection
      1.4.3 Portal hypertension
      1.4.4 Congenital heart diseases
      1.4.5 Schistosomiasis
      1.4.6 Chronic hemolytic anemia
   1.5 Persistent pulmonary hypertension of the newborn
1′. Pulmonary veno-occlusive disease and/or pulmonary capillary hemangiomatosis
2. Pulmonary hypertension due to left-sided heart disease
   2.1 Systolic dysfunction
   2.2 Diastolic dysfunction
   2.3 Valvular disease
3. Pulmonary hypertension due to lung diseases and/or hypoxia
   3.1 COPD
   3.2 Interstitial lung disease
   3.3 Other pulmonary diseases with mixed restrictive and obstructive pattern
   3.4 Sleep-disordered breathing
   3.5 Alveolar hypoventilation disorders
   3.6 Chronic exposure to high altitude
   3.7 Developmental abnormalities
4. Chronic thromboembolic pulmonary hypertension
5. Pulmonary hypertension with unclear or multifactorial causes
   5.1 Hematologic disorders: myeloproliferative disorders, splenectomy
   5.2 Systemic disorders: sarcoidosis, pulmonary Langerhans cell histiocytosis: lymphangioleiomyomatosis, neurofibromatosis, vasculitis
   5.3 Metabolic disorders: glycogen storage disease, Gaucher disease, thyroid disorders
   5.4 Others: tumoral obstruction, fibrosing mediastinitis, chronic kidney failure on dialysis

ALK1 = activin receptor-like kinase type 1; BMPR2 = bone morphogenetic protein receptor type II; PAH = pulmonary arterial hypertension.

Reprinted from Journal of the American College of Cardiology, 62(25 Suppl), Simonneau G, Gatzoulis MA, Adatia I, et al, Updated clinical classification of pulmonary hypertension, D34-41, 2014, with permission from Elsevier.

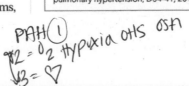

clinical presentation, and approach to treatment. All five groups can be termed PH, but group 1 is distinguished by disease localized to small pulmonary arterioles resulting in high pulmonary vascular resistance and is referred to as pulmonary arterial hypertension (PAH). Groups 2 through 5 refer to important secondary causes of PH and include left-sided heart disease, respiratory disorders (COPD, interstitial lung disease, and sleep-disordered breathing), and chronic venous thromboembolic disease. Groups 1 (PAH) and 4 (chronic thromboembolic pulmonary hypertension [CTEPH]) are discussed separately from the other causes of PH (see Pulmonary Arterial Hypertension and Chronic Thromboembolic Pulmonary Hypertension sections).

PAmean >25 (handwritten margin note)

> **KEY POINT**
> - Pulmonary hypertension is defined by a resting mean pulmonary artery pressure of 25 mm Hg or greater.

Pathophysiology

The pathophysiology of PH is determined by the specific cause, with the vast majority of cases of PH attributed to left-sided heart disease (group 2) and hypoxic respiratory disorders (group 3). With group 2 disease, left ventricular (LV) dysfunction and valvular disease lead to PH by volume and pressure overload. In group 3, vasoconstriction brought on by alveolar hypoxia is an important mechanism in patients with chronic respiratory disorders, eventually leading to pulmonary vascular remodeling. With all causes of PH, RV hypertrophy and dilatation develop over time in response to pulmonary artery pressure overload, at which point mismatch of myocardial oxygen supply and demand can result in ischemia, arrhythmias, and RV failure.

> **KEY POINT**
> - The vast majority of cases of pulmonary hypertension are attributed to left-sided heart disease and hypoxic respiratory disorders.

Diagnosis

PH is easily overlooked because early signs and symptoms, such as exertional dyspnea and fatigue, are nonspecific. In patients with chronic LV dysfunction or lung disease, symptoms due to PH may be minimal and difficult to distinguish from the underlying condition. As the disorder progresses, RV impairment may be heralded by exertional chest pain, syncope, and peripheral edema. Findings on physical examination depend on the severity of disease. The cardiovascular examination may show jugular venous distention, a prominent jugular venous *a* wave, parasternal heave, a widened split S$_2$ with a prominent pulmonic component, or right-sided regurgitant murmurs as the RV dilates. As RV dysfunction progresses, hepatomegaly, ascites, and peripheral edema develop.

Echocardiography is a useful initial tool in the evaluation of suspected PH, as it allows an estimation of pulmonary artery pressures and right heart function as well as an assessment of the left heart. Because echocardiography may underestimate true pulmonary artery pressures, the evaluation should not end with an unrevealing echocardiogram if the index of suspicion for PH is high. In such cases, right heart catheterization may be confirmatory.

Once PH is confirmed, further testing, guided by clinical history, helps determine identifiable causes. Left heart catheterization can assess coronary flow and LV function. Diagnostic tests for respiratory diseases might include pulmonary function tests, chest imaging, ventilation-perfusion (V/Q) scanning, and overnight pulse oximetry. Laboratory studies to explore group 1 disease may include HIV serology, liver chemistry studies, and autoantibody titers. Prior to treatment, exercise testing such as the 6-minute walk test should be performed to determine functional impairment and to serve as a baseline with which to compare therapeutic response.

> **KEY POINTS**
> - Echocardiography is a useful initial tool in the evaluation of suspected pulmonary hypertension, as it provides a noninvasive estimation of pulmonary artery pressures and right heart function as well as an assessment of the left heart.
> - Because echocardiography may underestimate true pulmonary artery pressures, right heart catheterization should be considered after a normal echocardiogram if the index of suspicion for pulmonary hypertension is high.

Treatment

Therapy for PH groups 2 through 5 is typically directed at the underlying condition. Strategies may include medical optimization of LV systolic and diastolic function, optimal inhaler therapy for COPD, supplemental oxygen for documented hypoxemia, and positive airway pressure therapy for sleep-disordered breathing. Anticoagulation and possible surgery is indicated for CTEPH (group 4). Advanced therapy (vasodilators) is generally reserved for PAH (group 1) and does not have a clear role in groups 2 through 5 PH. Advanced therapy may, in fact, be harmful in patients with PH due to LV dysfunction (group 2) or lung disease (group 3) because of the potential for pulmonary vasodilators to overload a compromised LV and to worsen V/Q mismatching, respectively.

> **KEY POINTS**
> - Therapy for pulmonary hypertension groups 2 through 5 (disease resulting from left-sided heart disease, respiratory disorders, or chronic venous thromboembolic disease) is directed at the underlying condition.
> - Advanced therapy for pulmonary hypertension with vasodilators should be reserved for patients with pulmonary arterial hypertension (group 1) as they have not been shown to be efficacious and may be harmful in this group.

HVC

Chronic Thromboembolic Pulmonary Hypertension

A small subset (<5%) of patients who experience an acute pulmonary embolism go on to develop CTEPH. For a discussion of pulmonary embolism, see MKSAP 17 Hematology and Oncology. In CTEPH, the organized thrombus incorporates into the pulmonary artery endothelium, thereby increasing pulmonary vascular resistance and pressures and eventually leading to right-sided heart failure. A hypercoagulable state is sometimes, but not always, proved by laboratory investigations in such patients, whose endogenous fibrinolytic system that would normally break down acute clot is overcome.

Diagnosis

CTEPH usually presents with progressive exertional dyspnea that correlates with the extent of hemodynamic derangement and RV involvement. Because this symptom is nonspecific and a substantial proportion of patients (>25%) do not report a history of pulmonary embolism, CTEPH remains an underappreciated cause of PH. There are two diagnostic criteria: (1) documentation of PH (pulmonary artery pressure ≥25 mm Hg) by right heart catheterization in the absence of left heart pressure overload and (2) compatible imaging evidence of chronic thromboembolism. CT pulmonary angiography (CT-PA), a commonly utilized test in the evaluation of exertional dyspnea, may demonstrate proximally located abnormalities such as vascular webs, intimal irregularities, and luminal narrowing but has limited sensitivity in more distal lesions. V/Q scanning is a more sensitive indicator of CTEPH and is generally the preferred first imaging modality. Once CTEPH is suggested by V/Q scanning or possibly CT-PA, conventional pulmonary angiography should be performed to best characterize the extent and distribution of organized thrombus and to determine suitability for surgical intervention.

KEY POINTS

- There are two diagnostic criteria for chronic thromboembolic pulmonary hypertension: (1) documentation of pulmonary hypertension (pulmonary artery pressure ≥25 mm Hg) by right heart catheterization in the absence of left heart pressure overload and (2) compatible imaging evidence of chronic thromboembolism.

HVC
- Ventilation-perfusion scanning is a sensitive indicator of chronic thromboembolic pulmonary hypertension and is generally the preferred first imaging modality.

Management

Anticoagulant therapy is indicated in all patients to help prevent further thromboembolism and, generally, duration of treatment is lifelong. In patients with coexisting clot in the lower extremities, inferior vena cava interruption can be considered to help prevent further thromboembolism; however, its role in long-term outcomes is not known. Surgery in the form of pulmonary thromboendarterectomy is the only definitive

therapy for CTEPH. Because even mild disease may irreversibly progress, surgical evaluation at an experienced center is warranted in all patients with CTEPH regardless of disease severity. Pulmonary thromboendarterectomy can result in normalization of pulmonary hemodynamics in about one third of patients who undergo surgery; however, only about half of patients will be surgical candidates and fewer than that will opt for surgery.

KEY POINT

- Pulmonary thromboendarterectomy is the only definitive therapy for chronic thromboembolic pulmonary hypertension.

Pulmonary Arterial Hypertension

Group 1 PAH is defined by a proliferative vasculopathy originating in the pulmonary artery endothelium, driven by imbalances in substances that affect vascular tone and endothelial/smooth muscle cellular growth. These pathways (nitric oxide, prostacyclin, and endothelin) are targets for therapy. PAH is classified as (1) idiopathic (previously referred to as primary pulmonary hypertension), (2) heritable, or (3) associated with other conditions.

Heritable forms, which are autosomal dominant with incomplete penetrance, demonstrate mutations in the transforming growth factor-β (TGF-β) signaling system, with most occurring in bone morphogenetic protein receptor type II (*BMPR2*). Because *BMPR2* is a gene that normally contributes to the apoptotic process, mutations might explain the propensity for cellular proliferation in PAH. Heritable disease comprises a minority of PAH cases but appears to confer a worse prognosis than sporadic disease.

PAH is most commonly encountered in association with other conditions, including connective tissue diseases, portal hypertension, HIV infection, illicit drug use, toxin exposure, and congenital heart disease.

Connective tissue diseases (classically systemic sclerosis) obliterate pulmonary arterioles and capillaries by direct proliferative effects on the vascular wall as well as by fibrosis of the surrounding lung interstitium. The association with PAH is stronger in limited cutaneous systemic sclerosis than in diffuse cutaneous disease. Rheumatoid arthritis can also affect the pulmonary vascular bed, as can systemic lupus erythematosus.

Patients with chronic liver disease and portosystemic shunting can develop a form of PAH referred to as portopulmonary hypertension (see MKSAP 17 Gastroenterology and Hepatology). The mechanism might relate to the diseased liver's inability to clear vasoactive substances that subsequently act on the pulmonary vasculature.

Patients with HIV infection have an approximately 10-fold higher risk of PAH compared with patients without HIV infection. The mechanism is not known but likely relates to both viral and host factors.

CONT.

Drugs implicated in PAH include fenfluramine, phentermine, and dexfenfluramine. The association with anorectic drugs may also suggest a link between PAH and obesity. Reports exist of PAH associated with tyrosine kinase inhibitors (dasatinib and imatinib) as well as with interferon alfa. Illicit drugs linked to PAH include cocaine and amphetamines (smoked or injected).

PAH in patients with congenital heart disease is attributable to pulmonary vessel blood volume overload due to intracardiac shunting typical of ventricular or atrial septal defects.

Younger patients with PAH are more commonly female; gender distribution is similar in older age groups. Variables associated with worse outcomes include increasing age, advanced functional limitation, and elevated levels of cardiac biomarkers such as N-terminal pro B-type natriuretic peptide. Echocardiographic findings of pericardial effusion, right atrial enlargement, and poor RV contractile reserve during stress testing also portend a worse prognosis. **H**

KEY POINT

- Pulmonary arterial hypertension is most commonly encountered in association with other conditions, including connective tissue diseases, portal hypertension, HIV infection, illicit drug use, toxin exposure, and congenital heart disease.

Diagnosis

The diagnostic evaluation of PAH usually includes testing similar to that described for other forms of PH, with the exception that right heart catheterization is required to confirm pulmonary hemodynamics as well as to determine whether there is a specific response to vasodilator infusion, which may help guide therapy. Although PAH is defined by typical pathology of the pulmonary arterial bed, lung biopsies in this population are risky and are generally not performed in practice. The role of genetic testing is not yet defined. **H**

KEY POINT

- In pulmonary arterial hypertension, right heart catheterization is required to confirm pulmonary hemodynamics as well as to determine whether there is a specific response to vasodilator infusion, which may help guide therapy.

Treatment

There are no curative treatments for PAH, but the use of targeted vascular therapies has improved survival rates. The goals of therapy are to reduce vascular pressures, control symptoms, and improve or maintain quality of life. Supportive measures should be considered in all patients with PAH. Such interventions might include diuretic therapy to combat volume overload and supplemental oxygen for hypoxemia at rest or with exercise. Because PAH predisposes to in-situ pulmonary vascular thrombosis and embolism,

anticoagulation is recommended. Digoxin appears to improve RV function in some patients with PAH and, owing to its vagal properties, may be a useful adjunct in managing supraventricular dysrhythmias that are common in this population. Exercise training has been shown to improve functional limitations.

Vascular-targeted treatments are directed at reducing vasoconstriction and/or interrupting the pathways mediating cellular proliferation. Calcium channel blockers, used for decades prior to the availability of current advanced therapy agents, are still prescribed but only for patients demonstrating a vasodilator response on right heart catheterization. Close follow-up is required because the effect may not be durable. Use of advanced agents (**Table 36**) may be guided by disease severity. Oral agents (phosphodiesterase-5 inhibitors, such as sildenafil or tadalafil, or endothelin-1 receptor antagonists, such as bosentan or ambrisentan) are reasonable initial therapies for mild to moderate disease. Iloprost, an inhaled prostanoid, can be used but requires frequent administration. A parenteral prostacyclin analogue such as epoprostenol, administered by a continuous central venous infusion, is first-line therapy for severe disease and for those in whom disease progresses despite oral therapy. Combining drugs with different mechanisms may enhance efficacy. Given the complexity of management and the steady increase in the number of drugs available to treat PAH, some of which can cost more than $100,000 per year, careful initiation and follow-up by an experienced specialist is warranted. Lung or heart-lung transplantation should be considered for patients in whom drug treatment is unsuccessful. **H**

TABLE 36. Pharmacologic Therapy for Pulmonary Arterial Hypertension

Class	Comments
Calcium channel blockers	Only for patients with acute vasodilator response at catheterization; acute response does not assure chronic response
Prostanoids (epoprostenol, treprostinil, iloprost)	Supplements endogenous levels of prostacyclin (PGI$_2$), a vasodilator with anti-smooth muscle proliferative properties
Endothelin-1 receptor antagonists (bosentan, ambrisentan)	Blocks action of endogenous vasoconstrictor and smooth muscle mitogen endothelin; class-wide risk of liver injury and teratogenicity; liver chemistry testing and pregnancy testing for reproductive-aged women are required[a]
Phosphodiesterase-5 inhibitors (sildenafil, tadalafil)	Prolongs effect of intrinsic vasodilator cyclic GMP by inhibiting hydrolysis by phosphodiesterase-5

GMP = guanosine monophosphate.

[a]Although not required for ambrisentan, some experts suggest that it is prudent to perform liver chemistry tests at the outset of treatment for pulmonary arterial hypertension and at periodic intervals thereafter at the discretion of the managing physician.

Lung Tumors

Pulmonary Nodule Evaluation

A solitary pulmonary nodule (SPN) is defined as a lesion less than 3 cm in size surrounded by normal lung parenchyma. The causes of SPNs include malignancy (primary lung and metastatic cancer) as well as benign causes such as granulomata, hamartomas, or vascular malformations.

A SPN 8 mm or smaller is considered a subcentimeter pulmonary nodule and is managed differently than a larger nodule. The risk of malignancy in an individual patient's subcentimeter pulmonary nodule is divided into low and high risk based on the patient's age (older than 50 years of age confers higher risk), history of past or present smoking, and other risk factors for lung cancer, such as environmental or occupational exposures (for example, asbestos and radon), a diagnosis of COPD, a history of radiation therapy, and possibly a family history of lung cancer. The clinician should establish if prior imaging studies are available for comparison. If long-term stability cannot be established from prior imaging studies, serial interval imaging is recommended. The Fleischner criteria (**Table 37**) are commonly used to determine the timing and duration of imaging follow-up for subcentimeter nodules.

For nodules larger than 8 mm but less than 30 mm, the first step in management is also to assess the pretest probability of malignancy. Clinical prediction models, such as the Veterans Affairs Cooperative or the Mayo Clinic models, are available to categorize the risk as low (<5%), moderate (5% to 65%), and high (>65%). These models typically incorporate several risk factors for malignancy: older age, smoking history, nodule size, history of prior malignancy, upper lobe location, and the presence of spiculation; clinicians frequently add findings of nodule attenuation on CT to help determine the risk for malignancy. Low-attenuation nodules (subsolid) are less dense on imaging, allowing normal parenchymal structures to be visualized through them. Subsolid nodules are less common but are actually more likely to be malignant.

As with subcentimeter nodules, the availability of prior imaging of the chest to assess the stability or growth of these lesions is helpful. An enlarging pulmonary nodule warrants more aggressive evaluation with tissue diagnosis or excision depending on the nodule's pretest probability of malignancy. If prior imaging is not available or the nodule is stable in size, further management is based on the pretest probability (**Table 38**). Additionally, if imaging reveals multiple pulmonary nodules, guidelines recommend evaluating the risk of malignancy for each individual nodule to determine the best management strategy. If solid pulmonary nodules remain stable in size for 24 months, most clinicians no longer recommend surveillance imaging. However, given the higher probability of malignancy with ground-glass and partly solid nodules, these patients may warrant longer, if not lifelong, surveillance.

A pulmonary mass, defined as greater than 3 cm in diameter, is highly suspicious for malignancy in a patient with risk factors. Biopsy for tissue diagnosis (in the absence of suspected metastases) or surgical resection (if no evidence of metastatic disease is found) is typically the first step in the evaluation.

TABLE 37. Fleischner Criteria for Surveillance Imaging of Subcentimeter Solitary Solid Pulmonary Nodules		
Nodule Size (mm)[a]	**Low Pretest Probability[b]**	**High Pretest Probability[c]**
≤4	No follow-up needed[d]	Follow-up CT at 12 months; if unchanged, no further follow-up[e]
>4 to 6	Follow-up CT at 12 months; if unchanged, no further follow-up[e]	Initial follow-up CT at 6 to 12 months then at 18 to 24 months if no change[e]
>6 to 8	Initial follow-up CT at 6 to 12 months then at 18 to 24 months if no change	Initial follow-up CT at 3 to 6 months then at 9 to 12 months and 24 months if no change
>8	Follow-up CT at around 3, 9, and 24 months; dynamic contrast-enhanced CT, PET, and/or biopsy	Same as for low-risk patient

[a]Average of length and width.

[b]Minimal or absent history of smoking and of other known risk factors.

[c]History of smoking or of other known risk factors.

[d]The risk of malignancy in this category (<1%) is substantially less than that in a baseline CT scan of an asymptomatic smoker.

[e]Nonsolid (ground glass) or partly solid nodules may require longer follow-up to exclude indolent adenocarcinoma.

Reprinted from MacMahon H, Austin JH, Gamsu G, et al; Fleischner Society. Guidelines for management of small pulmonary nodules detected on CT scans: a statement from the Fleischner Society. Radiology. 2005 Nov;237(2):395-400. [PMID: 16244247], with permission from the Radiological Society of North America.

smoking squam central

TABLE 38. Management Recommendations for Solid Solitary Pulmonary Nodules Ranging from Greater than 8 mm to Less than 30 mm

Pretest Probability of Malignancy	Recommendation
Low (<5%)	Surveillance CT at 3 to 6, 9 to 12, and 18 to 24 months (re-evaluate for PET imaging, tissue diagnosis, or excision if evidence of growth)
Intermediate (5% to 65%)	PET/CT imaging:
	Tissue diagnosis or excision if the nodule demonstrates high metabolic activity, as defined by the concentration of uptake of the tracer (fluorodeoxyglucose)
	At least short-term surveillance if negative, but consider more aggressive evaluation depending on individual patient factors
High (>65%)	Surgical excision (consider PET/CT imaging for staging first)

Information from Alberts WM; American College of Chest Physicians. Diagnosis and management of lung cancer executive summary: ACCP evidence-based clinical practice guidelines (2nd Edition). Chest. 2007 Sep;132(3 Suppl):1S-19S. [PMID: 17873156]

KEY POINTS

- The first step in the management of a solitary pulmonary nodule is to assess the pretest probability of malignancy.

HVC
- If prior imaging of the chest is available, it should be reviewed as a low-risk and inexpensive way to assess the stability or growth of the solitary pulmonary nodule.

Lung Cancer

Lung cancer is the second most common cancer diagnosed in the United States but is the leading cause of cancer deaths. Approximately 80% to 90% of lung cancers can be attributed to cigarette smoking or exposure to second-hand smoke. Therefore, smoking prevention and cessation may be the most important steps in preventing lung cancer. Additional risk factors for lung cancer include exposure to asbestos, ionizing radiation, radon, and arsenic. The relative risk for developing lung cancer significantly increases when a smoker is exposed to another carcinogen or risk factor, such as asbestos. The incidence of lung cancer is also increased in patients with a history of HIV infection, increasing age, and a history of comorbid lung conditions, including emphysema and idiopathic pulmonary fibrosis. Although still poorly understood, a familial predisposition of primary lung cancer has been observed as well.

KEY POINTS

- Lung cancer is the second most common cancer diagnosed in the United States but is the leading cause of cancer deaths.

HVC
- Smoking prevention and cessation may be the most important steps in preventing lung cancer.

Lung Cancer Types

Lung cancers are classified by histologic type (**Table 39**). Most (80%) lung cancers are non–small cell lung cancers (NSCLC), with the most common type being adenocarcinoma of the lung. Adenocarcinoma typically presents in the periphery of the lung. Most squamous cell carcinomas, which represent the second most common form of NSCLC, are located in the central portions of the lung and are more common in patients with a smoking history. Current treatment options for both of these NSCLCs include surgical resection, radiation therapy, chemotherapy, and targeted therapies (see MKSAP 17 Hematology and Oncology). Small cell lung cancer (SCLC) tends to be more aggressive than NSCLC and is usually already disseminated at presentation but is usually more sensitive to chemotherapy and radiation therapy initially. It typically presents as a large hilar mass with bulky mediastinal lymphadenopathy.

Diagnosis and Staging

The evaluation of a patient with suspected lung cancer aims to confirm whether the patient indeed has lung cancer, to determine the pathology (NSCLC versus SCLC), and to assess the stage at presentation. Most patients typically undergo chest CT as the first imaging modality, either after an abnormal chest radiograph or as evaluation of a symptom. Initial chest CT imaging is used to determine the size and location of the primary tumor, the presence and location of regional lymph node involvement, and the presence of metastases, which include not only extrathoracic organs but also nodules within a contralateral lobe of the lung and pleural disease. The findings on the chest CT help determine whether a PET/CT is necessary. A PET/CT can help in staging and therefore also help guide where to biopsy. For example, if a patient has a solitary pulmonary nodule, a PET/CT may help determine if any lymph node involvement is present that was not visible on the chest CT.

TABLE 39. Histologic Classification of the Most Common Types of Lung Cancer

Histologic Type	Percentage of All Lung Cancers
Non-Small Cell Lung Cancer	
Adenocarcinoma	38%
Squamous cell carcinoma	20%
Large cell carcinoma	3%
Adenosquamous carcinoma	0.6% to 2.3%
Sarcomatoid carcinoma	0.3%
Neuroendocrine Tumors	
Small cell lung cancer	14%
Large cell lung cancer	3%
Typical carcinoid tumor	1% to 2%
Atypical carcinoid tumor	0.1% to 0.2%

The next step is to obtain tissue diagnosis. The choice of initial diagnostic testing should be aimed first at identifying potential lymph node involvement or metastatic disease. Tissue diagnosis should then be targeted at the lesion that would result in the highest potential staging. For example, a patient presenting with a concerning pulmonary mass and a pleural effusion would require diagnostic thoracentesis to provide accurate staging. The thoracentesis, however, may also provide a diagnosis if cytology is positive. If the patient underwent tissue diagnosis of the mass, a thoracentesis would still be required to provide staging information. The prognosis and treatment change based on the pathology and stage of the lung cancer. Consideration of both of these at the time of diagnosis can ultimately result in fewer tests for the patient. Conversely, in a patient who presents with an isolated pulmonary nodule or mass suspicious for NSCLC, biopsy or resection of this primary lesion is indicated. If the pretest probability of NSCLC is high, surgical resection may be the best strategy because this may be curative. Although SCLC can present as a SPN, this is incredibly rare. However, tissue biopsy to confirm the diagnosis of a NSCLC should be obtained prior to surgical resection if SCLC is a significant possibility (for example, in a patient with a hilar mass). If the pretest probability for NSCLC is low, CT-guided transthoracic needle aspiration or bronchoscopy with transbronchial biopsy could be considered depending on the location of the nodule.

Lung Cancer Screening

The National Lung Cancer Screening Trial (NLST) demonstrated a 20% reduction in lung cancer deaths at 6.5 years of follow-up in a specific group of high-risk patients who completed 3 years of annual chest imaging with low-dose CT compared with chest radiograph. Based on these data, the United States Preventive Services Task Force (USPSTF) recommends screening patients between the ages of 55 and 79 years who have a 30-pack-year or more history of smoking and who are currently smoking or quit within the last 15 years. Annual low-dose CT imaging should continue until comorbidity limits survival or the ability to tolerate surgical resection, or the patient reaches the age of 80 years. The USPSTF guidelines also recommend that annual screening be discontinued in patients who have stopped smoking for 15 years. If nodules are identified, clinicians should follow established guidelines on how to manage solitary pulmonary nodules for patients at high risk for lung cancer.

The risks of screening, especially the risk of potentially false-positive findings on imaging, outweigh the benefit in patients at low risk for lung cancer. Therefore, lung cancer screening is not currently recommended for patients who do not meet the above criteria.

The Centers for Medicare and Medicaid Services (CMS) recently began reimbursing low-dose CT for lung cancer screening in patients aged 55 to 77 years who meet the above criteria.

Preinvasive Lung Lesions

Both categories of NSCLC and SCLC include preinvasive lesions that warrant, at a minimum, ongoing surveillance. A 2011 change in the pathologic classification of lung cancer eliminated the previous term of bronchoalveolar cell carcinoma, previously considered a type of NSCLC. This entity is now divided into three categories or subtypes of adenocarcinoma: atypical adenomatous hyperplasia, adenocarcinoma in situ (AIS), and minimally invasive adenocarcinoma. AIS most commonly presents as an incidental finding of ground-glass opacification on chest CT (**Figure 15**). Ground-glass opacifications appear as gray subsolid lesions within the parenchyma of the lung that do not obscure the underlying blood vessels or airways. A less common variant is mucinous AIS, which appears as a solid nodule on imaging. Minimally invasive adenocarcinoma presents similarly to AIS but has a small area of invasion on pathology (≤5 mm). For all three subtypes, the 5-year survival rate is 100% after surgical resection. Current Fleischner criteria recommend that solitary ground-glass nodules larger than 5 mm should be monitored with repeat chest imaging. Initial imaging is recommended at 3 months and then annually for at least 3 years. The guidelines are the same for multiple ground-glass nodules when at least one is larger than 5 mm, whereas multiple ground-glass nodules of 5 mm or smaller should be monitored with repeat imaging at 2 and 4 years. Surgical resection should be considered if a nodule increases in size or the density increases.

Diffuse idiopathic pulmonary neuroendocrine cell hyperplasia is a rare potential precursor of neuroendocrine tumors of the lung and is defined as the presence of multiple carcinoid tumorlets (<0.5 cm) or widespread neuroendocrine cell hyperplasia.

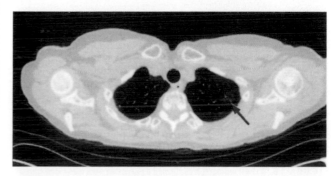

FIGURE 15. A large ground-glass opacification can be seen in the left lung apex on chest CT (*arrow*). It was later confirmed to be an adenocarcinoma in situ on surgical pathology.

Other Pulmonary Neoplasms

Bronchial Carcinoid Tumors

Although bronchial carcinoid tumors represent only a small percentage of all lung cancers, they are the most common lung cancer to present in children and adolescents. Most lesions involve the proximal airways, so patients may present with symptoms related to endobronchial narrowing or obstruction, including postobstructive pneumonia (**Figure 16**). Patients with peripheral lesions may be asymptomatic at the time of diagnosis. Only approximately 1% to 5% of patients present with symptoms of carcinoid syndrome, which is characterized by the release of vasoactive substances, including serotonin, and causes flushing, bronchospasm, and diarrhea. Carcinoid syndrome is associated with larger tumor size and the presence of liver metastases.

A typical carcinoid is considered a low-grade tumor with an excellent 5-year survival rate of 92% to 100%. Atypical carcinoid tumors are characterized by a higher number of observed mitoses or the presence of necrosis on pathology and are considered intermediate-grade malignancies. They have a higher tendency to metastasize and are associated with a lower 5-year survival rate of 61% to 88%. Although invasion of lymph nodes by typical carcinoid tumors may not decrease survival, it is associated with a worse prognosis in patients with atypical carcinoid tumors. Once a diagnosis is made, surgical resection is recommended for both types of bronchial carcinoid tumors even when lymph node involvement is documented. It may be beneficial to surgically resect affected lymph nodes and other areas of metastases as well. Carcinoids tend to be resistant to chemotherapy and radiation therapy. The routine use of adjuvant therapy is controversial but should be considered if residual disease is documented after attempted surgical resection or if patients present with either lesions not amendable to resection or progressive disease. Somatostatin analogs are reserved for patients who present with carcinoid syndrome and some patients with metastatic disease. Patients with a history of bronchial carcinoids should be monitored for recurrence.

KEY POINTS

- Most bronchial carcinoid tumors involve the proximal airways, so patients may present with symptoms related to endobronchial narrowing or obstruction, including postobstructive pneumonia.
- A typical carcinoid is considered a low-grade tumor with an excellent 5-year survival rate of 92% to 100%.

Mesothelioma

Malignant pleural mesothelioma is a very aggressive tumor that arises from the mesothelial cells of the pleura. Exposure to airborne asbestos fibers is the most significant risk factor for the development of mesothelioma. Patients most commonly present with symptoms of a slowly enlarging pleural effusion. Chest imaging typically shows a unilateral pleural effusion, but patients can also present with pleural thickening, nodules, or masses. This is usually accompanied by the presence of pleural plaques or calcifications (**Figure 17**). Cytologic diagnosis can often be established by thoracentesis or closed pleural biopsy. Video thoracoscopy may be required if initial attempts with less invasive sampling are nondiagnostic or if larger tissue samples are required for subtype classification. Patients with resectable disease still require chemotherapy and radiation therapy. If surgery is not possible, systemic chemotherapy is combined with symptom-driven treatments.

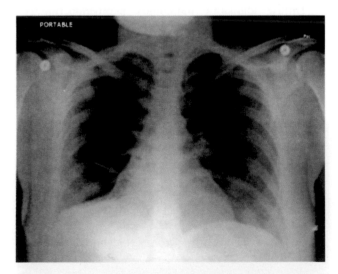

FIGURE 16. A chest radiograph confirmed a persistent right lower lobe consolidation (*arrow*) in a 20-year-old woman who presented with coughing and wheezing that persisted despite several courses of antibiotics. Bronchoscopy confirmed a typical bronchial carcinoid tumor obstructing the bronchus intermedius.

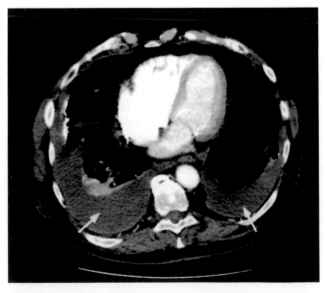

FIGURE 17. Chest CT shows bilateral pleural effusions (*yellow arrows*) with right-sided pleural plaques (*red arrow*).

For a discussion of other types of asbestos-related lung disease, see Occupational Lung Disease.

Pulmonary Metastases

Pulmonary metastases most commonly present as multiple, peripheral, or subpleural pulmonary nodules but can also present as solitary pulmonary nodules (**Figure 18**). Metastases are often identified on imaging obtained for staging of the primary cancer. Although many (80% in some reports) of the nodules identified during staging end up being benign, early detection and treatment of pulmonary metastases has improved survival in some patients, especially those with primary colon cancer or sarcomas. The most common primary malignancies to metastasize to the lung are carcinomas (colon, kidney, breast, testicle, and thyroid), sarcomas (bone), and melanoma. Endobronchial metastases are rare and are most commonly associated with renal cell carcinoma. Lymphangitic spread of tumor is most commonly associated with adenocarcinoma (lung, breast, and gastrointestinal tract), melanoma, lymphoma, and leukemia and should be considered if a peripheral interstitial abnormality is identified on high-resolution CT in a patient with one of these malignancies.

Mediastinal Masses

The mediastinum can be divided into three separate compartments (**Figure 19**), which can help narrow the differential diagnosis of a mediastinal mass. Each compartment normally contains separate and distinct anatomic structures that can lead to development of a mass. Patients may be asymptomatic and are diagnosed after obtaining a chest radiograph for another reason, whereas others present with symptoms related to compression of adjacent structures. For example, they may present with dyspnea if the airway is compressed from a nearby mass or with upper extremity edema if vascular structures are compressed.

Anterior Mediastinal Masses

In adults, anterior mediastinal thymomas are the most common mediastinal lesions, accounting for up to 20% of mediastinal masses. Thymomas are more common in the superior portion of the anterior compartment. Patients usually present as middle-age adults and may develop paraneoplastic syndromes. For example, myasthenia gravis can develop in 35% to 40% of patients with a thymoma. Other less common paraneoplastic syndromes include pure red blood cell aplasia, nonthymic cancers, and acquired hypogammaglobulinemia. The second most common cause is lymphoma (**Figure 20**); patients are typically younger at the time of presentation. Hodgkin lymphoma is the most common lymphoma to involve the mediastinum, followed by lymphoblastic lymphoma and primary mediastinal diffuse large B-cell lymphoma. Teratomas are the most common type of mediastinal germ cell tumors, and they typically present in the anterior mediastinum. They can contain fat, fluid, and even bone.

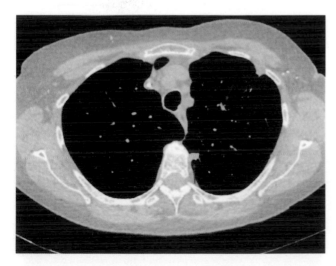

FIGURE 18. CT of the chest demonstrates two subcentimeter nodules (*arrows*) in the left upper lobe in a patient with known breast cancer.

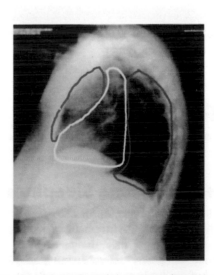

[handwritten: teratoma thymoma lymphoma = ant.]

FIGURE 19. A lateral chest radiograph demonstrates the anterior (*red*), middle (*yellow*), and posterior (*blue*) mediastinal compartments.

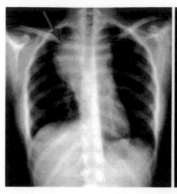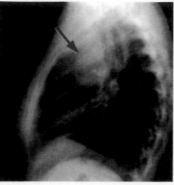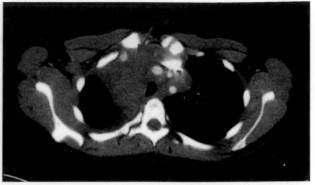

FIGURE 20. A 20-year-old woman presented with exertional dyspnea and was found to have an anterior mediastinal mass (*arrows*) on chest imaging. She was subsequently diagnosed with Hodgkin lymphoma.

Middle Mediastinal Masses

Lymphadenopathy is the most common cause of middle mediastinal masses. Several cystic structures can also develop in this compartment, including bronchogenic, pericardial, and esophageal duplication cysts. Although cysts can be followed, they may be resected if patients are symptomatic or the diagnosis is uncertain.

KEY POINT

- Lymphadenopathy is the most common cause of a middle mediastinal mass.

Posterior Mediastinal Masses

In children, posterior neurogenic tumors are the most common diagnosis of the mediastinum. These typically arise from the sympathetic ganglia (for example, neuroblastomas), whereas in adults, the neurogenic tumors tend to arise from the nerve sheaths (for example, schwannomas). Paraspinal extramedullary hematopoiesis may also involve this mediastinal compartment.

KEY POINT

- The most common cause of a posterior mediastinal mass is a neurogenic tumor.

Sleep Medicine

For a discussion of insomnia, see MKSAP 17 General Internal Medicine.

Excessive Daytime Sleepiness

Excessive daytime sleepiness (EDS), also referred to as hypersomnia, refers to the struggle to remain awake and alert during daytime hours. Patients may use terms like "tiredness," "fatigue," and "sleepiness" interchangeably to describe their symptoms, but the distinctions are important. Fatigue is a lack of energy that prevents mental or physical activity at the intensity and/or pace desired and is rarely the result of a primary sleep disorder.

Causes of excessive sleepiness can be categorized as extrinsic (circumstantial) or intrinsic (disease-related) processes (**Table 40**).

The most common cause of EDS is the overall lack of time devoted to the sleep period, referred to clinically as insufficient sleep syndrome.

The first step in the evaluation of EDS should include a thorough history of the sleep-wake schedule, with the goal of ensuring nightly opportunities for adequate sleep time (7.5 to 8.0 hours for most people). Sleep diaries maintained over a 1- or 2-week period are simple tools to track hours spent awake and asleep. For a more objective assessment, a wrist actigraph measures movement and ambient light and allows an estimation of the sleep period over a 1- or 2-week period. Subjective questionnaires such as the Epworth Sleepiness Scale may be helpful in quantifying EDS.

Laboratory-based polysomnography is generally indicated if there is suspicion of primary sleep disorders such

TABLE 40. Extrinsic and Intrinsic Causes of Excessive Daytime Sleepiness

Extrinsic Causes
Insufficient sleep duration (or inadequate opportunity for sleep)
Circadian rhythm disturbance (shift work sleep disorder, jet lag)
Drug-, substance-, or medical condition-related hypersomnia
Environmental sleep disorder (ambient noise, pets)

Intrinsic Causes
Sleep-disordered breathing syndromes, such as obstructive sleep apnea and central sleep apnea
Narcolepsy
Idiopathic hypersomnia
Restless legs syndrome and periodic limb movement disorder
Circadian rhythm sleep disorders

as sleep apnea, limb movement disorder, or a hypersomnia syndrome such as narcolepsy. Portable sleep monitoring devices can be used to diagnose obstructive sleep apnea (OSA). Occasionally, multiple sleep latency testing (MSLT) is used to provide an objective measure of sleepiness. MSLT requires a series of brief nap opportunities over the course of a full day in a sleep laboratory to determine the average time to fall asleep and is time and labor intensive; however, it is required to establish the diagnoses of narcolepsy and idiopathic hypersomnia. A mean sleep latency of less than 5 minutes is a clear indicator of pathologic sleepiness, whereas more than 15 minutes is considered normal.

Patients with EDS should be counseled to maintain a consistent sleep-wake schedule that allows for 8 hours of sleep and should be instructed about the dangers of driving or operating machinery while drowsy. Specific treatment depends on the underlying condition (for example, stimulant medications for narcolepsy). Strategic naps and/or caffeinated beverages may be helpful for short-term management of sleepiness.

> **KEY POINTS**
>
> - The most common cause of excessive daytime sleepiness is the overall lack of time devoted to the sleep period.
> - Patients with excessive daytime sleepiness should be counseled to maintain a consistent sleep-wake schedule that allows for 8 hours of sleep.

Common Conditions that Disrupt Circadian Rhythm

Jet Lag

Jet lag is a syndrome resulting from desynchronization of the internal circadian clock with the local destination time following air travel across multiple (usually more than five) time zones. Disruption of body rhythms occurs proportionally to the distance traveled. Symptoms may include insomnia, daytime sleepiness, and neuropsychiatric impairment. Because resynchronization takes on average 1.0 to 1.5 days for every hour change in time zone, lingering symptoms can be disruptive to business travel and family vacations. Management includes avoiding sleep deprivation prior to travel. For highly motivated travelers, a gradual shift in the sleep period over several days prior to travel to synchronize with the destination can ease the transition. Although hypnotic medications in flight may promote sleep, they pose a risk of parasomnias such as sleepwalking. Once at the destination, exposure to sunlight during the waking hours is the most powerful environmental cue to help reset the internal clock. Over-the-counter melatonin supplements, the timing of which depends upon the direction travelled, can also help resynchronization.

Shift Work Sleep Disorder

As many as one third of shift workers suffer from shift work sleep disorder (SWSD), characterized by insomnia during the daytime sleep period and resultant sleepiness during the nighttime work period. The first step in management is to address sleep-related behaviors and the sleep environment, referred to as sleep hygiene. Those who routinely work night shifts and suffer from SWSD should control exposure to bright light, promoting it in the evening before the night shift and avoiding it in the morning in anticipation of the daytime sleep period. Caffeinated beverages during work hours may enhance alertness. Planned napping during work breaks may also be useful. Modafinil, a novel stimulant approved for use in SWSD, should be considered only after conservative measures such as sleep hygiene counseling are tried. The long-term efficacy of hypnotic medications in those with chronic insomnia has not been proved.

Obstructive Sleep Apnea

OSA is a common condition defined by narrowing or occlusion of the upper airway during sleep, resulting in repetitive interruption of the sleep cycle. These disordered breathing events are classified as apneas (characterized by complete cessation of airflow) or hypopneas (reductions in airflow). They are typically accompanied by oxyhemoglobin desaturations and are terminated by an awakening from sleep. They may be quantified during diagnostic sleep testing by the apnea-hypopnea index (AHI). The AHI refers to the number of disordered breathing events per hour of sleep. An AHI of 5 to 15 is indicative of mild OSA, and an AHI of more than 30 reflects severe OSA.

> **KEY POINT**
>
> - Obstructive sleep apnea is a common condition defined by narrowing or occlusion of the upper airway during sleep, resulting in repetitive interruption of the sleep cycle.

Pathophysiology

An unstable upper airway is the hallmark of OSA. Neuromuscular mechanisms that maintain airway patency during sleep are overcome by forces that promote collapse (see Risk Factors). The same mechanisms are responsible for snoring. The upper airway is more prone to collapse due to gravitational forces during sleep in the supine position, as well as during rapid eye movement (REM), a stage of sleep characterized by atonia of most muscles of the body other than extraocular muscles and the respiratory diaphragm. During upper airway collapse, efforts to breathe against the occlusion continue, resulting in wide swings in intrathoracic pressure. Termination of disordered breathing events typically occurs with a brief awakening from sleep (called a microarousal), in which upper airway patency is restored, ventilation resumes, and reoxygenation occurs; this is followed by resumption of sleep.

Disruption of sleep architecture by repetitive micro-arousals is a primary contributor to the neurocognitive sequelae of OSA. Oxyhemoglobin desaturations can be pronounced, particularly in those who have coexistent cardiopulmonary disease. Disordered breathing events are associated with autonomic instability, increased vascular tone, and alterations in heart rate. Heart failure, cardiac arrhythmias, and diabetes mellitus are also associated with OSA, but because these conditions have similar underlying risk factors (such as obesity, aging, and male gender), cause and effect are difficult to establish.

Risk Factors

Obesity is the most important risk factor for OSA. Regional distribution of adipose tissue concentrated in the trunk and neck imparts the highest risk. Tonsillar hypertrophy, macroglossia, retrognathia/micrognathia, and upper airway mass lesions can cause upper airway narrowing. Cigarette smoking is a risk factor for OSA. OSA can be worsened by alcohol and sedative drugs. Endocrinopathies such as polycystic ovary syndrome and advanced hypothyroidism can increase the risk of OSA.

KEY POINT

- Obesity is the most important risk factor for obstructive sleep apnea.

Clinical Features and Diagnosis

Loud snoring, gasping, and breathing pauses observed by a bed partner are commonly the first indicators that bring patients with OSA to medical attention. Subjective symptoms include frequent awakenings, dry mouth, snoring, and non-restorative sleep. Nocturia is common in men with OSA.

EDS is the classic result of OSA. EDS is not a universal symptom, but the absence of self-reporting may not reflect the degree of impairment, which may be detectable on objective testing of alertness (such as MSLT). Other neuropsychiatric symptoms are common and include mood alterations, difficulty concentrating, and problems completing tasks at school or the workplace.

Occasionally, OSA first presents immediately following a surgical procedure involving general anesthesia and/or narcotic analgesia, where repeated apneas, acute respiratory failure, and even death unexpectedly occur. Screening questionnaires (STOP-Bang) are available to help identify OSA during pre-anesthesia evaluation and may reduce the increased rate of postoperative complications in these patients.

Objective testing is required for the diagnosis of OSA. The traditional gold standard of in-laboratory, technician-attended polysomnography (PSG) is being replaced in some regions of the country by portable technology designed for use by the unaccompanied patient, referred to as out-of-center sleep testing (OCST). This portable testing is typically limited to measurement of oronasal airflow, chest wall excursion, body position, and pulse oximetry, whereas in-laboratory PSG additionally measures brain waves (electroencephalography), muscle activity (electromyography), and heart rhythm (electrocardiography), all attended by a technician in case of technical issues. OCST performs comparably to PSG in patients without comorbid cardiopulmonary disease who have a high pretest probability of moderate to severe OSA.

Determining whether objective testing is indicated can be challenging. In general, any patient with unexplained EDS should undergo OSA testing. For less obvious cases, screening tools are available to aid in decision-making. Examples include the Sleep Apnea Clinical Score (SACS) and the Berlin questionnaire.

Overnight pulse oximetry alone has a high rate of false-positive and false-negative results and has not been validated as a screening tool for OSA. A normal-appearing overnight pulse oximetry may allow for avoidance of further testing in patients with a low pretest probability, those with few symptoms, or in those whose preference is to avoid treatment.

KEY POINTS

- Out-of-center sleep testing performs comparably to polysomnography in patients without comorbid cardiopulmonary disease who have a high pretest probability of moderate to severe obstructive sleep apnea.

- Overnight pulse oximetry alone has a high rate of false-positive and false-negative results and has not been validated as a screening tool for obstructive sleep apnea; its use should be limited to patients with low pretest probability, few symptoms, or in patients who prefer to avoid treatment. **HVC**

Treatment

The primary goal of OSA management is to resolve attributable symptoms, particularly EDS or daytime neurocognitive impairment. Positive airway pressure (PAP) therapy is generally the preferred treatment. Those who perform mission-critical work (truck drivers, pilots) warrant particular attention even when symptoms are limited. The role of treatment in asymptomatic, otherwise healthy individuals is debatable. Furthermore, treatment of OSA as a means to adjunctively manage comorbid cardiovascular disease such as hypertension, cardiac arrhythmias, and heart failure is controversial.

Behavioral Modifications

All patients with OSA should be counseled on behavior modifications, particularly weight loss in those who are overweight or obese. A weight loss program may be the primary therapy for minimally symptomatic patients with mild OSA. Studies of bariatric surgery have shown improvements in OSA, but surgery rarely leads to complete resolution of OSA. Additional lifestyle or conservative measures include reducing alcohol intake before bedtime and avoiding a supine posture if OSA is dependent on position.

- All patients with obstructive sleep apnea should be counseled on behavior modifications, particularly weight loss in those who are overweight or obese.

Positive Airway Pressure

PAP has proven efficacy in eliminating apneas and hypopneas, reducing symptoms, and enhancing quality of life. The mechanism by which PAP acts is primarily related to pressurization of the upper airway sufficient to overcome the collapsing forces of surrounding soft tissue, thereby eliminating upper airway collapse and airflow limitation.

There are a variety of modes by which PAP therapy is delivered (**Table 41**). Traditionally, PAP devices have been manually titrated by a trained technologist in the polysomnography laboratory to a fixed and constant pressure, referred to as continuous positive airway pressure (CPAP). However, the increasing use of OCST is coupled with autotitrating PAP (APAP), which uses a computer algorithm to detect and overcome upper airway resistance in real time, thereby eliminating the need for laboratory-based manual titration. Studies have shown APAP to be as effective as laboratory-derived CPAP at reducing the AHI and may have some advantages over CPAP in terms of patient comfort.

A variety of patient-device interfaces are available, including nasal pillows that sit at the nasal openings, nasal masks that cover the nose, and oronasal (full face) masks that cover the nose and mouth.

The effectiveness of PAP therapy is dependent on patient compliance, which can be compromised by lack of motivation or side effects such as rhinitis and nasal congestion. Data download from the machine provide objective measures of compliance (a minimum level of which is required for Medicare coverage) as well as information related to air leak that might indicate poor mask fit. Dedicated patient education programs can promote adherence. Proper mask fitting and a desensitization program (in which the patient gradually increases time wearing the mask while awake) can help manage claustrophobia. Nasal side effects can be alleviated with in-line heated humidification or anticholinergic or glucocorticoid nasal sprays.

- Positive airway pressure is the preferred therapy for nearly all patients with symptomatic obstructive sleep apnea.

Oral Appliances

Oral appliances are an alternative to PAP therapy for mild to moderate OSA. They act by one of two mechanisms to increase upper airway caliber: (1) advancement of the mandible by traction or (2) preventing posterior displacement of the tongue by suction. Oral appliances generally do not reduce the AHI as reliably as PAP; however, if patients treated with appliances are adherent to therapy over a greater total sleep time compared with PAP, as some data suggest, the "treatment dose" may be comparable between the two.

Upper Airway Surgery

Except for obstructing mass lesions of the upper airway, surgery is not recommended as initial therapy for OSA and should generally be preceded by a trial (as long as 3 months) of PAP.

Uvulopalatopharyngoplasty (UPPP), a soft-palatal procedure, results in very modest reductions in the AHI. Maxillomandibular advancement, which may be performed in conjunction with a soft-palatal procedure, may be more effective at reducing the AHI. Tonsillectomy is not generally curative in adults.

TABLE 41. Positive Airway Pressure Modes

Mode	Description	Indication
CPAP (continuous positive airway pressure)	Fixed pressure derived from an in-lab titration attended by a technician	OSA Occasionally CSA
APAP (auto-titrating positive airway pressure)	Range of pressure delivered to maintain upper airway patency, determined by a proprietary computer algorithm	OSA
BPAP (bilevel positive airway pressure, bilevel assisted ventilation)	Inspiratory pressure support delivered over and above a minimum expiratory pressure, derived from an in-lab titration	Hypoventilation syndromes OSA when CPAP fails (including when patient intolerant)
Auto-BPAP	Range of bilevel pressures determined by a proprietary computer algorithm	Same as BPAP
ASV	Breath-by-breath adjustment of inspiratory pressure support and back-up rate determined by proprietary computer algorithm; expiratory pressure set by a technician	CSA (including mixed CSA and OSA)
Auto-ASV	Inspiratory and expiratory pressures determined by a proprietary algorithm	Same as ASV

ASV = adaptive servoventilation; CSA = central sleep apnea; OSA = obstructive sleep apnea.

Central Sleep Apnea Syndromes

Classification and Pathophysiology

Central sleep apnea (CSA) syndromes share the common pathophysiologic mechanism of dysfunctional ventilatory control resulting in a tendency toward hyperventilation and hypocapnia.

CSA is defined by the loss of neural output originating from the respiratory centers in the central nervous system to the respiratory pump machinery, resulting in pauses in breathing. During sleep testing, CSA is manifested by the absence of respiratory effort associated with loss of airflow for at least 10 seconds.

Compared with wakefulness, ventilation normally decreases during sleep and is primarily determined by blood carbon dioxide tension (arterial P_{CO_2}), with a lesser influence from oxygen tension. There is a near-linear relationship between arterial P_{CO_2} and ventilation, particularly in non-REM sleep, when CSA is typically encountered. The stimulus to breathe decreases along with arterial P_{CO_2} until the apneic threshold is reached, at which point ventilation ceases. Common to all CSA syndromes is the propensity to intermittently cross the apneic threshold, which causes a pause in breathing that destabilizes further ventilation.

KEY POINT

- Central sleep apnea is manifested on sleep testing by the absence of respiratory effort associated with loss of airflow for at least 10 seconds.

Risk Factors

Comorbid illnesses that predispose to instability of the ventilatory control system are the most common risk factors for CSA. The most important and prevalent association is between CSA and heart failure, which classically manifests as the Cheyne-Stokes breathing pattern, characterized by a pattern of ventilation with periods of waxing and waning tidal volumes.

The association between opioid analgesics and CSA is increasingly recognized. Opioids are known for their respiratory depressant effects in high doses, but they also destabilize ventilation, resulting in CSA and a chaotic breathing rhythm.

Other risk factors for CSA include atrial fibrillation, stroke, brainstem lesions, and possibly kidney failure; high-altitude periodic breathing is a form of CSA. Primary or idiopathic CSA, in which no risk factors are identified, occurs in a small proportion of patients.

Symptoms and Diagnosis

Because symptoms of CSA may be difficult to distinguish from OSA (frequent awakenings, nonrestorative sleep, EDS), a high index of suspicion is needed, particularly in the clinical context of comorbid disease. In-laboratory polysomnography is required to accurately diagnose CSA; OCST is not indicated for non-OSA sleep disorders. Overnight pulse oximetry alone does not reliably distinguish between OSA and CSA.

Treatment

The strongest indication for treatment of CSA is the presence of sleep-related symptoms, and therapy should first target management of modifiable comorbid conditions or risk factors. For example, reduction or withdrawal of opioids improves CSA. Medical optimization of heart failure (with drugs, devices, or surgery such as valve repair or heart transplantation) has been shown to improve CSA and Cheyne-Stokes breathing.

CPAP may occasionally be useful, especially in patients with overlapping OSA; however, CSA may be exacerbated by CPAP (known as "complex sleep apnea" or "treatment-emergent CSA"). Adaptive servoventilation, a novel form of PAP therapy, often suppresses CSA during polysomnography, but has not yet been shown to improve important outcomes in those with heart failure. Consultation with a sleep specialist is recommended.

KEY POINT

- The strongest indication for treatment of central sleep apnea is the presence of sleep-related symptoms, and therapy should first target management of modifiable comorbid conditions or risk factors.

Sleep-Related Hypoventilation Syndromes

The sleep-related hypoventilation syndromes result from exacerbation of an underlying condition that impairs daytime gas exchange by the decreased ventilatory drive normally associated with sleep. The most common sleep-related hypoventilation syndromes are those associated with COPD, obesity, and restrictive lung diseases related to kyphoscoliosis or neuromuscular disorders (**Table 42**). Hypoventilation

TABLE 42. Sleep-Related Hypoventilation Syndromes
COPD
Obesity hypoventilation syndrome
Myxedema
Neuromuscular disease
Muscular dystrophy
Amyotrophic lateral sclerosis
Myasthenia gravis
Guillain-Barré syndrome
Phrenic nerve injury
Poliomyelitis, post-polio syndrome
Cervical spine injury
Kyphoscoliosis

is most marked during REM sleep, during which muscle atonia can result in severe oxyhemoglobin desaturations. Hypoventilation syndromes are diagnosed when there are sustained reductions in oxyhemoglobin saturations (<90% for at least 5 minutes or more than 30% total sleep time by pulse oximetry or polysomnography) in the context of a compatible medical condition. Obstructive disordered breathing events may or may not be an associated feature, and it is the sustained reductions in oxyhemoglobin saturations that distinguish hypoventilation syndromes from the brief, repetitive deoxygenation-reoxygenation cycles typical of OSA.

KEY POINT

- The most common sleep-related hypoventilation syndromes are those associated with COPD, obesity, and restrictive lung diseases related to kyphoscoliosis or neuromuscular disorders.

Chronic Obstructive Pulmonary Disease

Hypoventilation in COPD typically results from severe airflow obstruction. Treatment should include optimization of COPD therapy. Supplemental oxygen has been a mainstay of treatment for hypoxemia due to COPD. Nocturnal bilevel positive airway pressure (BPAP) can be used for hypercapnic respiratory failure due to COPD. OSA may be superimposed on these gas exchange abnormalities; this is referred to as the overlap syndrome. PAP has been found to improve important outcomes in the overlap syndrome, such as mortality and hospitalization rates.

Obesity Hypoventilation Syndrome

Daytime hypercapnia (arterial P_{CO_2} >45 mm Hg [6.0 kPa]) is a cardinal sign of obesity hypoventilation syndrome (OHS), reflecting reduced ventilation during wakefulness and sleep that is not attributed to another cause. It likely results from a combination of mechanical load owing to obesity and attenuation of both hypoxic and hypercapnic ventilatory drive. Cardiopulmonary morbidity in OHS is prevalent, with high rates of biventricular failure and pulmonary hypertension.

First-line therapy for OHS is PAP. Because OSA often coexists with OHS, patients with OHS have historically been treated with CPAP, with or without supplemental oxygen. However, because hypoventilation and hypoxemia often persist on CPAP, the paradigm is shifting towards BPAP devices. Weight loss (and possibly bariatric surgery) should be recommended.

KEY POINT

- Daytime hypercapnia is a cardinal sign of obesity hypoventilation syndrome, reflecting reduced ventilation during wakefulness and sleep that is not attributed to another cause.

Neuromuscular Diseases

Assisted breathing devices are often prescribed to alleviate sleep-related symptoms and support blood oxygen levels in patients with neuromuscular disorders (see Table 42). BPAP or volume-cycled devices with or without supplemental oxygen may be useful, particularly if the patient has associated pulmonary hypertension, right-sided heart failure, or polycythemia. Tracheostomy and home mechanical ventilation are effective and may be appropriate for some patients. Supplemental oxygen should generally not be prescribed without adjunctive ventilatory support because supplemental oxygen may further depress ventilation in patients with respiratory muscle weakness.

KEY POINT

- Assisted breathing devices are often prescribed to alleviate sleep-related symptoms and support blood oxygen levels in patients with neuromuscular disorders.

High-Altitude-Related Illnesses

Sleep Disturbances and Periodic Breathing

High-altitude illness (HAI) encompasses a number of disorders that can occur when a person residing at low altitude ascends to higher elevation. Although the proportion of air comprised of oxygen remains constant at 21% as altitude increases, diminishing barometric pressure reduces the amount of oxygen available for gas exchange, resulting in a condition known as hypobaric hypoxia. The response to hypobaric hypoxia is a common pathophysiologic mechanism underlying HAI.

In general, HAI is more common at elevations of 2500 meters (approximately 8200 feet) and above. Susceptibility to HAI is individualized and difficult to predict but is likely to recur in those who have experienced it previously. Young age and the level of physical fitness have not been shown to be protective. Two key risk factors are the destination altitude and the rate of ascent, with gradual ascension allowing acclimatization and a decreased risk for HAI.

One of the first responses to hypoxic stress associated with hypobaric hypoxia is an increase in ventilation, which is a key pathophysiologic mechanism in high-altitude periodic breathing (HAPB). Hypoxia-induced hyperventilation drives the arterial P_{CO_2} toward the apneic threshold, with a decrease in respiratory rate and eventual rise in arterial P_{CO_2}; this results in increased respiratory drive and recurrent hyperventilation. These cyclic apneas and hyperpneas are associated with repetitive arousals from sleep, often with paroxysms of dyspnea and usually occurring the first night at elevation.

HAPB and other HAIs can be prevented by gradually ascending, which can generally be accomplished by spending one night at an intermediate altitude to allow acclimatization. Acetazolamide accelerates the acclimatization process by inducing a slight metabolic acidosis to stimulate ventilation and enhance gas exchange; it can be used prophylactically in patients with a history of altitude illness. Supplemental oxygen can relieve symptoms of disrupted sleep and paroxysmal nocturnal dyspnea, but because most cases of HAPB are self-limited after a few nights, this is generally not indicated in otherwise healthy individuals.

KEY POINTS
- Gradual ascent allows acclimatization and attenuates symptoms of high-altitude illness.
- Acetazolamide accelerates the acclimatization process to high altitude by inducing a slight metabolic acidosis to stimulate ventilation and enhance gas exchange.

Acute Mountain Sickness and High-Altitude Cerebral Edema

Hypoxia and hypocapnia associated with altitude alter cerebral blood flow and oxygen delivery to the brain. When autoregulatory mechanisms are overcome, symptoms may be mild, as with acute mountain sickness (AMS), or severe, as with life-threatening cerebral edema. AMS, the most common HAI, is characterized by nonspecific symptoms such as headache, fatigue, nausea, and vomiting, in addition to disturbed sleep related to HAPB. Approximately 25% of unacclimatized visitors to an altitude of 2000 meters (approximately 6500 feet), the elevation at most major U.S. ski areas, will experience AMS. Heavy exertion and dehydration tend to amplify the symptoms, which are typically delayed for 6 to 12 hours after ascent and usually resolve within 24 to 48 hours, provided no further ascent occurs. As in HAPB, slow ascent helps prevent the syndrome. For mild symptoms, conservative treatment may include aspirin, NSAIDs, or antiemetics. Acetazolamide is best proven as a prophylactic for AMS but may be effective as a treatment by accelerating acclimatization. Dexamethasone reduces symptoms of AMS. Supplemental oxygen or hyperbaric therapies, when available, are also used to treat AMS.

High-altitude cerebral edema is a more extreme manifestation of AMS that tends to occur at elevations above 3000 to 4000 meters (approximately 9800 to 13,000 feet); prophylactic acetazolamide should be considered in patients planning to ascend to this level to decrease the risk of this significant complication. Vascular leak leads to brain swelling, resulting in manifestations that range from confusion and irritability to ataxic gait to coma and death. Recognition of cerebral edema mandates immediate intervention. Definitive treatment is immediate descent from altitude, particularly when the patient is still ambulatory, because evacuation is exponentially more complicated, if not impossible, when the patient is incapacitated. Dexamethasone, supplemental oxygen, and hyperbaric therapy may be used in addition to descent from altitude.

KEY POINTS
- Acute mountain sickness is the most common high-altitude illness and is characterized by headache, fatigue, nausea, vomiting, and disturbed sleep; acetazolamide may be used to prevent acute mountain sickness.
- High-altitude cerebral edema is a medical emergency resulting from vasogenic brain swelling and should prompt urgent descent from altitude.

High-Altitude Pulmonary Edema

As in cerebral edema, vascular leak driven by hypoxia appears to play a role in high-altitude pulmonary edema; the two conditions can coexist. The cascade of events seems to begin with a rise in pulmonary arterial pressures within 2 to 4 days of ascent to altitudes generally greater than 2500 meters (approximately 8200 feet). Symptoms of cough, dyspnea, and exertional intolerance are usually insidious but occasionally may occur abruptly and awaken a patient from sleep. Other features of AMS may or may not be present. A key feature of high-altitude pulmonary edema is dyspnea at rest. Tachypnea and tachycardia are typical, and crackles or wheezing can be auscultated. Pink frothy sputum or frank hemoptysis may occur, followed by worsening gas exchange and respiratory failure. The treatment of choice is supplemental oxygen along with rest, both of which will acutely reduce pulmonary arterial pressures. Descent should be considered, particularly if oxygen is not available. Salvage therapies in the absence of supplemental oxygen and descent include vasodilators such as nifedipine or phosphodiesterase-5 inhibitors (sildenafil or tadalafil). Conventional treatments for pulmonary edema in the setting of heart failure, such as diuretics and nitrates, are not recommended in this setting.

Air Travel in Pulmonary Disease

The principles of hypobaric hypoxia also apply to commercial airline travel, where cabins are pressurized to the equivalent of 1500 to 2500 meters (approximately 5000 to 8200 feet) in altitude, resulting in an inspired oxygen tension between 110 and 120 mm Hg (about 70% of the levels encountered at sea level). Although in healthy individuals this correlates with an arterial Po_2 of approximately 60 mm Hg (8.0 kPa), those with underlying pulmonary disease are at risk for significant hypoxemia during flight. For such patients, pulse oximetry is a useful screening tool. An oxyhemoglobin saturation of less than 92% at sea level indicates a likely need for in-flight supplemental oxygen. Two to three liters per minute of supplemental oxygen by nasal cannula is typically adequate. In those with sea-level oxyhemoglobin saturation between 92% and 95%, hypoxia altitude simulation testing, available at some centers, can be used to determine the need for oxygen supplementation. Patients considered high-risk for in-flight hypoxia and its complications include those with COPD with hypercapnia, a recent exacerbation of chronic lung disease, pulmonary hypertension, and restrictive lung disease, in addition to patients who have had previous in-flight symptoms. In patients who are already on long-term supplemental oxygen, doubling of the flow rate during flight is typically adequate.

Trapped air in any noncommunicating body cavity (lung bullae, blebs, or cysts) will expand under hypobaric conditions. However, the risk of pneumothorax associated with rupture of these cavities during flight is believed to be low, owing to the partial pressurization of airline cabins. Acute exacerbations of obstructive airways disease such as asthma or COPD, in which air trapping can be pronounced, might present a particular risk for pneumothorax and should prompt a delay in planned air travel. An existing pneumothorax has traditionally been considered a contraindication to flight owing to the potential risk of expansion and tension physiology; however, there is some evidence that travel may be safe in the presence of a small pneumothorax that has been radiographically stable.

KEY POINTS

- An oxyhemoglobin saturation of less than 92% at sea level indicates a likely need for in-flight supplemental oxygen to prevent hypoxia.
- In patients who are already on long-term supplemental oxygen, doubling of the flow rate during flight is typically adequate to prevent hypoxia.

Critical Care Medicine

Recognizing the Critically Ill Patient

Timely and directed care for critically ill patients is important for their recovery. Identifying critically ill patients can be challenging because disease presentations may be subtle and progressive. The initial history, vital signs, physical examination, and other supportive information, such as the oxygen saturation breathing ambient air and basic laboratory tests, establish a baseline for later comparison. General criteria for ICU admission vary among institutions depending on the type of specialty ICU, intermediate units, or support staff that are available. Indications for ICU admission include an unstable airway, unstable blood pressure, unstable mental status, life-threatening cardiac arrhythmias, respiratory failure, severe metabolic derangements, or the need for frequent (more than every 2 hours) measurement of vital signs.

In patients not initially admitted to the ICU, several parameters have been identified to assist in the identification of patients at risk for instability. The different scoring systems use different parameters and have variable sensitivities and specificities. The common parameters used in all scoring systems include changes in respiration rate, heart rate, systolic blood pressure, temperature, alertness, and oxygen saturation (with and without oxygen use). Patient age is an independent risk factor for increased risk of adverse events.

Rapid response teams (RRTs) were created to improve the care of hospitalized patients with deteriorating status; the goal is to reduce the incidence of cardiopulmonary arrest and hospital mortality. Unfortunately, clear criteria do not exist for activating RRTs. However, a number of indicators have been identified that are associated with increased risk of decompensation; when these indicators are present, rapid response intervention may be effective. These indicators include changes in vital signs (heart rate of <30/min or ≥139/min; systolic blood pressure <70 mm Hg or ≥200 mm Hg; respiration rate <9/min or >35/min, temperature <34.0 °C [93.2 °F] or ≥39.0 °C [102.2 °F]), oxygen saturation less than 85%, and development of altered mental status or coma.

Rapid response systems (RRSs) involve mechanisms to identify clinical criteria suggesting potential deterioration or instability in patients, along with methods for notifying and activating the RRT of this change in status. RRSs also provide analysis of the event data, feedback, quality review, and recommendations for improvement and periodic reassessment of the system. Whether electronic alerts (by prompts in the electronic medical record or by direct paging of different types of systems) will add to outcome improvement has not been determined. The effectiveness of RRSs is debated, but most RRSs are associated with reduced rates of cardiopulmonary arrest outside of the ICU. Delay in activation of the system is associated with higher mortality. The overall impact of RRSs on mortality of hospitalized adult patients depends on the individual hospital and its resources for recognizing and rescuing deteriorating patients. Several large studies have shown that the introduction of RRSs does not reduce mortality at hospital discharge in adult patients.

Telemedicine is a strategy that uses remote monitoring of patients in the ICU to improve the quality of health care. The information collected includes patient vital signs, electrocardiogram, other types of electrical data, and remote visualization of the patient by camera. Although this technology has been available for over 25 years, study results on patient outcomes are variable, ranging from no demonstrable clinical benefit or improvement in hospital mortality to reduced hospital mortality, reduced ICU length of stay, and reduced duration of mechanical ventilation. Differences between studies have been attributed to the uneven access of the patient to the different telemedicine teams, with some teams having primary versus consultant roles. Patients of telemedicine programs are more likely to receive evidence-based care to prevent ICU complications. Although interest in the use of this technology is growing, the cost of implementation and maintenance can be substantial. More data are needed to optimize the use and appropriate circumstances for implementation of this strategy (for example, rural versus suburban, small ICU versus large ICU, degree of illness).

Methods for assessing severity of illness in patients admitted to the ICU include the Acute Physiology and Chronic Health Evaluation (APACHE), the Mortality Probability Model (MPM), and the Simplified Acute Physiology Score (SAPS). However, severity scoring has limited usefulness in predicting individual patient outcomes. Therefore, their use is more commonly limited to assessing ICU performance and quality benchmarking. **H**

KEY POINT

- Indications for ICU admission include an unstable airway, unstable blood pressure, unstable mental status, life-threatening cardiac arrhythmias, respiratory failure, severe metabolic derangements, or the need for frequent (more than every 2 hours) measurement of vital signs.

Principles of Critical Care

General Ventilator Principles

Noninvasive (usually via face mask) and invasive (via endotracheal or cuffed tracheostomy tube) ventilators are available to support patients with respiratory failure. Before any ventilator is used, the purpose and goals of using the device should be identified; this is helpful in deciding which therapy is appropriate and the initial device settings to use (Table 43).

TABLE 43. Determination of the Purpose and Goals of Invasive or Noninvasive Ventilation in a Patient with Respiratory Failure

Considerations	Potential Answers
What is the cause of the failure?	Hypoxia, hypercapnia, or both
How quickly will the patient recover?	Noninvasive ventilation can be considered if recovery is quick (as long as there are no contraindications); otherwise use invasive ventilation
What is the best tidal volume for this patient?	6-8 mL/kg of ideal body weight is a safe starting point for most forms of respiratory failure (≤6 mL/kg for most patients with ARDS)
What should the minute ventilation be for this patient?	Minute ventilation equals tidal volume times the respiration rate; setting a normal minute ventilation of 6-8 L/min is a starting point; it may need to be higher for metabolic acidosis or catabolic states or in situations where dead space is increased; it may need to be higher when lung-protective strategies are used
How much oxygen is needed?	Start with an FIO$_2$ of 1.0 and quickly decrease while following pulse oximetry to target oxygen saturation at 92% to 95% for most patients; use PEEP at an initial setting of 5 cm H$_2$O; increase PEEP to decrease high FIO$_2$ need via alveolar recruitment and optimal airway pressures

ARDS = acute respiratory distress syndrome; PEEP = positive end-expiratory pressure.

Noninvasive Ventilation
Fundamental Concepts
Noninvasive ventilation (NIV) is the delivery of positive airway pressure using a cushioned face mask without the use of an invasive connection directly in a patient's airway, such as an endotracheal tube or tracheostomy. Similar to invasive mechanical ventilation, different ventilation modes can be used (see Invasive Mechanical Ventilation, Fundamental Concepts). Pressure is the most common means through which the primary breath is supported, with all breaths initiated by the patient. Similar to invasive mechanical ventilation, the inspiratory phase of respiration can be supported by delivering air pressure and the expiratory phase can occur with exhalation against positive end-expiratory pressure (PEEP). Physiologically, the positive inspiratory pressure (also known as pressure support) assists with the inspiratory effort to offset the work of breathing. PEEP slightly expands the airways; this recruits atelectatic or flooded alveoli and counters the increased workload of breathing associated with increased airway resistance. Continuous positive airway pressure (CPAP) uses a continuous pressure during inhalation and exhalation with the primary goal of providing PEEP on exhalation. Although there is positive pressure during the inspiratory phase of respiration with CPAP, this pressure is continuous during inspiration and expiration. Bilevel support is the term used when positive pressure is changed with the inspiratory and expiratory phase of respiration in NIV. Bilevel support allows for increased support of inspiration with PEEP and potentially results in higher total volume of ventilation, CO$_2$ clearance, and decreased work of breathing.

Indications and Patient Selection
NIV in critically ill patients can prevent use of intubation in several disease states. For example, NIV decreases the need for intubation in patients with moderate to severe exacerbations of COPD (see Chronic Obstructive Pulmonary Disease). Careful monitoring of response to NIV after 1 to 2 hours is important to avoid deterioration to respiratory arrest. Intubation is indicated if there is no clinical response or if arterial blood gases worsen after the start of NIV.

In cardiogenic pulmonary edema, NIV reduces the risk of intubation (using either CPAP or inspiratory pressure support with PEEP) and is associated with a faster resolution of respiratory distress and metabolic derangements. Mortality data for NIV in cardiogenic pulmonary edema vary, but all studies reveal some benefit, such as more rapid relief of respiratory distress, decreased mortality, or reduced intubation rate. CPAP is recommended initially; however, if the patient has evidence of hypercapnia or remains dyspneic, a switch to inspiratory pressure support with PEEP is indicated. Intubation is the next step if improvement is not seen on close monitoring.

NIV can be used to support patients in acute respiratory failure due to obesity hypoventilation syndrome (OHS). NIV

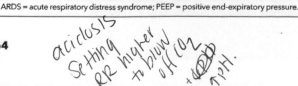

for OHS respiratory failure is associated with similar efficacy and better outcomes as compared with NIV for patients with COPD exacerbation.

In patients with hypoxic respiratory failure, such as severe pneumonia or acute respiratory distress syndrome (ARDS), the use of NIV is controversial. Select patients may benefit from short-duration NIV to avoid intubation, ventilation, and associated complications. These patients should be monitored closely in an ICU so that intubation can be performed if they do not improve or begin to deteriorate.

NIV is associated with decreased ICU mortality, intubation rates, and ICU length of stay in immunocompromised patients. Factors associated with failure of NIV include the need for vasopressors or kidney replacement therapy or the presence of ARDS.

The use of NIV after extubation to facilitate weaning from invasive mechanical ventilation for patients with COPD has yielded mixed results. A trial of NIV can be done if the reason for respiratory failure is quickly reversible; however, the threshold for reintubation should be low if the patient is not quickly improving.

NIV can be used after planned extubation for patients with a high risk of deterioration (>65 years of age, cardiac failure as a cause of intubation, COPD exacerbation, hypercapnia during a spontaneous breathing trial, or any combination of failure of weaning, heart failure, arterial P_{CO_2} of >45 mm Hg [6.0 kPa] after extubation, multiple comorbidities, or weak cough or stridor after extubation). In most patient populations, data suggest that NIV is not helpful in preventing reintubation in those with established respiratory failure after extubation.

Application

Starting NIV promptly is important for patients with respiratory failure who do not have contraindications to NIV use (Table 44). Waiting to start NIV until after the failure of medical treatment reduces its benefits. Patient selection is important, as the patient needs to have a level of mentation that will allow for both the placement of a tight mask and some ability to interact with the staff. The application of NIV requires trained personnel familiar with proper mask fitting and how to make adjustments of the pressure depending on the patient's condition and tolerance. Patients should be assessed for improvement of respiration rate, pH, P_{CO_2}, oxygen saturation, and mental status after an hour of NIV. If improvement is seen, NIV should be continued, and the patient should be subsequently weaned as tolerated. If there is no improvement but the patient is clinically stable, titration of NIV can be made with reassessment. Intubation is indicated when the patient's condition is unstable or deteriorating. Complications of NIV include mask pressure skin breakdown, sinus congestion, gastric distention, and eye irritation. Patients should be monitored in an ICU or an area equipped to respond to potential deterioration. **H**

TABLE 44. Potential Contraindications to Noninvasive Ventilation
Medical Instability
Respiratory or cardiac arrest
Severe acidosis (initial pH <7.25; failure to improve after 1-2 h)
Hemodynamic instability/severe cardiac arrhythmia
Active upper gastrointestinal bleeding
Inability to Protect Airway
Excessive secretions/inability to clear secretions
Severe bulbar dysfunction
Encephalopathy or agitated delirium
Mechanical Issues
Large air leak due to inability to fit mask
Recent facial trauma or surgery
Recent transsphenoidal surgery or high esophageal anastomosis
Upper airway obstruction
Intolerance to delivered pressure

KEY POINTS

- Noninvasive ventilation in critically ill patients can prevent intubation in those with respiratory failure associated with several disease states, including COPD exacerbation, heart failure, and obesity hypoventilation syndrome.

- Noninvasive ventilation is associated with decreased ICU mortality, intubation rate, and ICU length of stay in immunocompromised patients.

HVC

Invasive Mechanical Ventilation
Fundamental Concepts
Invasive mechanical ventilation refers to the administration of ventilation directly in the trachea via an endotracheal tube or tracheostomy. Indications for intubation include the failure to oxygenate despite supplemental oxygenation and/or the inability to maintain carbon dioxide levels in an appropriate range for a specific patient.

The ventilator uses a mode to define the interaction with the patient. There are numerous mode names (nearly 300 according to a recent review), and the same mode may have different labels depending on the ventilator manufacturer. Mode taxonomy has been described in the literature but has not been universally adopted.

Despite variable nomenclature, the different modes of mechanical ventilation consist of three basic components that may serve as a useful basis for classification:

1. Breath control: This refers to the method by which the mechanical breath is delivered. If the tidal volume and inspiratory flow are designated, the breath is classified as volume controlled (VC). Conversely, if the breath is delivered based on a preset inspiratory pressure, the breath is pressure controlled (PC).

breath = volume delivered or pressure

Handwritten margin notes:
breath sequence: spont + mandatory.
Mand = triggered by machine
Mand = assisted.
cycled = ended by machine
can be triggered by pt effort.
CMV - all breaths mandatory.
-pt may trigger @ higher rate but breaths are assisted.

2. Breath sequence: Spontaneous and mandatory are the two types of breaths. A mandatory breath is started (triggered) or ended (cycled) by the machine; ventilators may also be set to allow triggering of a mandatory breath coordinated with patient inspiratory effort. If the breath is both triggered and cycled by the patient, it is a spontaneous breath. By definition, a mandatory breath is always assisted (that is, the machine does some portion of the work of breathing), but a spontaneous breath may or may not be assisted. Therefore, there are three breath sequences:

• Continuous mandatory ventilation (CMV): All breaths are mandatory. A preset frequency represents the minimum number of mandatory breaths per minute; the patient may trigger breaths at a higher frequency.

• Intermittent mandatory ventilation (IMV): Spontaneous breaths are allowed between or during mandatory breaths. A preset frequency represents the maximum number of mandatory breaths per minute.

• Continuous spontaneous ventilation (CSV): All breaths are spontaneous.

3. Targeting scheme: This refers to a variety of ventilator algorithms that can be used to tailor mechanical ventilation to the patient's continuously changing lung characteristics and respiratory effort. These options are often proprietary, vary between ventilators, and range from simply maintaining a constant airway pressure during a pressure-controlled breath to use of artificial intelligence-based algorithms to achieve specific treatment goals.

Based on these variables, a ventilator mode may be classified by indicating the method of breath control followed by the breath sequence. For example, VC-IMV indicates volume-controlled, intermittent mandatory ventilation. The targeting scheme is then defined by a small letter at the end of the acronym. Because IMV may have two types of breaths, the two letters indicating the targeting scheme are separated by a comma. The most commonly used modes of mechanical ventilation are described in **Table 45**.

TABLE 45. Most Frequently Used Ventilator Modes				
Common Name	**Mode Classification**	**Breath Control Variable**	**Breath Sequence**	**Targeting Scheme**
Volume control and assist/control	VC-CMVs	VC: The ventilator controls the flow (volume) during the mandatory breath. If the patient's effort, lung compliance, or resistance changes, the ventilator will still deliver the set tidal volume (but the pressure will change).	CMV: All breaths are mandatory. The patient may or may not trigger the breath, but the ventilator always ends the breath when the tidal volume is delivered. The name "assist/control" is a misnomer from the past.	Set-point, s: The operator sets all the parameters of the breath (flow waveform, flow rate, and volume). The ventilator only delivers the breath and does not adjust anything to the patient effort or change in lung characteristics.
Pressure control and assist/control	PC-CMVs	PC: The ventilator controls the pressure during the mandatory breath. If the patient's effort, lung compliance, or resistance changes, the ventilator will still deliver the set inspiratory pressure (but the tidal volume delivered will change).	CMV: All breaths are mandatory. The patient may or may not trigger the breath, but the ventilator always ends the breath when the preset inspiratory time elapses.	Set-point, s: The operator sets all the parameters of the breath (inspiratory pressure and inspiratory time). The ventilator only delivers the breath and does not adjust to the patient effort or change in lung characteristics.
Pressure support, continuous positive airway pressure	PC-CSVs	PC: The ventilator controls the pressure during the breath.	CSV: All breaths are spontaneous. The patient triggers and cycles the breath.	Set-point, s: The operator sets all the parameters of the breath (inspiratory pressure). The ventilator delivers the breath and does not adjust to the patient effort or change in lung characteristics.
Synchronized intermittent mandatory ventilation	PC-IMVs,s or VC-IMVs,s	PC or VC: The mandatory breaths can be set to be volume or pressure controlled, not both. The breath may be volume or pressure controlled.	IMV: Preset mandatory breaths are given at a minimum set rate. Spontaneous breaths are permitted in between mandatory breaths. The triggering of the mandatory breath will be coordinated with the patient if the inspiratory effort occurs close to the scheduled time trigger (determined by the set frequency).	Set-point, s: One "s" refers to the mandatory breath and the other to the spontaneous breath. Generally, all spontaneous breaths in IMV are pressure supported (PC-CSVs).

CMV = continuous mandatory ventilation; CSV = continuous spontaneous ventilation; IMV = intermittent mandatory ventilation; PC = pressure controlled; VC = volume controlled.

[handwritten at top: → VC-CMV ie: 6 cc/kg in ARDS.]

CONT.

VC-CMV is commonly used in patients with ARDS, where the goal is to limit tidal volume. PC-CMV can also be used to ventilate in patients with ARDS, but close monitoring of the tidal volume should be maintained and adjustments of pressure should be performed as compliance improves.

The synchronized IMV mode was originally designed to gradually reduce support over time; however, clinical trials show it to be an inferior mode for weaning. Several modes that incorporate newer technology rely on the IMV breath sequence. This allows the patient to breathe spontaneously when able but to have the safety of a backup mandatory breath rate when needed. These modes require more sophisticated targeting schemes such as using artificial intelligence to run the ventilator.

Weaning

[handwritten: 30 min / RR<35, >90% / RSBI <80 <105]

Weaning from mechanical ventilation can start when the precipitating event or underlying condition that caused respiratory failure has resolved or is resolving. Patients should be assessed daily for their readiness to be removed from mechanical ventilation by performing a spontaneous breathing trial (SBT). Protocol-driven methods of assessing weaning readiness may reduce the duration of mechanical ventilation and the complications associated with longer ventilator stays. Sedation reduction or removal allows for a more accurate SBT. There are several methods used to assess if an SBT will be successful. The respiration rate to tidal volume ratio, or rapid shallow breathing index (RSBI), is the most familiar. A patient with an RSBI of less than 105 has an approximately 80% chance of being successfully extubated, whereas an RSBI of greater than 105 virtually guarantees weaning failure.

Other criteria that have been suggested for a successful weaning trial include (1) the ability to tolerate a weaning trial for 30 minutes (in most patients, SBT failure will occur within approximately 20 minutes), (2) maintain a respiration rate of less than 35/min, and (3) keep an oxygen saturation of 90% without arrhythmias; sudden increases in heart rate and blood pressure; or development of respiratory distress, diaphoresis, or anxiety. Once the SBT is tolerated, the ability to clear secretions, a decreasing secretion burden, and a patent upper airway are other criteria that should be met to increase extubation success. [H]

KEY POINT

- Patients should be assessed daily for their readiness to be weaned from mechanical ventilation by withdrawing sedation and performing a spontaneous breathing trial.

Ventilator-Associated Pneumonia

Ventilator-associated pneumonia (VAP) is defined as pneumonia that occurs at least 48 hours after endotracheal intubation. VAP is a serious, costly, and preventable condition associated with an increased mortality and length of ICU and hospital stay. VAP is difficult to diagnose but potential clues to its presence include temperature greater than 38.0 °C (100.4 °F), leukocytosis or leukopenia, increased purulent secretions, new or progressive pulmonary infiltrates, and worsening ventilation parameters, particularly after a period of improvement. Patients suspected of having VAP should undergo lower respiratory tract sampling, followed by microscopic analysis and culture of the specimen. Nonbronchoscopic sampling methods are simple suctioning of the endotracheal tube and mini–bronchoalveolar lavage, which involves use of a telescoping catheter (instead of a bronchoscope) to instill and aspirate physiologic saline for microbiologic analysis. Bronchoscopic methods use standard bronchoalveolar lavage and a protected specimen brush. Deep sampling methods may allow for narrower antibiotic choices and more rapid de-escalation of antibiotics. For further discussion of VAP, see MKSAP 17 Infectious Disease.

Invasive Monitoring

Invasive monitoring using a pulmonary artery catheter (PAC) to determine the stroke volume and cardiac output (CO) by thermodilution was a common method to determine volume status in critically ill patients and is the standard to which current noninvasive CO devices are compared. Owing to the lack of benefit in many studies using PACs, indications for the use of a PAC are now more selective. These indications now focus on cardiac conditions, such as cardiogenic shock requiring supportive therapy, severe heart failure requiring vasoactive therapy, differentiating high-output heart failure from sepsis, and differentiating and/or treating causes of pulmonary hypertension. Because of the potential harms and difficulty in interpretation associated with invasive CO measurement, noninvasive devices are more attractive for use in unstable patients. In resuscitating hemodynamically unstable patients, the ability to predict intravascular volume status and responsiveness to fluids (defined as an increase of cardiac output ≥15% following an adequate fluid challenge) is important. Bedside ultrasound to assess vena caval dimensions induced by positive-pressure ventilation appears to be highly predictive of volume responsiveness and is a noninvasive alternative to PAC. Likewise, the use of bedside ultrasound to assess global cardiac function has gained acceptance. However, like PACs, there are limited data showing that any of the noninvasive monitoring devices improve patient outcomes, and all have limitations. The accurate prediction of intravascular volume status and subsequent fluid response remains clinically difficult and lacks an accepted standard testing methodology.

Blood Pressure Support

Blood pressure support is important for all forms of shock (see Shock), with a goal mean arterial pressure of

CONT.

approximately 65 mm Hg. Lower values may be tolerated as long as kidney perfusion is maintained. Fluid resuscitation to ensure adequate intravascular volume is a necessary initial intervention (see Sepsis, Management, Initial Resuscitation), with timely addition of vasopressors through central access if hypotension persists despite volume challenge. Multiple comparative studies of vasopressors in septic shock suggest norepinephrine as a first-line agent, followed by epinephrine. Dopamine should be reserved for select patients; tachycardia is a major side effect, making this agent useful to increase cardiac output in the presence of a relative bradycardia. Vasopressin is considered a second-line agent (although it has been shown to be effective in less severe sepsis) that can be added to decrease the dose and side effects of norepinephrine. Indications, physiologic actions, side effects, and contraindications of vasopressors are described in **Table 46**.

Intravenous Access

A large-caliber intravenous (IV) peripheral access is standard for administering resuscitation fluids and remains the preferred initial IV route in resuscitation. When blood pressure remains low and infusion of vasoconstricting agents is needed to improve the mean arterial pressure, central access is required. The four broad categories of central access are (1) peripherally inserted central catheter (PICC), (2) temporary nontunneled, (3) long-term tunneled, and (4) implanted port (**Table 47**). However, when IV access cannot rapidly be obtained, intraosseous (I/O) access is an immediate alternative. Sites for I/O access in adults include 1 to 2 cm below the tibial tuberosity and the humeral head. Alternative access should replace the I/O within approximately 24 hours of placement to minimize complications.

Ultrasound-guided central line insertion is recommended for the placement of central lines to reduce failure of catheter placement and vessel injury, as well as prevention of pneumothorax for approaches above the diaphragm.

KEY POINTS

- Bedside ultrasound to assess vena caval dimensions induced by positive-pressure ventilation appears to be highly predictive of volume responsiveness and is a noninvasive alternative to a pulmonary artery catheter. **HVC**

- A large-caliber intravenous peripheral access is standard for administering resuscitation fluids and remains the preferred initial intravenous route in resuscitation.

- Ultrasound-guided central line insertion is associated with a reduction in failure of catheter placement and vessel injury, as well as prevention of pneumothorax. **HVC**

Comprehensive Management of Critically Ill Patients

Once a patient in the ICU has been stabilized, comprehensive management includes identifying goals of care, preferably with the patient's input. However, most critically ill patients are unable to participate in decisions regarding their care, so the person best able to represent the patient's interests must be identified. If there is a health care power of attorney (POA), any and all decisions regarding the patient can be made by the appointee once the patient is unable to make decisions on his or her own. In the absence of a POA, a health care representative should be identified. Each state differs in the defined hierarchy to be followed in identifying the health care representative. The decisions that can be made by the health care representative are more restricted than those of a POA, and regulations vary from state to state. Ultimately, clear communication with all participants involved in the care of the patient is needed for optimal care decisions.

TABLE 46.	Vasopressor Agents and Their Physiologic Effects		
Agent (Dose)	**Receptors**	**Clinical Use**	**Common Side Effects or Contraindications**
Norepinephrine	$\alpha_1 > \beta_1$	First-line in septic shock, other refractory shock	Some arrhythmias, digital ischemia
Dopamine (low)	$DA > \beta_1$	Historically used for kidney failure, but no evidence of effectiveness for this indication	Arrhythmias, ischemia
Dopamine (medium)	$\beta_1 > \beta_2$	Septic or cardiogenic shock	Arrhythmias, ischemia
Dopamine (high)	$\alpha_1 > \beta_1$	First-line for septic shock, other refractory shock	Arrhythmias, ischemia
Epinephrine (low)	$\beta_1 > \beta_2$	Second-line for septic or cardiogenic shock	Arrhythmias, ischemia
Epinephrine (high)	$\alpha_1 = \beta_1$	Second-line for septic shock, other refractory shock	Arrhythmias, ischemia
Phenylephrine	α_1	Milder shock states, least risky through peripheral IV line	Lowest arrhythmia risk, not as powerful as other vasopressors
Vasopressin	Vasopressin receptors	Second vasopressor for septic shock only, add to catecholamine vasopressor	Splanchnic, mesenteric, and digital ischemia

$\alpha_1 = \alpha_1$ adrenergic receptor; $\beta_1 = \beta_1$ adrenergic receptor; $\beta_2 = \beta_2$ adrenergic receptor; DA = dopaminergic receptor; IV = intravenous.

TABLE 47. Types of Central Access

Type	Indications	Duration	Potential Complications	Contraindications
Peripheral IV central catheter	Delivery of potentially caustic medications such as vasoactive agents, sedatives or antibiotics; central venous access	Few days up to 1 year	Low risk overall, avoiding pneumothorax and fewer infections; clot formation or occlusion due to smaller vessel diameter	Current or pending dialysis; not for rapid infusion of blood products
Temporary nontunneled central venous access	Same as above; short-term dialysis; central venous pressure monitoring	Usually not more than 6 weeks	Infection; site-specific complications such as pneumothorax for subclavian or low intrajugular approach	Not for rapid infusion of blood products owing to small diameter of catheter
Long-term tunneled central venous access (valved tip and nonvalved tip)	Long-term TPN; chemotherapy; long-term antibiotic; dialysis	More than 6 weeks	Infection; valves prevent back bleeding but have an increased risk of catheter malfunction	Not for rapid infusion of blood products owing to small diameter of catheter
Ports or totally implanted central venous access	Long-term intermittent access such as chemotherapy	More than 6 weeks	Lowest risk of infection but more difficult to implant with more costs; hidden extravasation beneath skin	Not for rapid infusion of blood products owing to small diameter of catheter
Intraosseous (tibia or humeral head [adults])	When IV access otherwise not obtained and need for emergency fluids and/or medications	About 24 hours	Low risk of infection; flow rates may be slower; if pain with infusion can use 2% preservative-free lidocaine injected slowly to control it	Do not place in a bone with a fracture or recent (24-48 h) intraosseous access attempt

IV = intravenous; TPN = total parenteral nutrition.

Sedation and Sedation Interruption

Pain, agitation, and delirium are interrelated, and current recommendations suggest a comprehensive view of all three for critically ill patients. For a discussion of delirium, see MKSAP 17 Neurology. Light sedation (defined as a drowsy or calm and cooperative patient), rather than deep sedation (where the patient is barely awake or unarousable) is recommended unless contraindicated (severe ARDS, ventilator dyssynchrony). Either daily sedation interruption or light sedation targeted titration should be used routinely in mechanically ventilated adult patients in the ICU. Using a lighter sedation goal reduces ICU-related posttraumatic stress disorder, time on the ventilator, and mortality.

Strategies using nonbenzodiazepine-based sedatives are preferred owing to the increased ICU delirium associated with benzodiazepine use. Analgesia-based sedation is an alternative method to benzodiazepine-based sedation that does not result in an increase in days on the ventilator or in the ICU. Opioids are considered the drug class of choice for treatment of non-neuropathic pain in critically ill patients, including mechanically ventilated adult patients in the ICU. An opioid analgesic should be given as an interrupted infusion.

KEY POINT

- When compared with deep sedation, light sedation (a drowsy and cooperative patient) reduces ICU-related posttraumatic stress disorder, time on the ventilator, and mortality.

Early Mobilization

Early mobilization strategies range from simple range of motion of extremities to standing and walking. Mobilization is recommended within 48 hours of admission to the ICU and improves physical function of ICU survivors. Early mobilization, along with careful attention to pain, agitation, and delirium management, has been shown to reduce ICU and hospital length of stay, shorten return to independent functional status, and improve survival.

KEY POINT

- Mobilization within 48 hours of admission, along with careful attention to pain, agitation, and delirium management, reduces ICU and hospital length of stay, shortens return to independence, and improves survival.

ICU–Acquired Weakness

ICU-acquired weakness includes critical illness polyneuropathy (with axonal nerve degeneration) and critical illness myopathy (with muscle myosin loss), resulting in profound weakness. The pathophysiologic mechanisms are postulated to be multifactorial; they include dysfunctional microcirculation that leads to neuronal and axonal injury, inactivation of sodium channels, myonecrosis secondary to the catabolic state, acute muscle wasting of critical illness, and mitochondrial dysfunction of skeletal muscles. ICU-acquired weakness is associated with long-term functional disability, prolonged ventilation, and in-hospital mortality. Cited risk factors include hyperglycemia, sepsis, multiple organ dysfunction, and systemic inflammatory response. Exposure to glucocorticoids and neuromuscular blocking agents was not found to be consistently associated with ICU-acquired weakness; however, limited use is recommended if these medications are required in the care of critically ill patients.

Long-Term Cognitive Impairment

Long-term cognitive impairment is now recognized in patients recovering from critical illness. Delirium is frequently seen in patients in the ICU, and longer durations of delirium are associated with worse executive function and global cognition at 3 and 12 months. A strong association is also noted with ICU hypoxemia when cognition is assessed at 1 year. Hypoglycemic periods have also been associated with mood disorders after discharge. These findings have raised interest in understanding longer-term outcomes in patients in the ICU, and they are considered part of the postintensive care syndrome.

Postintensive Care Syndrome

Postintensive care syndrome is a term used to describe new or worsening physical, cognitive, or mental health problems arising after a critical illness that persist beyond the initial hospital discharge. This term can be applied to either the patient or family member, as both report a wide range of impairment after hospital discharge. There is a paucity of data available to provide direction on the most effective interventions for the patient and family. The use of ICU diaries and clear communication by the ICU team with the family appear to have a beneficial effect on the family.

> **KEY POINT**
>
> - ICU-acquired weakness (polyneuropathy and myopathy) is associated with long-term functional disability, prolonged ventilation, and in-hospital mortality; risk factors include hyperglycemia, sepsis, multiple organ dysfunction, and systemic inflammatory response.

Nutrition

Nutrition is an essential part of management for patients in the ICU and can be given enterally or parenterally, with the enteral route preferred. Initiation of enteral nutrition is recommended at 24 to 48 hours following admission if the patient is hemodynamically stable, with advancement to goal by 48 to 72 hours. The presence of abdominal distention, decreased passage of stool or flatus, or vomiting indicates that the patient may have gut ischemia or another gastrointestinal problem, and tube feeds should be discontinued or slowed. Studies examining gastric residual volumes suggest that volumes of 200 to 500 mL are safe; however, increasing residual volumes may signal a need to hold or reduce the feeding volume. The caloric goals of nutrition should be clearly identified and determined by the energy requirement of the patient. The energy requirement can be calculated by any of a number of predictive equations or more accurately by indirect calorimetry, although this may not be widely available. The simple formula of 25 to 35 kcal/kg/d, based on actual body weight, can also be used to estimate caloric need in patients in the ICU (or approximately 30 mL/kg/d of a 1 kcal/mL formula). If less volume is needed, more concentrated formulas can be used. Medications such as propofol add fat calories and should be considered in the calculation of total calories. Providing enteral calories and protein close to goals improves outcomes. For patients who cannot tolerate enteral feeding, parenteral nutrition in the form of total parenteral nutrition should not be started before day 7 of an acute illness; studies show that late feeding (after 7 days) is associated with faster recovery and fewer complications as compared with early feeding (within 48 hours).

> **KEY POINT**
>
> - Initiation of enteral nutrition is recommended at 24 to 48 hours following ICU admission if the patient is hemodynamically stable, with advancement to goal by 48 to 72 hours.

ICU Care Bundles

ICU care bundles are a set of treatment goals that, when grouped together, should promote optimal outcomes for a patient in the ICU. The Institute for Healthcare Improvement supports the use of bundles to ensure the minimal standard of care for each patient. Unfortunately, not all care bundles consist of the same components, and the effectiveness of all aspects of the bundle and the overall benefits of bundles in ICU care have not yet been established.

High-Value Care in the ICU

The cost of care in the ICU is often extremely high. Despite the level of severity of illness in the ICU, providing high-value care should remain a primary consideration in managing patients in this setting. Several critical care organizations have joined with the American Board of Internal Medicine Foundation to provide five tests or procedures whose necessity should be questioned or discussed. The five selected for patients in the ICU are listed in **Table 48.**

Common ICU Conditions

Upper Airway Emergencies

Delayed recognition and management of severe upper airway obstruction is often catastrophic given the difficulty of

TABLE 48.	ICU Choosing Wisely Top Five
Don't order diagnostic tests at regular intervals (such as every day), but rather in response to specific clinical questions.
Don't transfuse erythrocytes in hemodynamically stable, nonbleeding patients in the ICU who have a hemoglobin concentration greater than 7 g/dL (70 g/L).
Don't use parenteral nutrition in adequately nourished critically ill patients within the first 7 days of an ICU stay.
Don't deeply sedate mechanically ventilated patients without a specific indication and without daily attempts to lighten sedation.
Don't continue life support for patients at high risk for death or severely impaired functional recovery without offering patients and their families the alternative of care focused entirely on comfort.

Reprinted with permission of the American Thoracic Society. Copyright © American Thoracic Society.

endotracheal intubation in this setting and the risks associated with emergent surgical cricothyrotomy. Maintaining a low threshold to secure a safe airway with early intubation, as well as close respiratory monitoring of at-risk patients not undergoing immediate intubation, is vital. The presence of drooling, stridor, and voice change helps identify patients with significant airway compromise. Endoscopic visualization of the upper airway is helpful for identifying the cause, severity, and progression over time. Epiglottitis is an important infectious cause of obstruction and is associated with sore throat and odynophagia in nearly all patients. The diagnosis is confirmed by direct visualization of the epiglottis or by the presence of epiglottal edema on lateral neck radiographs. Abscesses in the peritonsillar, retropharyngeal, and parapharyngeal space, as well as Ludwig angina (bilateral infection of the submandibular space), can present with similar symptoms and cause life-threatening upper airway obstruction. In addition to ensuring airway patency, treatment consists of antibiotics along with surgical drainage of abscesses when present. Noninfectious causes of upper airway obstruction include trauma, foreign body, external compression from tumor or thyroid disease, inhalational injuries (see Acute Inhalational Injuries), and angioedema (see Anaphylaxis).

Shock

Shock is defined as a general deficiency in vascular perfusion, leading to tissue ischemia and dysfunction. The term shock is generic and denotes a condition that can arise from a wide range of causes and manifest in a variety of ways clinically, depending on the duration and severity of ischemia and the sensitivity to hypoxia of affected organs. Signs of shock relate to hypoperfusion, such as low blood pressure and prolonged capillary refill time, and other signs and symptoms relate to organ dysfunction due to oxygen deprivation (Table 49).

Blood pressure measurements and responses may be variable in shock. Not all hypotension is shock, and not all

shock states may present initially with hypotension. The blood pressure of a patient in shock may be within normal parameters, but it may be relatively low compared with baseline pressure for that individual. Such a situation will sometimes lead to organ dysfunction, in which case the organ-specific manifestations may be the key to early diagnosis of the shock state. Nonetheless, blood pressure and its physiologic components are essential to understanding and managing shock (Figure 21).

Shock can be classified into three basic types depending on the principal reason for decreased tissue perfusion. Hypovolemic shock is due to inadequate perfusion in the setting of decreased blood volume (for example, from hemorrhage or dehydration). Cardiogenic shock refers to poor perfusion from decreased cardiac function, such as from an exacerbation of heart failure or from acute heart failure following a coronary event. Distributive shock results from a loss of vascular tone, as in sepsis or anaphylaxis, leading to redistribution of the blood volume and poor circulation. Obstructive shock is a subset of cardiogenic shock in which there is mechanical blockage in the central circulation, as can occur with massive pulmonary embolism or tension pneumothorax.

The basic goals of management in shock, regardless of type, are to restore perfusion as quickly as possible and to reverse the disease process leading to the shock state. Understanding which type of shock a patient has is critically important, as interventions may differ dramatically for one type versus another. The mainstays of shock treatment include fluid administration, vasopressors (see Blood Pressure Support), inotropes, and blood transfusion. Each of these therapies may have a role in any kind of shock, but they should be used carefully in each specific patient to avoid creating

TABLE 49. Signs and Symptoms of Shock	
Evidence of Hypoperfusion	**Evidence of Organ Dysfunction**
Low blood pressure	Lightheadedness
SBP <90 mm Hg	Altered mental status
MAP <65 mm Hg	Diaphoresis
Decrease in SBP >40 mm Hg	Decreased urine output
Lack of BP response to fluid bolus	Increased serum creatinine level
Prolonged capillary refill time	Chest pain or other ischemic pain

BP = blood pressure; MAP = mean arterial pressure; SBP = systolic blood pressure.

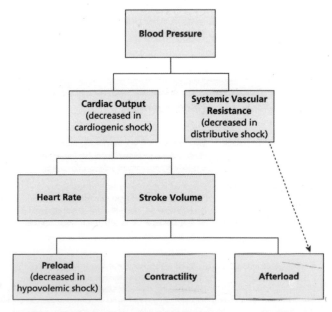

FIGURE 21. Key hemodynamic parameters of shock.

iatrogenic harm. Although these measures mitigate the effects of poor perfusion in a patient experiencing shock, diagnosing and reversing the underlying cause of shock is just as important and may involve a variety of interventions specific to the situation (**Table 50**).

KEY POINTS

- Shock is classified into three types: (1) hypovolemic (due to inadequate perfusion in the setting of decreased blood volume), (2) cardiogenic (due to poor perfusion from decreased cardiac function), and (3) distributive (due to loss of vascular tone).

- The basic goals of management in shock, regardless of its type, are to restore perfusion as quickly as possible and to reverse the disease process leading to the shock state.

- The mainstays of shock treatment include fluid administration, vasopressors, inotropes, and blood transfusion; however, diagnosing and reversing the underlying cause of shock is as important as restoring perfusion.

Hypoxemic Respiratory Failure

Hypoxemic respiratory failure is one of the major types of respiratory insufficiency and results from a disease process leading to inadequate oxygenation of arterial blood. Severe hypoxemia is generally defined as an arterial P_{O_2} of 60 mm Hg (8.0 kPa) or less or an oxygen saturation of 89% or less while breathing ambient air, and/or an arterial P_{O_2}/F_{IO_2} ratio of 200 mm Hg (26.6 kPa) or less. When hypoxia does not immediately respond to supplemental oxygen, there is risk of ischemic organ damage, and aggressive measures to improve oxygenation of the blood and the organs it perfuses may be needed.

The most common causes of hypoxemic respiratory failure are conditions that lead to mismatch of the ventilation (V) by inspired air in the alveoli and perfusion (Q) of adjacent alveolar capillaries by blood with the capacity to carry and circulate the oxygen to body tissues (called V/Q mismatch, in which the ratio of V to Q may be "high" if the unbalance is toward more ventilation than perfusion, or "low" if unbalanced toward more perfusion and less ventilation). Conditions such as pulmonary embolism lead to high V/Q mismatch, where ventilation is normal and perfusion is impaired in the lungs. More common are low V/Q conditions (also called intrapulmonary shunt) such as pneumonia or atelectasis, in which blood flows through capillaries adjacent to alveoli that are not ventilated, so the blood does not pick up any oxygen. Hypoxia due to low V/Q (shunt) will not improve with supplemental oxygen because inspired gas does not interface with the shunted blood in the lungs. In contrast, high V/Q is generally more responsive to oxygen therapy.

KEY POINTS

- Hypoxemic respiratory failure is usually characterized by an arterial P_{O_2} of 60 mm Hg (8.0 kPa) or less or an oxygen saturation of 89% or less while breathing ambient air, and/or an arterial P_{O_2}/F_{IO_2} ratio of 200 mm Hg (26.6 kPa) or less.

- Hypoxemic respiratory failure is commonly caused by low ventilation-perfusion (V/Q) mismatch conditions (also called intrapulmonary shunt), in which blood flows through capillaries adjacent to alveoli that are not ventilated.

Acute Respiratory Distress Syndrome

ARDS is a clinical syndrome that can result from a variety of insults to the lungs, leading to alveolar and interstitial inflammation and edema, with a complex milieu of inflammatory cells and protein. There is heterogeneous but often widespread damage to the alveolar epithelium and vascular endothelium, as well as surfactant dysfunction leading to alveolar instability and collapse. The pathologic description of this process is diffuse alveolar damage (**Figure 22**). All of these features worsen gas exchange, and the result can be profound hypoxia due to

TABLE 50.	Characteristics of the Types of Shock		
Type of Shock	**Pathophysiology**	**Measures to Restore Perfusion**	**Measures to Reverse the Cause of Shock**
Hypovolemic shock	Decreased effective circulating volume diminishes preload and the heart is unable to maintain adequate output	IV fluids Blood transfusion	Control sites of bleeding Control other fluid loss (e.g., diarrhea)
Cardiogenic shock	Cardiac function is impaired, either because of damage or disease to the heart muscle, arrhythmia, or obstruction of the central circulation or heart valves	IV fluids or diuresis to optimize preload Inotropic medications Maintenance of an appropriate heart rate	Coronary revascularization Thrombolysis Treatment of underlying rhythm disturbance Relief of obstruction
Distributive shock	Loss of vascular tone leads to pooling of blood in capacitance spaces, decreasing the circulating volume	IV fluids Vasopressors	Antibiotics Control of infectious source

IV = intravenous.

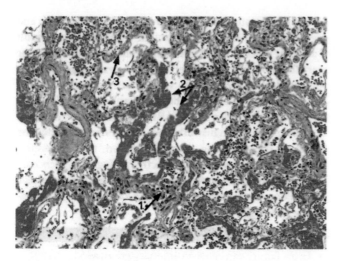

FIGURE 22. Diffuse alveolar damage. 1 = interstitial edema (thickened cellular space between airspace and vasculature); 2 = hyaline membranes (proteinaceous alveolar exudates that accumulate along the alveolar surfaces and impair gas exchange); 3 = denuded epithelium (usually numerous type 1 alveolar cells have undergone apoptosis and been replaced by hyaline membrane or fibrosis).

H
CONT.

low V/Q mismatch. The changes can severely reduce lung compliance, making adequate ventilation difficult and further worsening hypoxia. Pulmonary artery pressure is also increased, which can worsen oxygen delivery by decreasing overall cardiac output.

ARDS is diagnosed when the following Berlin definition criteria are met:

- Presentation within 1 week of known insult, or with worsening respiratory symptoms

- Pao_2/Fio_2 ≤300 mm Hg (40.0 kPa) with PEEP ≥5 cm H_2O

- Bilateral otherwise unexplained opacities seen on frontal chest imaging

In 2012, the classification scheme for ARDS was modified to include three severity levels based on oxygenation:

- Mild: Pao_2/Fio_2 ≤300 mm Hg (40.0 kPa) but >200 mm Hg (26.6 kPa)

- Moderate: Pao_2/Fio_2 ≤200 mm Hg (26.6 kPa) but >100 mm Hg (13.3 kPa)

- Severe: Pao_2/Fio_2 ≤100 mm Hg (13.3 kPa)

In addition, the term acute lung injury for milder cases of ARDS was eliminated, and pulmonary artery occlusion pressure was no longer included as part of the diagnostic criteria.

ARDS may be caused by a wide variety of diseases, conditions, or insults, some of which lead to direct injury to the lung and some of which cause indirect injury. Pulmonary causes include pneumonia, aspiration, inhalational injury, near drowning, and drugs. Nonpulmonary causes include sepsis, pancreatitis, and transfusion reactions. In some cases, different causes are associated with different prognoses for recovery; however, after treatment for the underlying cause, the management of all forms of ARDS is the same. Importantly, some cases of ARDS may be caused or made worse by

mechanical ventilation, especially if lung-protective strategies are not used.

Ventilatory Management

Ventilator management (see Invasive Mechanical Ventilation) is required for most patients with ARDS; however, mechanical ventilation has the potential to cause and/or worsen the condition. When this happens, it is known as ventilator-induced lung injury (VILI) and is especially likely if the mode or settings lead to overdistention of alveoli (volutrauma), repeated opening and closing of alveoli (atelectrauma), or release of inflammatory mediators in the lung or systemic circulation (biotrauma). Even patients who had no evidence of lung injury at the time of intubation can develop ARDS quickly if the ventilator settings are injurious. Those whose lungs are already injured or who have risk factors for developing injury are even more likely to have damage from VILI.

Because of this, lung-protective ventilator strategies have been developed and have led to improved outcomes for patients with ARDS. These parameters generally include limiting the tidal volume given in mechanical ventilation to 6 mL/kg of ideal body weight, limiting the plateau pressure in the respiratory cycle to no more than 30 cm H_2O, and use of adequate PEEP to prevent the collapse of unstable alveolar units in the expiratory phase of the cycle. There is evidence that even lower tidal volumes may be better for the lungs and that higher levels of PEEP than those previously recommended may be more protective. Current recommendations are to use a PEEP level that achieves adequate oxygenation with an Fio_2 of less than 0.6 and does not cause hypotension. With emphasis on minimizing the mechanical stress to injured lung tissue, the currently recommended approach is to limit volume and pressure as much as patients can tolerate, even allowing blood levels of CO_2 to rise somewhat in exchange for more protective volumes and pressures; this is known as permissive hypercapnia. In the absence of evidence-based guidelines, a pH of 7.25 or even lower may be acceptable in order to ventilate the lungs as gently as possible. **H**

KEY POINT

- Patients with acute respiratory distress syndrome should be ventilated using lung-protective ventilator strategies, which consist of limiting the tidal volume to 6 mL/kg of ideal body weight, limiting the plateau pressure to no more than 30 cm H_2O, and using adequate positive end-expiratory pressure to prevent the collapse of unstable alveolar units in the expiratory phase.

Nonventilatory Management

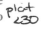

Decades of research on potential treatments for ARDS have produced no approved pharmacologic therapies, although some molecular targets are still under investigation and may lead to effective interventions. Some controversy still exists regarding the use of glucocorticoids, but trial results have been inconsistent and mostly negative, and published guidelines do not recommend them for use in ARDS.

Although there is some evidence that neuromuscular blockade may be helpful in decreasing mortality associated with ARDS, it is not an established therapy in treating ARDS.

Conservative fluid management has been shown to affect clinical outcomes in ARDS; the goal is to keep the lungs as dry as possible during the period of injury and susceptibility to additional damage. Limiting intravenous fluids and using diuretics to keep central venous pressures at lower targets has been associated with a more rapid improvement in lung function, shorter duration of mechanical ventilation, and shorter ICU length of stay, but no effect on mortality.

Studies of other adjunct therapies such as inhaled vasodilators (nitric oxide or prostacyclin) and glucocorticoids have generally shown improved oxygenation but no survival benefit.

In 2013 a randomized controlled trial of prone positioning showed an impressive mortality benefit for patients placed in the prone position for 16 hours per day until their oxygenation improved to an arterial Po_2/Fio_2 ratio of at least 150 mm Hg (20.0 kPa). Based on this evidence, prone positioning is recommended for all patients with severe ARDS for whom the risk/benefit ratio of such positioning is low. Some patients cannot be placed prone owing to their weight or other comorbid conditions. The process of placing critically ill patients prone may be technically challenging; it can be done manually or in specialized beds that rotate the patient between the prone and supine positions.

16 hrs

In patients with refractory hypoxemia, extracorporeal membrane oxygenation (ECMO) is a rescue therapy that can be considered to improve oxygenation while the lungs heal. The ability to oxygenate selected patients with this technology has improved markedly, but still only a relatively small number of patients with ARDS are candidates for ECMO (usually those with no other organ systems in failure and a reasonably good prognosis for lung recovery with time and treatment). Additionally, only a few large medical centers offer ECMO. If this therapy is to be considered, patients should be transferred to such a center as early as possible in their illness. **H**

KEY POINTS

- Patients with acute respiratory distress syndrome should receive conservative fluid management, which consists of limited intravenous boluses and using diuretics to keep central venous pressures at lower targets.

- Prone positioning may result in a mortality benefit for selected patients with acute respiratory distress syndrome on mechanical ventilation.

H Heart Failure

Heart failure is a common cause of hypoxemic respiratory failure. Unlike in ARDS, in which the edema is part of a complex process with tissue damage, inflammatory cells, and other changes, pulmonary edema from heart failure is usually transudative fluid in the pulmonary interstitium and alveolar spaces. Fluid can accumulate in the lungs as a result of acute or chronic impairment of either systolic or diastolic heart function. It can interfere with gas exchange dramatically, but it usually improves with noninvasive positive airway pressure ventilation and diuresis. Cardiogenic pulmonary edema can appear identical to ARDS on imaging, so diagnostic measures to distinguish the two entities are essential and should be considered in a timely fashion; these measures include clinical presentation, electrocardiography, echocardiography, and measurement of biomarkers for cardiac ischemia or strain (troponin, creatine kinase, B-type natriuretic peptide). **H**

KEY POINT

- Heart failure can cause pulmonary edema and interfere with gas exchange; however, it usually improves with noninvasive positive airway pressure ventilation and diuresis.

Atelectasis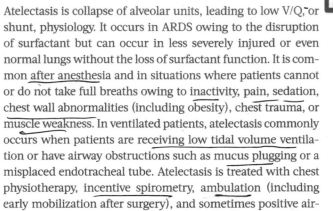

Atelectasis is collapse of alveolar units, leading to low V/Q, or shunt, physiology. It occurs in ARDS owing to the disruption of surfactant but can occur in less severely injured or even normal lungs without the loss of surfactant function. It is common after anesthesia and in situations where patients cannot or do not take full breaths owing to inactivity, pain, sedation, chest wall abnormalities (including obesity), chest trauma, or muscle weakness. In ventilated patients, atelectasis commonly occurs when patients are receiving low tidal volume ventilation or have airway obstructions such as mucus plugging or a misplaced endotracheal tube. Atelectasis is treated with chest physiotherapy, incentive spirometry, ambulation (including early mobilization after surgery), and sometimes positive airway pressure, such as PEEP on a ventilator or noninvasive CPAP. **H**

KEY POINT

- Atelectasis is treated with chest physiotherapy, incentive spirometry, ambulation (including early mobilization after surgery), and sometimes positive airway pressure.

Pneumonia

Pneumonia is infection filling the alveolar space, and it often causes consolidation on lung imaging studies. Because infected alveoli are not aerated, this creates shunt, which can lead to hypoxemia if widespread. Pneumonia is also a common cause of ARDS. The two processes may coexist and can be difficult to differentiate from each other. When pneumonia or any other alveolar filling process in the lung is heterogeneous, the affected areas can be difficult to recruit using PEEP, since added pressure will expand the unaffected, more compliant areas of the lungs much more easily and can lead to injury (volutrauma) to these healthier segments before the diseased segments improve. **H**

Hypercapnic (Ventilatory) Respiratory Failure

Hypercapnic, or ventilatory, respiratory failure occurs when alveolar ventilation is inadequate to clear the CO_2 produced by cellular metabolism, and the level of CO_2 increases in the blood. The imbalance can be due to increased CO_2 production associated with an increased metabolic rate or due to decreased alveolar ventilation. Unlike hypoxemic respiratory failure, ventilatory failure is not usually due to gas exchange abnormalities, since CO_2 is more soluble than oxygen and therefore diffuses more readily between the alveolar air space and pulmonary capillary blood. Because oxygenation also depends on ventilation of the alveoli with fresh inspired gas, patients in ventilatory failure are often hypoxic as well. However, these patients' hypoxia will improve with supplemental oxygen more readily than those with V/Q mismatch.

Decreased alveolar ventilation is caused by one or more of three abnormalities: (1) decreased respiratory drive; (2) restrictive defects of the lung, chest wall, or respiratory muscles; or (3) conditions that increase dead space in the lungs so that much of the inspired air does not reach areas of gas exchange with the blood.

Decreased Respiratory Drive

Decreased respiratory drive is most often due to sedative and analgesic drugs that suppress the respiratory center in the brainstem. Overdoses of both medicinal and recreational agents can be lethal by this mechanism. Opiates are especially potent inhibitors of respiratory drive, but benzodiazepines, barbiturates, and any other sedating medication can have the same effect if taken in sufficient doses (see Toxicology, Toxicity of Drugs of Abuse). Strokes do not usually suppress respiratory drive unless they increase intracranial pressure, which can lead to brainstem herniation. Metabolic conditions such as hypoglycemia and hypothyroidism can also sometimes suppress respiratory drive. Whenever respiratory drive is impaired, the respiration rate is decreased, often with decreased tidal volume as well. Interventions include ventilatory support and reversal of effects of any known or suspected suppressive agents.

KEY POINT

- In patients with hypercapnic respiratory failure due to decreased respiratory drive, interventions consist of ventilatory support and reversal of effects of any known or suspected suppressive agents.

Restrictive Lung Disease

Restrictive ventilatory defects are defined by a decrease in the total lung capacity or the vital capacity. Such limitation may be seen in three types of disease: (1) parenchymal lung disease, in which fibrotic or infiltrated lung tissue loses its mechanical compliance; (2) extrapulmonary restriction due to chest wall disease, in which the spine, ribs, or other thoracic structures limit lung expansion; and (3) neuromuscular weakness, in which the lungs can be passively expanded to normal volume but the patient's ability to take a full breath is limited by weakness of the respiratory muscles.

Diffuse Parenchymal Lung Disease

Diffuse parenchymal lung disease is discussed in the Diffuse Parenchymal Lung Disease chapter. It may be distinguished from the other two types of restrictive disease by the presence of fibrotic changes on high-resolution CT, reduced lung volumes, and a reduction in the diffusing capacity of the lungs, which is usually normal in chest wall disease and muscular weakness. Because of the diffusion abnormality, hypoxia is often more severe than hypercapnia in these patients, but they may develop ventilatory failure, especially in the setting of an exacerbation or other superimposed acute process such as infection or aspiration.

Extrapulmonary Restriction

Extrapulmonary restriction may be caused by deformities or diseases of the chest wall, spine, or abdomen. These conditions increase the work of breathing by placing the respiratory muscles at a mechanical disadvantage or by physically limiting the extent to which the lungs can expand with inhalation. In the ICU setting, chronic conditions of this type are usually only significant when combined with another acute condition that impairs breathing. Positive-pressure ventilation, either invasive or noninvasive, can be helpful in supporting patients through the acute condition that led to ventilatory failure. When extrapulmonary restriction is severe, patients have very limited ventilatory reserve, and they may go into respiratory failure frequently and after minimal provocation.

KEY POINT

- Hypercapnic respiratory failure due to extrapulmonary restriction may be caused by deformities or diseases of the chest wall, spine, or abdomen, which increase the work of breathing.

Neuromuscular Weakness

Neuromuscular weakness is a special case of extrapulmonary restriction, in which the lungs are usually normal, capable of normal gas exchange and expansion, but are limited by the patient's inability to fill them without assistance during inspiration. In patients with generalized weakness syndromes, pulmonary function tests show restriction on spirometry and lung volume measurement but normal diffusing capacity. Symptoms of dyspnea and especially orthopnea are common because the supine position impairs accessory respiratory muscles and leaves the weakened diaphragm with most of the work of breathing. Signs on physical examination may include paradoxical inward motion of the abdomen with inspiration and other signs of accessory muscle use for breathing. Some neuromuscular weakness syndromes (for example, amyotrophic lateral sclerosis) also affect bulbar function, resulting in slurred speech, trouble swallowing liquids, choking, and coughing. It is often complications from these related difficulties that result in acute respiratory failure and ICU admission for these patients. Aspiration pneumonia is common and poorly tolerated.

Patients with spinal cord injury may have respiratory muscle weakness as a result of their injury. The phrenic nerves originate from cervical spinal roots C3, C4, and C5. Patients with complete injury above the level of C3 will require lifelong mechanical ventilation assistance. Other patients with incomplete or lower injury may recover some function with time. Injuries below C5 will not directly impair muscles of inspiration but may impair forceful expiration and cough, making secretion management difficult and increasing the risk of atelectasis and infection.

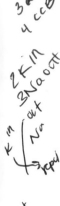

One of the challenges of caring for patients with neuromuscular weakness, especially those with progressive syndromes, is in knowing when to recommend mechanical ventilation and/or tracheostomy placement. Considerations include risk of aspiration and other complications, based on patients' respiratory muscle strength, but also on bulbar function and other impairments. Other factors affecting the quality of life include speech, mobility, and the ability to eat and drink. Patients with altered mental status, severe respiratory distress, or profound hypoxia or hypercapnia clearly need immediate ventilatory support. In patients with less dramatic presentation, pulmonary function testing and arterial blood gas analysis can help determine when ventilatory support is needed (Table 51). However, no single test can predict the ideal time to initiate ventilatory support for a given patient, so the decision should be made based on all available data, patient values and preferences, and clinical judgment. In patients requiring ventilator support, noninvasive positive pressure ventilation is the usual initial method used, typically on an intermittent, nocturnal basis.

KEY POINT

- In patients with generalized neuromuscular weakness syndromes, pulmonary function tests show restriction on spirometry and lung volume measurement but normal diffusing capacity.

Obstructive Lung Disease

Obstructive lung disease is defined by increased resistance to airflow, usually of small airways during expiration. This may be transient and reversible, as in asthma, or fixed, as in advanced COPD. Less commonly, obstruction may be caused by obstruction of the large airways due to tumors, abscesses, trauma, angioedema, or inhalational injury. Obstructive conditions can lead to ventilatory failure as the resistance to expiratory flow causes air trapping. This occurs when airway resistance to flow causes incomplete exhalation before the next breath is initiated by the mechanical ventilator. This "trapped" volume of air may be small with each breath, but it can build up over many breaths to a significant volume of unexpired air in the chest. This leads to elevated intrathoracic pressure, also called auto-PEEP or intrinsic PEEP, which hyperinflates the chest and reduces fresh gas entry into the alveoli. This converts normally functional alveolar units to dead space, which increases the work of breathing and decreases the effective alveolar ventilation, leading to a rise in CO_2. These patients may also be hypoxic but usually respond readily to supplemental oxygen. If hypoxia is profound or refractory to oxygen therapy, it is reasonable to consider another concurrent disease process.

KEY POINTS

- Obstructive lung disease can cause ventilatory failure as the resistance to expiratory flow causes air trapping, leading to elevated intrathoracic pressure known as auto–positive end-expiratory pressure (auto-PEEP) or intrinsic PEEP.

- Patients with ventilatory failure from obstructive lung disease may be hypoxic but usually respond readily to supplemental oxygen; if hypoxia is profound or refractory to oxygen therapy, alternative diagnoses should be considered.

Critical Care Management of Severe Asthma Exacerbation

Patients with severe asthma exacerbation may present with tachypnea, inability to speak in full sentences, accessory respiratory muscle use, and diminished air entry with pulsus paradoxus due to hyperinflation; however, not all patients presenting with serious exacerbation initially appear ill. Arterial blood gas analysis often shows hypocapnia, but a normal or mildly elevated CO_2 level can be a sign of respiratory

TABLE 51.	Signs of Respiratory Failure in Patients with Neuromuscular Weakness	
Test	**Findings Indicating Respiratory Failure**	**Comments**
Vital capacity	<50% of predicted	Lower values predict higher risk of respiratory failure
Maximal inspiratory pressure	−60 cm H_2O	If less negative, indicates diaphragm weakness and inadequate accessory muscle compensation leading to high risk of respiratory failure; this is the qualifying threshold for noninvasive ventilation
Maximal expiratory pressure	+40 cm H_2O	If less positive, indicates inadequate expiratory muscles, including abdominal muscles; may lead to impaired cough and secretion management
Arterial PCO_2	>45 mm Hg (6.0 kPa)	Most useful in initial assessment, less useful for following trends toward needing mechanical ventilation

[handwritten annotations: "breath", "↓RR ↓V_t or ↑insp flow rate", "auto PEEP > dont exhale fully", "air trap"]

CONT.

muscle fatigue and impending failure. FEV_1 or peak expiratory flow (PEF) may be measured if the patient can tolerate the maneuvers. If the FEV_1 and PEF do not increase to above 40% of predicted in response to aggressive bronchodilator and glucocorticoid therapy, the patient should be admitted to the ICU for close monitoring and continued aggressive therapy. If the patient is unable to perform FEV_1 or PEF maneuvers or has altered mental status, increasing work of breathing, or agonal respiration, immediate intubation is usually indicated.

Patients with severe asthma requiring admission to the ICU can be among the most challenging to manage, even with invasive mechanical ventilation. The problems of air trapping or auto-PEEP may be even worse while ventilated compared with when the patient was breathing spontaneously. If auto-PEEP is not recognized, pressure within the chest can build, mimicking the physiology of tension pneumothorax, with diminished air entry as well as decreased venous return to the heart, resulting in cardiovascular instability. If this is observed in a patient with asthma on mechanical ventilation, the immediate response is to disconnect the ventilator circuit from the patient's endotracheal tube to allow for a prolonged exhalation to release auto-PEEP. The ventilator settings should then be adjusted to allow for more effective exhalation to avoid further air trapping. Slowing the respiration rate, decreasing the tidal volume, and increasing the inspiratory flow rate while tolerating respiratory acidosis are ways to increase the exhaled volume with each cycle.

Glucocorticoids and bronchodilators remain the mainstay of pharmacologic therapy. Empiric antibiotics are recommended only when suspicion for a specific infection is high. Various adjunctive therapies exist for very severe asthma and may contribute to effective ventilation and resolution of the exacerbation; however, most of these lack strong evidence to recommend their use. These include high-dose magnesium sulfate, helium-oxygen mixtures (heliox, often in a ratio of 80:20 or 60:40), sedation with ketamine, and general anesthesia. **H**

[handwritten annotation: "→ blow off CO_2"]

KEY POINTS

- Arterial blood gas analysis often shows hypocapnia in patients with severe asthma exacerbation, but a normal or mildly elevated CO_2 level can be a sign of respiratory muscle fatigue and impending failure.
- If the FEV_1 and peak expiratory flow do not respond to aggressive bronchodilator and glucocorticoid therapy to above 40% of predicted, patients with severe asthma exacerbation should be admitted to the ICU for close monitoring and aggressive therapy.

Critical Care Management of COPD Exacerbation
Patients with severe COPD exacerbation present similarly to patients with asthma, with respiratory muscle fatigue from increased work of breathing. Their CO_2 levels are usually high, with a pH indicating an acute respiratory acidosis. If hypoxic, they should be given supplemental oxygen even if CO_2 is

elevated at baseline. Some of these patients rely on arterial Po_2 for respiratory drive; in these individuals, a reasonable oxygen saturation goal is 90% to 92%. If patients display signs of respiratory failure, ventilatory support is needed; noninvasive support is often effective in this situation. If a trial of noninvasive ventilation with bilevel PAP is not effective in reducing the work of breathing or the patient develops significant hypercapnia (usually meaning a level of CO_2 higher than the patient's normal level, which is worsening or not improving with therapy), the patient should be intubated and mechanically ventilated. Patients with COPD exacerbation have the same risk for air trapping and auto-PEEP as patients with asthma; therefore, the same ventilatory strategies should be used to avoid these issues. Patients intubated for COPD are unique in that when their respiratory parameters are improved, they are often extubated directly to bilevel noninvasive PAP, which is not usually done for other intubated patients. The same pharmacologic strategies that are used in less severe COPD exacerbations, including glucocorticoids, bronchodilators, and empiric antibiotics, should be continued (see Airways Disease, Chronic Obstructive Pulmonary Disease). **H**

KEY POINTS

- If patients with a COPD exacerbation display signs of respiratory failure, ventilatory support is needed; noninvasive support is often effective in this situation.
- If a trial of noninvasive ventilation is not effective to reduce the work of breathing in patients with COPD exacerbation, the patient should be intubated and mechanically ventilated.

Sepsis

Definition, Pathophysiology, and Clinical Presentation **H**

Sepsis is an intense host inflammatory response to a known or suspected infection that causes systemic manifestations remote from the site of infection. The sepsis response causes generalized vasodilation, increased microvascular permeability, and widespread cellular injury that result in multiorgan dysfunction. Severe sepsis is defined as sepsis that causes inadequate organ perfusion or outright organ dysfunction, and the term septic shock refers to sepsis-related hypotension that persists despite fluid resuscitation. In addition to demonstrating evidence of infection, patients with these advanced forms of sepsis present with characteristic derangements in their vital signs, physical examination findings, and laboratory studies (Table 52).

Early recognition of sepsis is based on signs of developing end-organ failure. However, signs and symptoms in early sepsis may be subtle and nonspecific, and timely diagnosis can be confounded by baseline comorbidities (for example, dementia) and medications (for example, β-blockers). Therefore, evidence of organ dysfunction in suspected sepsis should be actively sought (for example, evaluation for mild cognitive impairment or low urine output) since delays in treatment of

TABLE 52. Diagnostic Criteria for Sepsis[a]

Infection, documented or suspected, and some of the following:

General variables

Fever (>38.3 °C [100.9 °F])

Hypothermia (core temperature <36.0 °C [96.8 °F])

Heart rate >90/min or >2 SD above normal value for age

Tachypnea

Altered mental status

Significant edema or positive fluid balance (>20 mL/kg over 24 h)

Hyperglycemia (plasma glucose >140 mg/dL [7.8 mmol/L]) in absence of diabetes

Inflammatory variables

Leukocytosis (leukocyte count >12,000/μL [12 × 10⁹/L])

Leukopenia (leukocyte count <4000/μL [4 × 10⁹/L])

Normal leukocyte count with >10% immature forms

Plasma C-reactive protein >2 SD above normal value

Plasma procalcitonin >2 SD above normal value

Hemodynamic variables

Arterial hypotension (SBP <90 mm Hg, MAP <70 mm Hg, or SBP decrease >40 mm Hg in adults or <2 SD below normal for age)

Organ dysfunction variables

Arterial hypoxemia (Po$_2$/Fio$_2$ <300 mm Hg [39.9 kPa])

Acute oliguria (urine output <0.5 mL/kg/h for >2 h despite adequate fluid resuscitation)

Serum creatinine increase >0.5 mg/dL (44.2 μmol/L)

Coagulation abnormalities (INR >1.5 or aPTT >60 s)

Ileus (absent bowel sounds)

Thrombocytopenia (platelet count <100,000/μL [100 × 10⁹/L])

Hyperbilirubinemia (plasma total bilirubin >4 mg/dL [68.4 μmol/L])

Tissue perfusion variables

Hyperlactatemia (>1 mEq/L [1 mmol/L])

Decreased capillary refill or mottling

aPTT = activated partial thromboplastin time; INR = international normalized ratio; MAP = mean arterial pressure; SBP = systolic blood pressure; SD = standard deviation.

[a]Diagnostic criteria for sepsis in the pediatric population are signs and symptoms of inflammation plus infection with hyper- or hypothermia (rectal temperature >38.5 °C [101.3 °F] or <35.0 °C [95.0 °F]), tachycardia (may be absent in hypothermic patients), and at least one of the following indications of altered organ function: altered mental status, hypoxemia, increased serum lactate level, or bounding pulses.

Springer and Intensive Care Medicine, Volume 39, 2013, 165-228, 2012 Surviving Sepsis Campaign: international guidelines for management of severe sepsis and septic shock 2012, Dellinger RP, Levy MM, Rhodes A, et al, Table 1, with kind permission from Springer Science and Business Media.

 early sepsis are associated with higher mortality. Unlike most shock states, early sepsis typically produces bounding pulses and warm rather than cool extremities. Measurement of plasma lactate may identify early sepsis in normotensive patients in need of aggressive fluid resuscitation despite having a normal blood pressure. **H**

KEY POINTS

- Early recognition of sepsis is based on signs of developing end-organ failure.
- Delays in treatment of early sepsis are associated with higher mortality.

Epidemiology

Not only is the annual incidence of sepsis increasing worldwide, but severe sepsis and septic shock account for a growing proportion of all cases. These more severe forms carry a 25% mortality risk. Absence of baseline comorbidities, urinary tract site of infection, community-acquired infection, early administration of appropriate antibiotics, and aggressive hemodynamic support predict lower mortality.

Management

Successful treatment of severe sepsis and septic shock depends on the rapid institution of hemodynamic support, empiric treatment of infection, and diagnostic studies. To that end, the following interventions should be performed concomitantly rather than sequentially.

KEY POINT

- Successful treatment of severe sepsis and septic shock depends on the rapid institution of hemodynamic support, empiric treatment of infection, and diagnostic studies.

Initial Resuscitation

Morbidity and mortality in patients with sepsis are heavily influenced by the care delivered during the first several hours after sepsis onset. Multiple clinical trials have established the critical role of timely recognition of sepsis and early goal-directed therapy (EGDT), defined as aggressive management of specific clinical parameters to specified targets, in improving clinical outcomes. Once sepsis is recognized, EGDT interventions focus on adequate fluid resuscitation with intravenous fluid and vasopressors to support blood pressure and avoid organ hypoperfusion and multiorgan injury, as well as early treatment of infection.

Patients with severe sepsis and septic shock usually have clinically apparent evidence of end-organ injury due to hypoperfusion. Hypotension is often the most evident manifestation of hypoperfusion and has been defined as serial systolic blood pressure readings less than 90 mm Hg or mean arterial pressure less than 70 mm Hg. Lactic acidosis also supports organ injury due to hypoperfusion and is used to identify patients with severe sepsis and septic shock.

Crystalloid infusion (normal [0.9%] saline or lactated Ringer solution) to support circulating intravascular volume should be administered to all patients with severe sepsis and septic shock. Crystalloid is recommended at a volume of 30 mL/kg body weight, with most patients receiving between 2 to 4 L as the initial intervention to treat shock due to sepsis.

Recent evidence has shown that chloride-rich fluids increase the risk of acute kidney injury in sepsis, and switching from normal saline to lower chloride alternatives such as lactated Ringer solution may reduce the risk of kidney failure in patients requiring large-volume resuscitation. Multiple trials indicate albumin and crystalloids are equally effective for fluid resuscitation in patients with sepsis, although albumin may be advantageous in the subset of patients with low oncotic pressure and persistently low intravascular filling pressures. Crystalloids are less expensive and considered first-line therapy. The synthetic colloid hydroxyethyl starch increases the risk of kidney failure in patients with sepsis and is not recommended.

The optimal targets to measure adequacy of resuscitation are not clear. A commonly used measure is central venous pressure (CVP) with a goal of 8 to 12 mm Hg. Although CVP does not consistently reflect volume status, a low CVP generally can be relied on as a marker of fluid responsiveness. Urine output of 0.5 mL/kg/h or greater is also indicative of adequate fluid resuscitation, but this marker may not be feasible in patients with acute kidney injury associated with hypoperfusion. Central venous oxygen saturation ($Scvo_2$) is used as an indicator of adequacy of oxygenation, reflecting the balance between oxygen delivery and consumption. A $Scvo_2$ greater than or equal to 70% has been recommended as a target for adequacy of resuscitation.

The current Surviving Sepsis Campaign guidelines recommend measurement of CVP and serial measurement of $Scvo_2$ to assess the adequacy of resuscitation, with failure to achieve the target $Scvo_2$ during the first 6 hours of resuscitation being an indication for initiation of inotropes and blood transfusion. However, several recent studies that did not use CVP or $Scvo_2$ monitoring to guide resuscitation had similar outcomes compared with patients managed with EGDT using these endpoints. Therefore, the utility of CVP and $Scvo_2$ monitoring compared with clinical judgment and other measures of fluid responsiveness is unclear, and further study of methods for assessing adequacy of resuscitation are ongoing.

Current Surviving Sepsis Campaign guidelines also recommend serial plasma lactate measurements to assess the adequacy of resuscitation. Among patients with elevated lactate levels, resuscitation is targeted to reduce levels by 10% to 20% over the first 6 hours. While aggressive fluid resuscitation is efficacious in the first several hours of sepsis management, judicious fluid administration is warranted thereafter, as intravascular volume overload can contribute to pulmonary edema and pleural effusions.

If hypotension does not rapidly correct with fluids, vasopressors should be titrated to maintain a mean arterial pressure of 65 mm Hg or greater. Norepinephrine is considered first-line therapy. Dopamine is known to cause tachyarrhythmia and should be reserved for selected patients with hypoperfusion and relative bradycardia. Vasopressin, epinephrine, and phenylephrine typically are added when norepinephrine alone is insufficient.

KEY POINT

- Early fluid resuscitation in sepsis warrants close monitoring and often entails serial measurements of blood pressure, central venous pressure, urine output, central venous oxygen saturation, serial plasma lactate measurements, and a variety of noninvasive assessments of fluid responsiveness.

Antibiotic Therapy

In septic shock, mortality increases with each hour that appropriate antibiotic therapy is delayed. Two sets of blood cultures should be obtained before antibiotic infusion, in addition to cultures from the suspected infection site. However, antibiotics should ideally be administered within 1 hour of diagnosis, even if full cultures have not been obtained. Empiric antimicrobial treatment should cover all suspected pathogens, with special attention to risk factors for resistant or opportunistic organisms, including methicillin-resistant *Staphylococcus aureus* and *Pseudomonas* species. The latter organisms merit empiric combination antibiotic therapy. Indications for empiric coverage of *Candida* species include recent antibiotic exposure, use of total parenteral nutrition, colonization in multiple sites, and impaired immune function. Allowable speed of administration, penetration into the infected site, drug-drug interactions, recent antibiotic exposure, local anti-infective resistance patterns, allergies, and comorbidities such as hepatic failure and acute kidney injury are important considerations in antimicrobial selection. De-escalation of empiric coverage should be considered daily depending on culture results and clinical course. Treatment should be narrowed to coverage of the causative organism alone if identified.

KEY POINT

- Broad, empiric antimicrobial coverage should be initiated within 1 hour of diagnosis of sepsis, even if obtaining cultures is incomplete.

Source Control

Identification and control of the source of infection are critical steps in managing sepsis; this ideally should be achieved within 12 hours using the highest yield and lowest risk diagnostic intervention available. Respiratory and skin sources of sepsis are usually readily identified by history, examination, and chest radiography. In contrast, the diagnosis of abdominal sepsis can be challenging, particularly in obtunded or sedated patients (see Acute Abdominal Surgical Emergencies). Antibiotics alone may be insufficient to control infection in a variety of scenarios, such as severe colitis, necrotizing fasciitis, and ascending cholangitis.

Adjunctive Therapies

Although hydrocortisone improves hypotension in septic shock, the bulk of evidence suggests no mortality reduction. Patients with persistent shock despite fluids and vasopressors may be an exception, and the current Surviving Sepsis

Campaign guidelines recommend a daily total dose of 200 mg of intravenous hydrocortisone in this setting. Addition of a mineralocorticoid is unnecessary, and cortisol stimulation testing to identify patients with relative adrenal insufficiency is not recommended. However, stress-dose hydrocortisone is indicated for persistently hypotensive patients with baseline adrenal insufficiency, as well as in at-risk patients, such as those on chronic, low-dose systemic glucocorticoids.

Hyperglycemia is common in critically ill patients and is associated with increased morbidity and mortality. A study of intensive insulin therapy, which targeted plasma glucose levels between 80 and 110 mg/dL (4.4 and 6.1 mmol/L), found reduced mortality in postsurgical patients. However, in the subsequent landmark NICE-SUGAR trial, intensive insulin therapy resulted in higher mortality among patients in the medical and surgical ICU compared with maintaining plasma glucose levels between 144 and 180 mg/dL (8.0 and 10.0 mmol/L). The American College of Physicians guideline recommends that, following initial stabilization, patients with severe sepsis and hyperglycemia who are admitted to the ICU should receive insulin therapy to achieve a plasma glucose level between 140 and 200 mg/dL (7.8 and 11.1 mmol/L). Some guidelines use a threshold of two consecutive plasma glucose levels greater than 180 mg/dL (10.0 mmol/L) for initiating intravenous insulin.

Indications for invasive mechanical ventilation in patients with sepsis include hypoxemia, increased work of breathing, and encephalopathy with compromised airway protection. A lung-protective ventilator strategy that utilizes low tidal volumes is recommended when ARDS is present. The role of noninvasive ventilation in ARDS is limited, given a lack of efficacy in clinical trials and the high prevalence of concomitant encephalopathy.

Thrombocytopenia often complicates septic shock. In the absence of active bleeding, the Surviving Sepsis Campaign guidelines recommend a threshold of less than 10,000/µL (10×10^9/L) for platelet transfusion but a threshold of less than 20,000/µL (20×10^9/L) in the presence of risk factors, which include fever, recent minor hemorrhage, rapid decline in platelet count, and concomitant coagulation abnormalities. The 2012 American College of Chest Physicians guidelines on thrombosis prevention recommend mechanical, rather than pharmacologic, deep venous thrombosis prophylaxis in critically ill patients with platelet counts less than 50,000/µL (50×10^9/L).

Acute Inhalational Injuries

Smoke Inhalation

Smoke inhalation is the leading cause of fire-related deaths, with mortality and morbidity occurring through three distinct pathways: thermal injury to the upper airway, irritant-mediated injury to the tracheobronchial tree, and poisoning from carbon monoxide and hydrogen cyanide (see Carbon Monoxide Poisoning and Cyanide Poisoning). Ensuring upper airway patency is the first priority in patients with significant smoke exposure. Intense heat can cause edema and blistering from the mouth to the larynx; subglottic thermal injury is uncommon. Patients with a visibly damaged airway or stridor are at high risk of complete upper airway obstruction due to swelling and require immediate intubation. In less severe cases, fiberoptic laryngoscopy can identify laryngeal edema that may warrant prophylactic intubation. Patients who are not immediately intubated should be monitored closely, especially those requiring massive fluid resuscitation that may result in increased soft tissue edema surrounding the injured airway. Treatment is supportive but requires confirmation that upper airway patency has been restored before extubation. This typically entails assessing for the presence of a cuff leak when the endotracheal tube cuff is deflated, but direct endoscopic visualization of the vocal cords also may be helpful in ambiguous cases.

Patients with inhalational injury involving the lower airways typically present with a normal chest radiograph. Wheezing, cough, and dyspnea are early signs of tracheobronchial injury, generally manifesting 12 to 36 hours after exposure. Patients are at risk of subsequent airway necrosis, mucosal sloughing, bleeding, copious secretions, atelectasis, pneumonia, and ARDS. Fiberoptic bronchoscopy can reveal the extent of injury and facilitate clearance of airway debris and secretions. In patients requiring intubation owing to inhalational injury–associated ARDS, a low tidal volume strategy is appropriate. Bronchospasm is treated with bronchodilators. Limited data support the use of nebulized heparin and nebulized N-acetylcysteine to promote clearance of blood clots and secretions. Long-term respiratory outcomes are generally favorable among survivors. **H**

KEY POINTS

- Ensuring upper airway patency is the first priority in patients with significant smoke inhalation.
- Patients with tracheobronchial injury are at risk of subsequent airway necrosis, mucosal sloughing, bleeding, copious secretions, atelectasis, pneumonia, and acute respiratory distress syndrome.

Other Forms of Inhalational Injury

Upper airway and lung injury occur in a variety of settings, including occupational exposures (see Airways Disease, Asthma), use of recreational drugs, and exposure to chemical terrorism agents. Cocaine inhalation commonly causes bronchospasm and sputum production, but it can also precipitate pulmonary edema, pulmonary hemorrhage, pneumothorax, and thermal upper airway injury (in the case of free-basing cocaine and use of crack cocaine pipes). Inhalation of chlorine, ammonia, and riot-control agents causes rapid onset of upper airway irritation and respiratory distress. Phosgene gas can also cause life-threatening ARDS, but this typically manifests several hours after exposure.

Anaphylaxis

Anaphylaxis is defined as a severe, potentially life-threatening allergic or hypersensitivity reaction that occurs within seconds to a few hours of allergen exposure, most commonly food, medication, or an insect sting. Classically, anaphylaxis occurs when allergen-specific IgE coating the surface of mast cells and basophils comes in contact with the triggering allergen, thereby precipitating cellular degranulation. The resulting abrupt systemic release of a host of mediators has a variety of effects including vasoconstriction, vasodilatation, increased vascular permeability, and bronchoconstriction. The presentation is variable, and predicting the ultimate severity of the episode is difficult. Therefore, optimal management is contingent on prompt recognition and treatment. The diagnosis of anaphylaxis is dependent on the presence of multiorgan system involvement and/or exposure to a known or suspected allergen. Signs and symptoms according to organ system are summarized in **Table 53**. The nonspecific presentation makes recognition particularly difficult in critically ill patients already experiencing respiratory distress, hypotension, or anxiety.

In addition to eliminating exposure to the inciting agent, treatment entails early administration of epinephrine, either intramuscularly or as a continuous intravenous infusion. H$_1$ antihistamines relieve skin symptoms, whereas systemic glucocorticoids reduce the risk of recurrent or persistent symptoms. Repeat epinephrine administration may be needed until antihistamines or glucocorticoids become effective. Severely affected patients may require fluid resuscitation, vasopressors, and intubation due to upper airway edema. Following recovery, patients should maintain home access to an epinephrine autoinjector and may benefit from evaluation for anaphylactic triggers.

It is important to differentiate anaphylactic from nonallergic causes of upper airway edema, as the treatment differs substantially. Compared with anaphylaxis, nonallergic angioedema generally is not associated with pruritus or urticaria and usually has a more gradual onset. Medications, most commonly ACE inhibitors, can trigger angioedema via elevation of bradykinin levels. In these patients, management is primarily supportive and includes discontinuation of the offending medication and prompt intubation if the airway becomes compromised. The treatment of hereditary and acquired causes of angioedema, such as C1 inhibitor deficiency, centers on therapies to counter aberrant bradykinin and complement activation.

KEY POINTS

- The diagnosis of anaphylaxis is dependent on the presence of multiorgan system involvement and/or exposure to a known or suspected allergen; skin or mucosal involvement is present in 85% of affected patients.

- In addition to eliminating exposure to the inciting agent, treatment of anaphylaxis entails early administration of epinephrine, either intramuscularly or as a continuous intravenous infusion.

Hypertensive Emergencies

Hypertensive emergency refers to elevation of systolic blood pressure greater than 180 mm Hg and/or diastolic blood pressure greater than 120 mm Hg that is associated with end-organ damage; however, in some conditions such as pregnancy, more modest blood pressure elevation can constitute an emergency. An equal degree of hypertension but without end-organ damage constitutes a hypertensive urgency, the treatment of which requires gradual blood pressure reduction over several hours. Patients with hypertensive emergency require rapid, tightly controlled reductions in blood pressure that avoid overcorrection. Management typically occurs in an ICU with continuous arterial blood pressure monitoring and continuous infusion of antihypertensive agents. An expedited evaluation for the cause of hypertension as well as assessing for the presence of end-organ failure, including encephalopathy, focal neurologic deficits (including vision changes), myocardial ischemia, heart failure, and acute kidney injury, should be performed. Diagnostic studies should be driven by clinical suspicion (**Table 54**).

A paucity of treatment trials exists for hypertensive emergencies. However, the choice of antihypertensive medication and the degree of acute blood pressure reduction are guided by a strong pathophysiologic rationale for any given clinical scenario (see Table 54).

TABLE 53. Organ System Involvement in Anaphylaxis

Organ System	Symptoms	Signs	% of Patients with Organ Involved
Skin and mucosa	Pruritus of skin, oropharynx, genitals, palms, soles	Flushing, urticaria, angioedema	85%
Respiratory	Dyspnea, chest and throat tightness, stridor, cough, hoarseness, sneezing, rhinorrhea	Wheeze, stridor, respiratory distress	70%
Cardiovascular	Lightheadedness, chest pain, palpitations	Hypotension, tachycardia > bradycardia	45%
Gastrointestinal	Pain, nausea, vomiting, diarrhea		45%
Neurologic	Sense of impending doom, headache	Encephalopathy	15%

TABLE 54. Presentation and Treatment of Hypertensive Emergencies

Emergency	Presentation	Initial Diagnostic Studies	Target Blood Pressure (mm Hg)	First-Line Agents	Notes
Hypertensive encephalopathy	Confusion, headache, vision changes	Head CT to exclude stroke and hemorrhage	↓ by 15%-20% or DBP to 100-110	Nicardipine Labetalol Nitroprusside	Risk of cyanide toxicity with nitroprusside
Ischemic stroke	Focal deficit, CNS depression, seizure	Head CT	Treat if SBP >220 or DBP >120; ↓ by 15%	Nicardipine Labetalol Nitroprusside	Target BP <185/110 mm Hg if a candidate for thrombolytic therapy
Hemorrhagic stroke	Focal neurologic deficit, CNS depression, seizure	Head CT	BP 160/90 or MAP 110	Nicardipine Labetalol	+/- intracranial pressure monitor to target BP
Aortic dissection	Chest, back pain; asymmetric BP; acute aortic regurgitation	Chest radiograph with wide mediastinum CT angiogram	SBP 100-120	Esmolol or labetalol first, add nitroprusside as needed	Target HR <65/min
Myocardial infarction	Chest pain, dyspnea, nausea	Electrocardiogram Troponin	MAP 60-100	Nitroglycerin β-Blocker	Avoid hydralazine
Acute left-sided heart failure	Dyspnea, crackles	Chest radiograph	MAP 60-100	Nitroglycerin and/or nitroprusside	Caution with calcium and β-blockers, hydralazine
Acute kidney injury	Usually no symptoms	↑ Cr, proteinuria	↓ by 20%-25%	Fenoldopam Nicardipine β-Blocker	ACE if scleroderma renal crisis
Preeclampsia, eclampsia	SBP >160 mm Hg or DBP >110 mm Hg, edema, seizure	Proteinuria ↑ liver chemistry studies, ↑Cr ↓ platelets	SBP 130-150 DBP 80-100	Labetalol Hydralazine	Avoid ACE inhibitor and nitroprusside Delivery = "cure"
Sympathomimetic drug use	Diaphoresis, mydriasis, ↑ BP	History Urine drug screen	↓ by 20%-25%	Nicardipine Nitroprusside	Benzodiazepine first Avoid β-blocker
Pheochromocytoma	↑ HR, diaphoresis, headache	Urine and plasma metanephrines	↓ by 20%-25%	Phentolamine Nitroprusside	Avoid β-blocker

ACE = angiotensin-converting enzyme; BNP = B-type natriuretic peptide; BP = blood pressure; CNS = central nervous system; Cr = serum creatinine; DBP = diastolic blood pressure; HR = heart rate; MAP = mean arterial pressure; SBP = systolic blood pressure.

KEY POINTS

- Hypertensive emergency refers to elevation of systolic blood pressure greater than 180 mm Hg and/or diastolic blood pressure greater than 120 mm Hg that is associated with end-organ damage.
- Patients with hypertensive emergency require rapid, tightly controlled reductions in blood pressure that avoid overcorrection.

Hyperthermic Emergencies

Severe hyperthermia is a life-threatening elevation of core body temperature to greater than 40.0 °C (104.0 °F). Unlike fever, which stems from an inflammatory response, hyperthermia is due to a failure of normal thermoregulation.

Heat Stroke

Heat stroke occurs with high ambient temperature and humidity and is defined by the presence of temperature greater than 40.0 °C (104.0 °F) and encephalopathy. It is often associated with hypotension, gastrointestinal distress, and weakness. Patients with advanced heat stroke exhibit shock, multiorgan failure, rhabdomyolysis, and myocardial ischemia. Exertional heat stroke typically occurs in healthy individuals undergoing vigorous physical activity in warm conditions. In contrast, the majority of patients with nonexertional heat stroke are older than 70 years or have chronic medical conditions that impair thermal regulation. Medications and recreational drugs with anticholinergic, sympathomimetic, and diuretic effects, including alcohol, pose added risk.

CONT.

The diagnosis typically is made based on the clinical context and physical examination. The differential diagnosis includes other causes of hyperthermia (**Table 55**), infection, stroke, seizures, and toxin ingestions. Rapid, sustained improvement in temperature with cooling interventions strongly suggests heat stroke. The primary treatment for nonexertional heat stroke is evaporative, external cooling. This involves removing all clothing and spraying the patient with a mist of lukewarm water while continuously blowing fans on the patient. Ice packs on the neck, axillae, and groin augment cooling. Ice water immersion is recommended for exertional heat stroke in young patients if intubation or close monitoring is unnecessary. Cooling should be continued until the rectal temperature falls to approximately 38.5 °C (101.3 °F). The usual response is sufficiently rapid enough that invasive interventions are largely unneeded. Antipyretic agents and dantrolene are not effective. 🅷

KEY POINTS

- Rapid, sustained improvement in temperature with cooling interventions strongly suggests heat stroke.
- Exertional heat stroke is often treated with ice water immersion, whereas nonexertional heat stroke is typically managed with evaporative external cooling.

🅷 **Malignant Hyperthermia**

Malignant hyperthermia is an uncommon cause of severe hyperthermia that occurs in genetically susceptible individuals upon exposure to a volatile anesthetic such as halothane or isoflurane. Features include mixed respiratory and metabolic acidosis, muscle rigidity, hyperkalemia, and rhabdomyolysis. Treatment includes prompt discontinuation of the triggering agent, increase in minute ventilation, bicarbonate infusion, correction of hyperkalemia, and dantrolene.

Neuroleptic Malignant Syndrome

Neuroleptic malignant syndrome (NMS) is associated with the use of neuroleptic medications and is characterized by the presence of encephalopathy, muscle rigidity, autonomic instability, and fever. Although most frequently described with older agents such as haloperidol, NMS can occur with atypical neuroleptics, including olanzapine, quetiapine, and risperidone. Antiemetic medications (including metoclopramide) and dose reduction of antiparkinson medications are also associated with NMS. The features of NMS overlap substantially with severe serotonin syndrome (see Table 55). Serotonin syndrome can be distinguished from NMS by the presence of hyperreflexia and myoclonus.

Accidental Hypothermia

Accidental hypothermia stereotypically affects young outdoor enthusiasts in cold climates, but in reality it occurs worldwide, in all seasons, often without outdoor exposure, and disproportionately among the elderly. Risk factors in addition to advanced age include chronic medical conditions, malnutrition, psychiatric illness, homelessness, and chemical dependency. The clinical manifestations of hypothermia vary depending on the severity (**Table 56**). Osborne or J waves (**Figure 23**) appear at temperatures less than 33.0 °C (91.4 °F) and should not be confused with myocardial ischemia. J waves can be present in the absence of known disease.

A critical first step in management is initiating passive external rewarming, which entails removing wet clothing and covering the patient with insulating material, especially the head and neck. Owing to a paucity of rewarming trials in accidental hypothermia, institutional resources and expertise play a major role in treatment selection. However, for mildly hypothermic, healthy individuals capable of shivering, passive external rewarming alone suffices. Active external rewarming using warm blankets or a forced heated air blanket is commonly used in hemodynamically stable patients with moderate hypothermia, when passive external rewarming proves

TABLE 55.	Causes of Severe Hyperthermia			
Diagnosis	**Suggestive History**	**Key Examination Findings**	**Treatment**	**Notes**
Heat stroke	Environmental exposure	Encephalopathy and fever	Evaporative cooling Ice water immersion	Avoid ice water immersion if nonexertional heat stroke
Malignant hyperthermia	Exposure to volatile anesthetic	Masseter muscle rigidity; ↑ arterial P_{CO_2}	Stop inciting drug Dantrolene	Monitor and treat ↑ K+ and ↑ arterial P_{CO_2}
Neuroleptic malignant syndrome	Typical > atypical antipsychotic agent; onset over days to weeks	Altered mentation, severe rigidity, ↑ HR, ↑ BP, no clonus, hyporeflexia	Stop the inciting drug Dantrolene Bromocriptine	Resolves over days to weeks Mentation change first
Severe serotonin syndrome[a]	Onset within 24 h of initiation or increasing drug dose, gastrointestinal prodrome	Agitation, clonus, ↑ reflexes, rigidity	Stop inciting drug Benzodiazepines Cyproheptadine	Resolves in 24 h

BP = blood pressure; HR = heart rate; K+ = potassium.

[a]Not routinely considered a cause of severe hyperthermia but commonly confused with neuroleptic malignant syndrome.

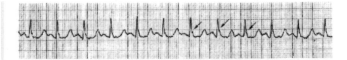

TABLE 56. Presentation of Hypothermia by Severity

Severity	Temperature	Findings
Mild	32.0-35.0 °C (89.6-95.0 °F)	↑HR, ↑BP, ↑RR, shivering, alert, poor judgment
Moderate	28.0-32.0 °C (82.4-89.6 °F)	↓HR, ↓BP, ↓RR, ↓CO, ↓O_2 consumption, ↓kidney function, somnolence, no shivering, supraventricular arrhythmia
Severe	<28.0 °C (82.4 °F)	Coma, absent reflexes, ventricular arrhythmia, asystole, apnea

BP = blood pressure; CO = cardiac output; HR = heart rate; RR = respiration rate.

FIGURE 23. Electrocardiogram showing Osborne waves (arrows). Hypothermia may be associated with sinus bradycardia or with atrial fibrillation, and the appearance of the classic Osborne waves at the QT interval. They are best seen in the inferior and lateral chest leads. Osborne waves are defined by the shoulder or "hump" between QRS and ST segments.

CONT.

inadequate in mild hypothermia, or as an adjunct in severe hypothermia. Administering warmed intravenous fluids (42.0 °C [107.6 °F]) transfers only a modest amount of heat but at least prevents further temperature declines associated with infusing large volumes of room-temperature fluids. Body cavity lavage with warm fluids is an option for patients with hypothermia that is severe or does not respond to external warming, particularly if there is no access to intravascular rewarming devices. The colon, bladder, and stomach are readily accessible for irrigation but have a small surface area for heat exchange. Rewarming by peritoneal or pleural space irrigation is supported by case reports. Although reported experience is limited, endovascular warming devices, which are routinely used for therapeutic hypothermia, are an attractive option for severely affected but hemodynamically stable patients. Extracorporeal support, including cardiopulmonary bypass, is recommended for patients in cardiac arrest because it maximizes the rewarming rate and can provide hemodynamic support. Conventional treatment of ventricular arrhythmias and asystole is often ineffective until the temperature is raised to greater than 30.0 °C (86.0 °F). Because severe hypothermia may appear clinically similar to death, aggressive rewarming is appropriate in all patients in a suggestive clinical situation in the absence of obvious irreversible signs of death. **H**

KEY POINT

- Mild cases of hypothermia in healthy patients generally respond to passive external rewarming, whereas unstable patients with severe hypothermia are best treated with invasive measures, including cardiopulmonary bypass.

H **Toxicology**

Treatment of patients with poisoning may require aggressive measures to stabilize extremes of blood pressure, in addition to endotracheal intubation for inadequate ventilation or airway protection, particularly if vomiting is present. Initial empiric treatment of patients with encephalopathy includes thiamine to prevent Wernicke encephalopathy and dextrose for hypoglycemia unless these diagnoses can be rapidly excluded. In addition to fingerstick glucose testing, the initial evaluation generally includes measurement of the acetaminophen level and salicylate level, analysis of QRS and QT intervals on electrocardiogram, and pregnancy testing in women of childbearing age. Urine toxicology screen is warranted in patients with severe symptoms or when the cause remains unclear after initial evaluation. Early consultation with a regional poison control center should be done in the case of severe or unfamiliar poisonings.

Alcohol Poisoning

A key early step in suspected alcohol toxicity is determining whether alcohol ingestion entirely accounts for the patient's presentation. The initial evaluation should consider infectious, neurologic, metabolic, and endocrinologic causes of central nervous system depression, as well as coingestion of other substances. Determination of the specific alcohol consumed is also a priority, as toxicity and treatment vary substantially between ethanol, isopropyl alcohol, ethylene glycol, and methanol poisoning (**Table 57**). In addition to venous or arterial blood gas measurement, initial laboratory evaluation includes measurement of the serum ethanol level, glucose, electrolytes, ketones, kidney function, and osmolality. Calculation of the anion and plasma osmolal gaps aids in the diagnosis (see Table 57).

Anion gap elevation can be more severe in methanol and ethylene glycol poisoning than is typically seen with salicylate poisoning, lactic acidosis, and ketosis. Ethanol and isopropyl alcohol do not directly increase the anion gap.

A plasma osmolal gap greater than 10 is abnormal and is characteristic of all alcohols, but it lacks sensitivity and specificity. For example, an osmolal gap greater than 25 is highly compatible with early severe methanol or ethylene glycol poisoning, but the gap may normalize with delayed presentation.

Early administration of the alcohol dehydrogenase inhibitor fomepizole prevents breakdown of methanol and ethylene glycol into toxic metabolites. This may require empiric therapy while awaiting laboratory confirmation. Ethanol can be used to compete for alcohol dehydrogenase activity when fomepizole is unavailable, but titration can be difficult.

For information on alcohol withdrawal, see MKSAP 17 General Internal Medicine. **H**

TABLE 57. Presentation and Treatment of Alcohol Poisoning

Alcohol	Common Sources	Major Findings	Anion Gap	Osmolal Gap[a]	Treatment
Ethanol	Alcoholic beverages	CNS depression Nausea, emesis	No	NA	Supportive care
Isopropyl alcohol	Rubbing alcohol Disinfectants Antifreeze	CNS depression Ketone elevation	No	Yes	Supportive care
Methanol	Windshield wiper fluid De-icing solutions Solvents "Moonshine"	CNS depression Vision loss Hypotension	Yes	Yes	Fomepizole Ethanol (second-line) Dialysis (if severe) Folic acid
Ethylene glycol	Antifreeze De-icing solutions Solvents	CNS depression Acute kidney injury Hypocalcemia Hypotension	Yes	Yes	Fomepizole Ethanol (second-line) Dialysis (if severe)

BUN = blood urea nitrogen; CNS = central nervous system; Na = sodium; NA = not applicable.

[a]The osmolal gap represents the difference between the measured osmolality and calculated osmolality. The calculated osmolality = $(2 \times [Na]) + [glucose (mg/dL)]/18 + [BUN (mg/dL)]/2.8$.

KEY POINT

- Ethylene glycol and methanol poisoning cause an elevated anion gap and an elevated osmolal gap; treatment is with fomepizole.

Carbon Monoxide Poisoning

Carbon monoxide poisoning causes thousands of deaths annually in the United States, with smoke inhalation as the leading cause of inadvertent exposure. Inhaled carbon monoxide has a much higher affinity for hemoglobin binding sites than oxygen and readily forms carboxyhemoglobin, which is an ineffective oxygen transporter and results in reduced tissue oxygen content. Symptoms of carbon monoxide poisoning vary and include headache, confusion, nausea, vomiting, and, in severe cases, loss of consciousness. It is important to understand that carboxyhemoglobin does not lower oxygen saturation measured by standard pulse oximetry or reduce arterial Po_2 determined by blood gas analysis. Co-oximetry, which measures carboxyhemoglobin levels, is used to make the diagnosis. Carboxyhemoglobin levels normally are less than 3% but can be 10% to 15% in heavy smokers. Myocardial ischemia is common in patients with carbon monoxide poisoning, and delayed onset of cognitive dysfunction, focal neurologic deficits, and movement disorders can arise even months after exposure.

Carbon monoxide is removed by competitive binding of oxygen to hemoglobin. The initial treatment is administration of 100% oxygen, which reduces the half-life of carboxyhemoglobin from 5 hours to 90 minutes. Hyperbaric oxygen therapy yields an even higher alveolar partial pressure of oxygen, thereby reducing the half-life to 30 minutes while substantially increasing the amount of oxygen directly dissolved in blood. Consensus is lacking on the use of hyperbaric therapy in carbon monoxide poisoning, but commonly cited indications include carboxyhemoglobin levels greater than 25% (or >20% in pregnant patients), persistent organ ischemia, and loss of consciousness. Carbon monoxide poisoning resulting from smoke inhalation should prompt consideration of concomitant cyanide poisoning.

KEY POINT

- Carbon monoxide poisoning presents with normal oxygen saturation as measured by standard pulse oximetry, is diagnosed with co-oximetry, and is treated with 100% oxygen and/or hyperbaric oxygen therapy.

Cyanide Poisoning

Acute cyanide poisoning primarily occurs through fire and occupational exposures and rarely from medications such as sodium nitroprusside. Cyanide disrupts oxidative phosphorylation, forcing cells to convert to anaerobic metabolism despite adequate oxygen supply. The result in severe cases is multiorgan failure with coma, seizures, and cardiovascular symptoms, including hypotension, bradycardia, heart block, and ventricular arrhythmias. Early manifestations are nonspecific. Diagnostic clues include lactic acidosis and inappropriately elevated $Scvo_2$, which manifests as bright red venous blood. Cherry-red skin color, a classic finding, is infrequently encountered. Cyanide levels are not readily available and since toxicity is rapidly fatal, prompt empiric treatment is imperative in suspected cases. Recommended treatment includes sodium thiosulfate in combination with either hydroxocobalamin or nitrites, depending on availability. Hydroxocobalamin effectively binds intracellular cyanide to form cyanocobalamin, which poses no harm. Nitrites induce production of methemoglobin, which then avidly binds cyanide to form the much less toxic cyanomethemoglobin. Finally, sodium thiosulfate is a sulfur donor that promotes conversion of cyanide to thiocyanate, which is well tolerated in the absence of acute kidney injury. When concomitant carbon monoxide poisoning is suspected, nitrites should be avoided because methemoglobinemia can further impair oxygen delivery.

Toxicity of Drugs of Abuse

The clinical presentation and toxic effects of commonly used sympathomimetic, opioid, sedative, and hallucinogenic drugs are described in **Table 58**. Coingestion of more than one psychoactive drug or alcohol is common, and such patients often have overlapping or indistinct toxicologic syndromes. Obtaining a history of ingestion and chronic medical issues helps narrow an exceedingly broad differential diagnosis that includes therapeutic drug toxicity, infection, extremes of temperature, benzodiazepine or ethanol withdrawal, and a myriad of brain disorders and metabolic disturbances. **Table 59** summarizes distinguishing features of opioid, sympathomimetic, anticholinergic, and cholinergic toxicologic syndromes.

Initial stabilization includes endotracheal intubation for airway protection in patients with a depressed level of consciousness. However, an early empiric trial of the opioid antagonist naloxone is warranted when opioid overdose is suspected. Serial escalating doses may be necessary, and patients who respond may require a continuous naloxone infusion. Chronic opioid users require close monitoring for withdrawal. In contrast, the use of flumazenil, a γ-aminobutyric acid (GABA)–receptor antagonist for benzodiazepine overdose is controversial. Although a response can be helpful in confirming the diagnosis and can obviate the need for additional diagnostic studies, flumazenil can precipitate seizures in chronic benzodiazepine users. Its short half-life makes it challenging to use in patients requiring sustained reversal of long-acting benzodiazepines, and given the overall low risk of benzodiazepine overdose, only selective use under the guidance of a toxicologist is recommended. Intubation is appropriate for patients with inadequate ventilation or an inability to handle their secretions. In general, treatment of benzodiazepine overdose is supportive with assurance of adequate ventilation.

Management of sympathomimetic overdose centers on controlling agitation with benzodiazepines, evaluating for end-organ injury, and treating persistent hypertension. Cocaine and other stimulants have β-adrenergic activity that produces

TABLE 58. Presentation and Toxicity of Drugs of Abuse

Drug Class	Examples	Examination Findings	Antidote
Opioids	Heroin, oxycodone, fentanyl analogs	↓ HR, ↓ temp, ↓ BP, ↓ RR, miosis	Naloxone
Benzodiazepines	Lorazepam	CNS depression, usually normal vital signs and eye examination	Flumazenil
Sympathomimetics		Shared findings: ↑ HR, ↑ BP, ↑ temp, diaphoresis, mydriasis, agitation, seizure, ↑ CK, ↑ liver chemistry studies, ↑ Cr	Benzodiazepines are first line for agitation Avoid β-blockers for hypertension Haloperidol may worsen hyperthermia
	Cocaine	30-minute duration, myocardial infarction prominent	
	Methamphetamine	Violent agitation prominent, duration 20 h	
	MDMA ("ecstasy")	↓ Na, serotonin syndrome	
	Bath salts ("plant food")	Hallucinations, violent agitation common, duration up to 48 h, negative urine drug screen	
Hallucinogens	Dextromethorphan	↑ HR, ↑ BP, agitation, coma	Benzodiazepines are first line for agitation Haloperidol is second line
	LSD	Mild ↑ HR, ↑ BP; rare ↑ temp and hemodynamic instability	
	PCP	Variable mental status, agitation > CNS depression, nystagmus	
	Synthetic cannabinoids ("Spice", "K-2")	↑ HR, agitation > marijuana, ↑ Cr, negative urine drug screen	

BP = blood pressure; CK = creatine kinase; CNS = central nervous system; Cr = creatinine; ECG = electrocardiogram; HR = heart rate; LSD = lysergic acid diethylamide; MDMA = 3,4-methylenedioxymethamphetamine; Na = sodium; PCP = phencyclidine; RR = respiration rate; temp = temperature.

TABLE 59. Toxic Drug Syndromes and Their Manifestations

Syndrome	Manifestations	Representative Drugs
Sympathomimetic	Tachycardia	Cocaine
	Hypertension	Amphetamines
	Diaphoresis	Ephedrine
	Agitation	Caffeine
	Seizures	
	Mydriasis	
Cholinergic	"SLUDGE"	Organophosphates (insecticides, sarin)
	Confusion	Carbamates
	Bronchorrhea	Physostigmine
	Bradycardia	Edrophonium
	Miosis	Nicotine
Anticholinergic	Hyperthermia	Antihistamines
	Dry skin and mucous membranes	Tricyclic antidepressants
	Agitation, delirium	Antiparkinson agents
	Tachycardia, tachypnea	Atropine
	Hypertension	Scopolamine
	Mydriasis	
Opioids	Miosis	Morphine and related drugs
	Respiratory depression	Heroin
	Lethargy, confusion	
	Hypothermia	
	Bradycardia	
	Hypotension	

SLUDGE = Salivation, Lacrimation, increased Urination and Defecation, Gastrointestinal upset, and Emesis.

pill bottles, substantially enhances providers' ability to institute optimal early treatment and anticipate problems. The physical examination is useful for ascertaining the class of drugs involved (**Table 60**) and identifying alternative causes of illness such as infection. Cholinergic syndromes most often occur with accidental exposure to organophosphate insecticides rather than ingestion of medications with cholinergic properties. Early treatment focuses on preventing absorption of additional medication, administration of antidotes, and measures to accelerate drug elimination such as hemodialysis. For most medications, administering activated charcoal may reduce drug levels, but it should be withheld if the patient is at risk of aspirating or more than 1 to 2 hours have elapsed since the time of ingestion.

For a discussion of acetaminophen toxicity, see MKSAP 17 Gastroenterology and Hepatology. For a discussion of salicylate toxicity, see MKSAP 17 Nephrology.

KEY POINT

- Coingestion commonly complicates the presentation and management of recreational and therapeutic drug toxicities.

Acute Abdominal Surgical Emergencies

Advanced age, immunosuppression, and use of systemic glucocorticoids are not only risk factors for severe abdominal disease but are associated with atypical clinical presentation. A host of relatively common (for example, acute myocardial infarction, diabetic ketoacidosis) and uncommon (for example, sickle cell disease, vasculitides) diseases that do not require surgical intervention may present with abdominal pain. Despite the large number of possible causes, it is important to achieve early differentiation of medically managed conditions from surgical emergencies. Early surgical intervention can be lifesaving (**Table 61**), and prompt surgical consultation is imperative. Abdominal imaging is not always necessary in determining the need for surgery, and CT scans in particular may cause harmful delays.

For a discussion of abdominal compartment syndrome, see MKSAP 17 Nephrology.

KEY POINT

- Early surgical consultation can be life-saving in patients with possible acute surgical abdomen.

Anoxic Brain Injury

Temperature management and therapeutic hypothermia are the standard of care for improving neurologic outcomes in resuscitated individuals who remain unresponsive following cardiac arrest. Benefit appears to be greatest in patients who are not responding appropriately to verbal commands after return of spontaneous circulation following ventricular fibrillation or pulseless ventricular tachycardia. Arrest due to asystole and pulseless electrical activity is associated with poor neurologic outcomes and the benefit of cooling in

vascular smooth muscle relaxation. Use of β-blockers in this setting therefore may exacerbate hypertension and should be avoided, although the actual risk is not well characterized.

Management of hallucinogenic overdose is supportive, as there are no antagonists to reverse the effects of these drugs. Patients with overdose of hallucinogens may be violent and combative and may require chemical and/or physical restraint while providing respiratory and hemodynamic support.

Therapeutic Drug Overdose

Critical illness can result from intentional or inadvertent overdose of a myriad of medications. Coingestion of medications or alcohol is particularly common with intended self-harm. Eliciting a detailed history from the patient, bystanders, first responders, and the patient's pharmacist, as well as retrieval of

TABLE 60. Presentation and Treatment of Therapeutic Drug Toxicities

Medication	Key Clinical Findings	Treatment	Notes
Nonopioid analgesics			
Acetaminophen	↑ liver chemistry studies, ↑Cr, ↑ INR, cerebral edema, vomiting	N-acetylcysteine	Transfer to liver transplant center if severe
Salicylates	Mixed respiratory alkalosis/anion gap metabolic acidosis, tinnitus, agitation, confusion	Bicarbonate infusion, dextrose	Target urine pH 7.5 to 8.0; hemodialysis if acute kidney injury or severe toxicity
Cardiovascular			
β-Blocker, calcium channel blocker	↓HR, ↓ BP, heart block, altered mental status if β-blocker	Atropine 1 mg IV up to 3 doses, glucagon, calcium chloride, vasopressors, cardiac pacemaker (if indicated), high-dose insulin and glucose, IV lipid emulsion	Treatments may be added sequentially or initiated simultaneously depending on severity of case and response to treatment
Digoxin	↓ HR, arrhythmia, nausea, emesis, abdominal pain, confusion, weakness	Digoxin-specific antibody	Use of antibody lowers K+; hemodialysis not effective
Anticholinergics			
Tricyclic antidepressants	↓ BP, sedation, seizure, anticholinergic signs, arrhythmia	Bicarbonate infusion titrated to QRS duration; benzodiazepines for seizure	Physostigmine contraindicated
Antihistamines	Anticholinergic signs including agitation and seizures	Benzodiazepines; physostigmine if isolated anticholinergic overdose	Physostigmine use requires continuous cardiac monitor and bedside atropine
Hypoglycemic			
Sulfonylurea	↓ glucose, confusion, seizure, anxiety, diaphoresis, tremor	Dextrose + octreotide, glucagon IM = temporizing	Monitor for ↓ glucose for 48 hours if large ingestion
Metformin	↑ lactate, abdominal pain	Hemodialysis for severe ↓ pH or acute kidney injury	Glucose usually normal if isolated metformin ingestion
Others			
Lithium	GI distress, confusion, ataxia, tremor, myoclonic jerks, diabetes insipidus	Hemodialysis if lithium level >4 mEq/L or severe symptoms	Serum level can guide need for hemodialysis, confirm diagnosis
SSRI/SNRI	Agitation, clonus, ↑ reflexes, rigidity, fever, ↑ HR	Benzodiazepines, cyproheptadine if severe	Venlafaxine has ↑ cardiac toxicity

BP = blood pressure; Cr = creatinine; GI = gastrointestinal; HR = heart rate; IM = intramuscular; IV = intravenous; K+ = potassium; SNRI = serotonin-norepinephrine reuptake inhibitor; SSRI = selective serotonin reuptake inhibitor.

these settings is unclear. However, temperature management is widely implemented regardless of the type of arrhythmia or whether the event was primarily cardiac or respiratory in origin.

Aside from advance directives limiting the aggressiveness of care, there are no absolute contraindications, and therapy should be initiated as soon as possible following arrival to the hospital. Intravascular cooling catheters, cooling blankets, cooling vests, and ice packs are commonly used to lower the temperature. Initial trials showing benefit cooled patients to 32.0 to 34.0 °C (89.6 to 93.2 °F) for 12 to 24 hours followed by gradual rewarming at 0.25 to 0.5 °C/hour (0.45 to 0.9 °F/hour). A recent, larger trial that compared cooling to 33.0 °C (91.4 °F) versus 36.0 °C (96.8 °F) for 28 hours found equivalent outcomes. In this study, temperatures were maintained below 37.5 °C (99.5 °F) until 72 hours post-arrest in both groups. Patients with ventricular fibrillation or ventricular tachycar-

dia, immediate high-quality cardiopulmonary resuscitation, and limited arrest time have the best opportunity for neurologic recovery. Cooling these patients to between 36.0 and 32.0 °C (96.8 to 89.6 °F) for 24 hours appears to benefit neurologic recovery and should be utilized in conjunction with comprehensive care and support. Avoidance of fever (<37.5 °C [99.5 °F]) for several days post-arrest is a reasonable strategy.

Prognosis in patients who do not awaken following rewarming is best determined by serial neurologic examinations combined with ancillary tests, including somatosensory evoked potentials.

KEY POINT

- Temperature management and therapeutic hypothermia are the standard of care for improving neurologic outcomes in resuscitated individuals who remain unresponsive following cardiac arrest.

TABLE 61. Causes and Presentation of Acute Abdominal Emergencies

Diagnosis	Presentation	Diagnostic Imaging	Notes
Acute cholecystitis and cholangitis	Persistent peritoneal RUQ or epigastric pain, fever, emesis, positive Murphy sign	Ultrasound EUS and ERCP for diagnosis and treatment of cholangitis	↑ alkaline phosphatase, ↑ bilirubin suggests cholangitis but typically not cholecystitis
Bowel obstruction	Cramping pain, emesis, distention, obstipation, dehydration	Radiograph: dilated loops of bowel with air-fluid levels CT scan: identifies cause, complications	Top causes: incarcerated hernia, adhesions, volvulus, intussusception
Acute appendicitis	Classic: periumbilical then RLQ pain, emesis, ↑ leukocyte count	Often unnecessary CT or ultrasound if unclear	Pain quality and location vary with appendix location
Peptic ulcer perforation	Abrupt peritoneal pain, later distention and hypovolemia	Radiograph: free air CT scan if unclear	Surgery necessary in majority of cases
Acute mesenteric ischemia	Pain > than examination findings, vomiting, hypotension, risk factors for clotting, embolism	CT angiography or conventional arteriography	Standard CT and serum lactate can be normal early in course
Toxic megacolon	Pain, diarrhea, ↑ temp, ↑ HR, ↑ BP, confusion	Radiograph: dilated colon, air-fluid levels in colon CT scan if unclear	Causes: inflammatory bowel disease, *Clostridium difficile* infection
Ruptured abdominal aortic aneurysm	↑ BP, abdominal and/or flank pain, pulsatile mass	Unnecessary if high suspicion and unstable CT or ultrasound if unclear	Risk factors: older age, male, smoking, hypertension, family history of aneurysm
Ectopic pregnancy with tubal rupture	↑ BP, ↑ Hb, ↑ hCG, abdominal pain, vaginal bleeding	Transvaginal ultrasound	High mortality without early surgery

BP = blood pressure; ERCP = endoscopic retrograde cholangiopancreatography; EUS = endoscopic ultrasound; Hb = hemoglobin; hCG = human chorionic gonadotropin; HR = heart rate; RLQ = right lower quadrant; RUQ = right upper quadrant; temp = temperature.

Bibliography

Pulmonary Diagnostic Tests

Casal RF, Ost DF, Eapen GA. Flexible bronchoscopy. Clin Chest Med. 2013 Sep;34(3):341-52. [PMID: 23993807]

Fielding DI, Kurimoto N. EBUS-TBNA/staging of lung cancer. Clin Chest Med. 2013 Sep;34(3):385-94. [PMID: 23993811]

Humphrey LL, Deffebach M, Pappas M, et al. Screening for lung cancer with low-dose computed tomography: a systematic review to update the US Preventive services task force recommendation. Ann Intern Med. 2013 Sep 17;159(6):411-20. [PMID: 23897166]

Katial RK, Covar RA. Bronchoprovocation testing in asthma. Immunol Allergy Clin North Am. 2012 Aug;32(3):413-31. [PMID: 22877619]

Miller MR, Hankinson J, Brusasco V, et al; ATS/ERS Task Force. Standardisation of spirometry. Eur Respir J. 2005 Aug;26(2):319-38. [PMID: 16055882]

Pellegrino R, Viegi G, Brusasco V, et al. Interpretative strategies for lung function tests. Eur Respir J. 2005 Nov;26(5):948-68. [PMID: 16264058]

Sarma A, Heilbrun ME, Conner KE, Stevens SM, Woller SC, Elliott CG. Radiation and chest CT scan examinations: what do we know? Chest. 2012 Sep;142(3):750-60. [PMID: 22948579]

Airways Disease

Barreiro E, Criner GJ. Update in chronic obstructive pulmonary disease 2013. Am J Respir Crit Care Med. 2014 Jun 1;189(11):1337-44. [PMID: 24881938]

Beghè B, Rabe KF, Fabbri LM. Phosphodiesterase-4 inhibitor therapy for lung diseases. Am J Respir Crit Care Med. 2013 Aug 1;188(3):271-8. [PMID: 23656508]

Chalmers JD, Smith MP, McHugh BJ, Doherty C, Govan JR, Hill AT. Short- and long-term antibiotic treatment reduces airway and systemic inflammation in non-cystic fibrosis bronchiectasis. Am J Respir Crit Care Med. 2012 Oct 1;186(7):657-65. [PMID: 22744718]

Chung KF, Wenzel SE, Brozek JL, et al. International ERS/ATS guidelines on definition, evaluation and treatment of severe asthma. Eur Respir J. 2014 Feb;43(2):343-73. Erratum in: Eur Respir J. 2014 Apr;43(4):1216. [PMID: 24337046]

Clancy JP, Jain M. Personalized medicine in cystic fibrosis: dawning of a new era. Am J Respir Crit Care Med. 2012 Oct 1;186(7):593-7. [PMID: 22723294]

Criner GJ, Bourbeau J, Diekemper RL, et al. Prevention of acute exacerbations of COPD: American College of Chest Physicians and Canadian Thoracic Society Guideline. Chest. 2015 Apr;147(4):894-942. [PMID: 25321320]

Cystic Fibrosis Foundation. Patient Registry Reports. Cystic Fibrosis Foundation Web Site. www.cff.org/livingwithcf/qualityimprovement/patientregistryreport/. Updated January 29, 2015. Accessed December 3, 2014.

Derichs N. Targeting a genetic defect: cystic fibrosis transmembrane conductance regulator modulators in cystic fibrosis. Eur Respir Rev. 2013 Mar 1;22(127):58-65. [PMID: 23457166]

Forno E, Celedón JC. Health disparities in asthma. Am J Respir Crit Care Med. 2012 May 15;185(10):1033-5. [PMID: 22589306]

Global Initiative for Chronic Obstructive Lung Disease (GOLD). Global Strategy for the Diagnosis, Management, and Prevention of Chronic Obstructive Pulmonary Disease. www.goldcopd.org/guidelines-global-strategy-for-diagnosis-management.html. Updated 2015. Accessed April 2, 2015.

Goldstein RS, Hill K, Brooks D, Dolmage TE. Pulmonary rehabilitation: a review of the recent literature. Chest. 2012 Sep;142(3):738-49. [PMID: 22948578]

Jain M, Goss CH. Update in cystic fibrosis 2013. Am J Respir Crit Care Med. 2014 May 15;189(10):1181-6. [PMID: 24832742]

Kerwin EM, Scott-Wilson C, Sanford L, et al. A randomised trial of fluticasone furoate/vilanterol (50/25 µg; 100/25 µg) on lung function in COPD. Respir Med. 2013 Apr;107(4):560-9. Erratum in: Respir Med. 2013 Dec;107(12):2094. [PMID: 23352226]

Lajunen TK, Jaakkola JJ, Jaakkola MS. The synergistic effect of heredity and exposure to second-hand smoke on adult-onset asthma. Am J Respir Crit Care Med. 2013 Oct 1;188(7):776-82. [PMID: 23981189]

Lee SD, Huang MS, Kang J, et al; Investigators of the Predictive Ability of CAT in Acute Exacerbations of COPD (PACE) Study. The COPD assessment test (CAT) assists prediction of COPD exacerbations in high-risk patients. Respir Med. 2014 Apr;108(4):600-8. [PMID: 24456695]

Martinez FD, Vercelli D. Asthma. Lancet. 2013 Oct 19;382(9901):1360-72. [PMID: 24041942]

Martínez-García MA, de la Rosa Carrillo D, Soler-Cataluña JJ, et al. Prognostic value of bronchiectasis in patients with moderate-to-severe chronic obstructive pulmonary disease. Am J Respir Crit Care Med. 2013 Apr 15;187(8):823-31. [PMID: 23392438]

McShane PJ, Naureckas ET, Tino G, Strek ME. Non-cystic fibrosis bronchiectasis. Am J Respir Crit Care Med. 2013 Sep 15;188(6):647-56. [PMID: 23898922]

Mogayzel PJ Jr, Naureckas ET, Robinson KA, et al; Pulmonary Clinical Practice Guidelines Committee. Cystic fibrosis pulmonary guidelines. Chronic medications for maintenance of lung health. Am J Respir Crit Care Med. 2013 Apr 1;187(7):680-9. [PMID: 23540878]

Müllerova H, Agusti A, Erqou S, Mapel DW. Cardiovascular comorbidity in COPD: systematic literature review. Chest. 2013 Oct;144(4):1163-78. [PMID: 23722528]

National Asthma Education and Prevention Program. Expert Panel Report 3 (EPR-3): Guidelines for the Diagnosis and Management of Asthma-Summary Report 2007. J Allergy Clin Immunol. 2007 Nov;120(5 Suppl):S94-138. Erratum in: J Allergy Clin Immunol. 2008 Jun;121(6):1330. [PMID: 17983880]

O'Sullivan BP, Freedman SD. Cystic fibrosis. Lancet. 2009 May 30; 373(9678):1891-904. [PMID: 19403164]

Parsons JP, Hallstrand TS, Mastronarde JG, et al; American Thoracic Society Subcommittee on Exercise-induced Bronchoconstriction. An official American Thoracic Society clinical practice guideline: exercise-induced bronchoconstriction. Am J Respir Crit Care Med. 2013 May 1;187(9):1016-27. [PMID: 23634861]

Pasteur MC, Bilton D, Hill AT; British Thoracic Society Bronchiectasis non-CF Guideline Group. British Thoracic Society guideline for non-CF bronchiectasis. Thorax. 2010 Jul;65 Suppl 1:i1-58. [PMID: 20627931]

Perret JL, Dharmage SC, Matheson MC, et al. The interplay between the effects of lifetime asthma, smoking, and atopy on fixed airflow obstruction in middle age. Am J Respir Crit Care Med. 2013 Jan 1;187(1):42-8. [PMID: 23155143]

Prieto-Centurion V, Markos MA, Ramey NI, et al. Interventions to reduce rehospitalizations after chronic obstructive pulmonary disease exacerbations. A systematic review. Ann Am Thorac Soc. 2014 Mar;11(3):417-24. [PMID: 24423379]

Sharif R, Cuevas CR, Wang Y, Arora M, Sharma G. Guideline adherence in management of stable chronic obstructive pulmonary disease. Respir Med. 2013 Jul;107(7):1046-52. [PMID: 23639271]

Short PM, Williamson PA, Elder DH, Lipworth SI, Schembri S, Lipworth BJ. The impact of tiotropium on mortality and exacerbations when added to inhaled corticosteroids and long-acting β-agonist therapy in COPD. Chest. 2012 Jan;141(1):81-6. [PMID: 21799028]

Tarlo SM, Lemiere C. Occupational asthma. N Engl J Med. 2014 Feb 13;370(7):640-9. [PMID: 24521110]

Tsai CL, Lee WY, Delclos GL, Hanania NA, Camargo CA Jr. Comparative effectiveness of noninvasive ventilation vs invasive mechanical ventilation in chronic obstructive pulmonary disease patients with acute respiratory failure. J Hosp Med. 2013 Apr;8(4):165-72. [PMID: 23401469]

Vestbo J, Agusti A, Wouters EF, et al; Evaluation of COPD Longitudinally to Identify Predictive Surrogate Endpoints Study Investigators. Should we view chronic obstructive pulmonary disease differently after ECLIPSE? A clinical perspective from the study team. Am J Respir Crit Care Med. 2014 May 1;189(9):1022-30. [PMID: 24552242]

von Mutius E, Hartert T. Update in asthma 2012. Am J Respir Crit Care Med. 2013 Jul 15;188(2):150-6. [PMID: 23855691]

Wechsler ME, Laviolette M, Rubin AS, et al; Asthma Intervention Research 2 Trial Study Group. Bronchial thermoplasty: Long-term safety and effectiveness in patients with severe persistent asthma. J Allergy Clin Immunol. 2013 Dec;132(6):1295-302. [PMID: 23998657]

Diffuse Parenchymal Lung Disease

Baughman RP, Culver DA, Judson MA. A concise review of pulmonary sarcoidosis. Am J Respir Crit Care Med. 2011 Mar 1;183(5):573-81. [PMID: 21037016]

Collard HR, Moore BB, Flaherty KR, et al; Idiopathic Pulmonary Fibrosis Clinical Research Network Investigators. Acute exacerbations of idiopathic pulmonary fibrosis. Am J Respir Crit Care Med. 2007 Oct 1;176(7):636-43. [PMID: 17585107]

King TE Jr, Bradford WZ, Castro-Bernardini S, et al; ASCEND Study Group. A phase 3 trial of pirfenidone in patients with idiopathic pulmonary fibrosis. N Engl J Med. 2014 May 29;370(22):2083-92. Erratum in: N Engl J Med. 2014 Sep 18;371(12):1172. [PMID: 24836312]

McCormack FX, Inoue Y, Moss J, et al; National Institutes of Health Rare Lung Diseases Consortium; MILES Trial Group. Efficacy and safety of sirolimus in lymphangioleiomyomatosis. N Engl J Med. 2011 Apr 28;364(17):1595-606. [PMID: 21410393]

Raghu G, Collard HR, Egan JJ, et al; ATS/ERS/JRS/ALAT Committee on Idiopathic Pulmonary Fibrosis. An official ATS/ERS/JRS/ALAT statement: idiopathic pulmonary fibrosis: evidence-based guidelines for diagnosis and management. Am J Respir Crit Care Med. 2011 Mar 15;183(6):788-824. [PMID: 21471066]

Richeldi L, du Bois RM, Raghu G, et al; INPULSIS Trial Investigators. Efficacy and safety of nintedanib in idiopathic pulmonary fibrosis. N Engl J Med. 2014 May 29;370(22):2071-82. [PMID: 24836310]

Tashkin DP, Elashoff R, Clements PJ, et al; Scleroderma Lung Study Research Group. Cyclophosphamide versus placebo in scleroderma lung disease. N Engl J Med. 2006 Jun 22;354(25):2655-66. [PMID: 16790698]

Travis WD, Costabel U, Hansell DM, et al; ATS/ERS Committee on Idiopathic Interstitial Pneumonias. An official American Thoracic Society/European Respiratory Society statement: Update of the international multidisciplinary classification of the idiopathic interstitial pneumonias. Am J Respir Crit Care Med. 2013 Sep 15;188(6):733-48. [PMID: 24032382]

Vassallo R. Diffuse lung diseases in cigarette smokers. Semin Respir Crit Care Med. 2012 Oct;33(5):533-42. [PMID: 23001806]

Washko GR, Hunninghake GM, Fernandez IE, et al; COPDGene Investigators. Lung volumes and emphysema in smokers with interstitial lung abnormalities. N Engl J Med. 2011 Mar 10;364(10):897-906. [PMID: 21388308]

Occupational Lung Disease

Markowitz SB, Levin SM, Miller A, Morabia A. Asbestos, asbestosis, smoking, and lung cancer. New findings from the North American insulator cohort. Am J Respir Crit Care Med. 2013 Jul 1;188(1):90-6. [PMID: 23590275]

Redlich CA, Tarlo SM, Hankinson JL, et al; American Thoracic Society Committee on Spirometry in the Occupational Setting. Official American Thoracic Society technical standards: spirometry in the occupational setting. Am J Respir Crit Care Med. 2014 Apr 15;189(8):983-93. [PMID: 24735032]

Rose C, Abraham J, Harkins D, et al. Overview and recommendations for medical screening and diagnostic evaluation for postdeployment lung disease in returning US warfighters. J Occup Environ Med. 2012 Jun;54(6):746-51. [PMID: 22588477]

Stayner L, Welch LS, Lemen R. The worldwide pandemic of asbestos-related diseases. Annu Rev Public Health. 2013;34:205-16. [PMID: 23297667]

Pleural Disease

Baumann MH, Strange C, Heffner JE, et al; AACP Pneumothorax Consensus Group. Management of spontaneous pneumothorax: an American College of Chest Physicians Delphi consensus statement. Chest. 2001 Feb;119(2):590-602. [PMID: 11171742]

Davies HE, Davies RJ, Davies CW; BTS Pleural Disease Guideline Group. Management of pleural infection in adults: British Thoracic Society Pleural Disease Guideline 2010. Thorax. 2010 Aug;65 Suppl 2:ii41-53. [PMID: 20696693]

Davies HE, Mishra EK, Kahan BC, et al. Effect of an indwelling pleural catheter vs chest tube and talc pleurodesis for relieving dyspnea in patients with malignant pleural effusion: the TIME2 randomized controlled trial. JAMA. 2012 Jun 13;307(22):2383-9. [PMID: 22610520]

Light RW. Clinical practice. Pleural effusion. N Engl J Med. 2002 Jun 20;346(25):1971-7. [PMID: 12075059]

MacDuff A, Arnold A, Harvey J; BTS Pleural Disease Guideline Group. Management of spontaneous pneumothorax: British Thoracic Society Pleural Disease Guideline 2010. Thorax. 2010 Aug;65 Suppl 2:ii18-31. [PMID: 20696690]

Maskell NA, Davies CW, Nunn AJ, et al; First Multicenter Intrapleural Sepsis Trial (MIST1) Group. U.K. Controlled trial of intrapleural streptokinase for pleural infection. N Engl J Med. 2005 Mar 3;352(9):865-74. Erratum in: N Engl J Med. 2005 May 19;352(20):2146. [PMID: 15745977]

Rahman NM, Maskell NA, West A, et al. Intrapleural use of tissue plasminogen activator and DNase in pleural infection. N Engl J Med. 2011 Aug 11;365(6):518-26. [PMID: 21830966]

Rahman NM, Mishra EK, Davies HE, Davies RJ, Lee YC. Clinically important factors influencing the diagnostic measurement of pleural fluid pH and glucose. Am J Respir Crit Care Med. 2008 Sep 1;178(5):483-90. [PMID: 18556632]

Roberts ME, Neville E, Berrisford RG, Antunes G, Ali NJ; BTS Pleural Disease Guideline Group. Management of a malignant pleural effusion: British Thoracic Society Pleural Disease Guideline 2010. Thorax. 2010 Aug;65 Suppl 2:ii32-40. [PMID: 20696691]

Tremblay A, Michaud G. Single-center experience with 250 tunnelled pleural catheter insertions for malignant pleural effusion. Chest. 2006 Feb;129(2):362-8. [PMID: 16478853]

Pulmonary Vascular Disease

Galiè N, Corris PA, Frost A, et al. Updated treatment algorithm of pulmonary arterial hypertension. J Am Coll Cardiol. 2013 Dec 24;62(25 Suppl):D60-72. [PMID: 24355643]

McGoon MD, Kane GC. Pulmonary hypertension: diagnosis and management. Mayo Clin Proc. 2009 Feb;84(2):191-207. Erratum in: Mayo Clin Proc. 2009 Apr;84(4):386. [PMID: 19181654]

Simonneau G, Gatzoulis MA, Adatia I, et al. Updated clinical classification of pulmonary hypertension. J Am Coll Cardiol. 2013 Dec 24;62(25 Suppl):D34-41. Erratum in: J Am Coll Cardiol. 2014 Feb 25;63(7):746. [PMID: 24355639]

Lung Tumors

Alberts WM; American College of Chest Physicians. Diagnosis and management of lung cancer executive summary: ACCP evidence-based clinical practice guidelines (2nd Edition). Chest. 2007 Sep;132(3 Suppl):1S-19S. [PMID: 17873156]

Aquino SL. Imaging of metastatic disease to the thorax. Radiol Clin North Am. 2005 May;43(3):481-95, vii. [PMID: 15847812]

Collins LG, Haines C, Perkel R, Enck RE. Lung cancer: diagnosis and management. Am Fam Physician. 2007 Jan 1;75(1):56-63. [PMID: 17225705]

Gould MK, Fletcher J, Iannettoni MD, et al; American College of Chest Physicians. Evaluation of patients with pulmonary nodules: when is it lung cancer?: ACCP evidence-based clinical practice guidelines (2nd edition). Chest. 2007 Sep;132(3 Suppl):108S-130S. [PMID: 17873164]

Henley SJ, Richards TB, Underwood JM, Eheman CR, Plescia M, McAfee TA; Centers for Disease Control and Prevention (CDC). Lung cancer incidence trends among men and women–United States, 2005-2009. MMWR Morb Mortal Wkly Rep. 2014 Jan 10;63(1):1-5. Erratum in: MMWR Morb Mortal Wkly Rep. 2014 Jan 17;63(2):45. [PMID: 24402465]

Murrmann GB, van Vollenhoven FH, Moodley L. Approach to a solid solitary pulmonary nodule in two different settings-"Common is common, rare is rare". J Thorac Dis. 2014 Mar;6(3):237-48. [PMID: 24624288]

National Lung Screening Trial Research Team, Church TR, Black WC, Aberle DR, et al. Results of initial low-dose computed tomographic screening for lung cancer. N Engl J Med. 2013 May 23;368(21):1980-91. [PMID: 23697514]

Scherpereel A, Astoul P, Baas P, et al; European Respiratory Society/European Society of Thoracic Surgeons Task Force. Guidelines of the European Respiratory Society and the European Society of Thoracic Surgeons for the management of malignant pleural mesothelioma. Eur Respir J. 2010 Mar;35(3):479-95. [PMID: 19717482]

Takahashi K, Al-Janabi NJ. Computed tomography and magnetic resonance imaging of mediastinal tumors. J Magn Reson Imaging. 2010 Dec;32(6):1325-39. [PMID: 21105138]

Travis WD. Advances in neuroendocrine lung tumors. Ann Oncol. 2010 Oct;21 Suppl 7:vii65-71. [PMID: 20943645]

Sleep Medicine

Caples SM, Rowley JA, Prinsell JR, et al. Surgical modifications of the upper airway for obstructive sleep apnea in adults: a systematic review and meta-analysis. Sleep. 2010 Oct;33(10):1396-407. [PMID: 21061863]

Chau EH, Lam D, Wong J, Mokhlesi B, Chung F. Obesity hypoventilation syndrome: a review of epidemiology, pathophysiology, and perioperative considerations. Anesthesiology. 2012 Jul;117(1):188-205. [PMID: 22614131]

Jordan AS, McSharry DG, Malhotra A. Adult obstructive sleep apnoea. Lancet. 2014 Feb 22;383(9918):736-47. [PMID: 23910433]

Phillips CL, Grunstein RR, Darendeliler MA, et al. Health outcomes of continuous positive airway pressure versus oral appliance treatment for obstructive sleep apnea: a randomized controlled trial. Am J Respir Crit Care Med. 2013 Apr 15;187(8):879-87. [PMID: 23413266]

Qaseem A, Dallas P, Owens DK, Starkey M, Holty JE, Shekelle P; Clinical Guidelines Committee of the American College of Physicians. Diagnosis of obstructive sleep apnea in adults: a clinical practice guideline from the American College of Physicians. Ann Intern Med. 2014 Aug 5;161(3):210-20. [PMID: 25089864]

Qaseem A, Holty JE, Owens DK, Dallas P, Starkey M, Shekelle P; for the Clinical Guidelines Committee of the American College of Physicians. Management of Obstructive Sleep Apnea in Adults: A Clinical Practice Guideline From the American College of Physicians. Ann Intern Med. 2013 Sep 24. [PMID: 24061345]

Rosen CL, Auckley D, Benca R, et al. A multisite randomized trial of portable sleep studies and positive airway pressure autotitration versus laboratory-based polysomnography for the diagnosis and treatment of obstructive sleep apnea: the HomePAP study. Sleep. 2012 Jun 1;35(6):757-67. [PMID: 22654195]

Sack RL. Clinical practice. Jet lag. N Engl J Med. 2010 Feb 4;362(5):440-7. [PMID: 20130253]

Yumino D, Bradley TD. Central sleep apnea and Cheyne-Stokes respiration. Proc Am Thorac Soc. 2008 Feb 15;5(2):226-36. [PMID: 18250216]

High-Altitude-Related Illnesses

Bärtsch P, Swenson ER. Clinical practice: Acute high-altitude illnesses. N Engl J Med. 2013 Jun 13;368(24):2294-302. [PMID: 23758234]

Silverman D, Gendreau M. Medical issues associated with commercial flights. Lancet. 2009 Jun 13;373(9680):2067-77. [PMID: 19232708]

West JB; American College of Physicians; American Physiological Society. The physiologic basis of high-altitude diseases. Ann Intern Med. 2004 Nov 16;141(10):789-800. [PMID: 15545679]

Critical Care Medicine

Ambrosino N, Carpenè N, Gherardi M. Chronic respiratory care for neuromuscular diseases in adults. Eur Respir J. 2009 Aug;34(2):444-51. [PMID: 19648521]

ARDS Definition Task Force, Ranieri VM, Rubenfeld GD, Thompson BT, et al. Acute respiratory distress syndrome: the Berlin Definition. JAMA. 2012 Jun 20;307(23):2526-33. [PMID: 22797452]

Barr J, Fraser GL, Puntillo K, et al; American College of Critical Care Medicine. Clinical practice guidelines for the management of pain, agitation, and delirium in adult patients in the intensive care unit. Crit Care Med. 2013 Jan;41(1):263-306. [PMID: 23269131]

Berg KM, Clardy P, Donnino MW. Noninvasive ventilation for acute respiratory failure: a review of the literature and current guidelines. Intern Emerg Med. 2012 Dec;7(6):539-45. [PMID: 23054404]

Brown DJ, Brugger H, Boyd J, Paal P. Accidental hypothermia. N Engl J Med. 2012 Nov 15;367(20):1930-8. Erratum in: N Engl J Med. 2013 Jan 24;368(4):394. [PMID: 23150960]

Carrillo A, Ferrer M, Gonzalez-Diaz G, et al. Noninvasive ventilation in acute hypercapnic respiratory failure caused by obesity hypoventilation syndrome and chronic obstructive pulmonary disease. Am J Respir Crit Care Med. 2012 Dec 15;186(12):1279-85. [PMID: 23103736]

Chatburn RL, Mireles-Cabodevila E. Closed-loop control of mechanical ventilation: description and classification of targeting schemes. Respir Care. 2011 Jan;56(1):85-102. [PMID: 21235841]

Churpek MM, Yuen TC, Edelson DP. Risk stratification of hospitalized patients on the wards. Chest. 2013 Jun;143(6):1758-65. [PMID: 23732586]

Dellinger RP, Levy MM, Rhodes A, et al; Surviving Sepsis Campaign Guidelines Committee including the Pediatric Subgroup. Surviving sepsis campaign: international guidelines for management of severe sepsis and septic shock: 2012. Crit Care Med. 2013 Feb;41(2):580-637. [PMID: 23353941]

Griffiths RD, Hall JB. Intensive care unit-acquired weakness. Crit Care Med. 2010 Mar;38(3):779-87. [PMID: 20048676]

Holstege CP, Borek HA. Toxidromes. Crit Care Clin. 2012 Oct;28(4):479-98. [PMID: 22998986]

Hudson LD, Milberg JA, Anardi D, Maunder RJ. Clinical risks for development of the acute respiratory distress syndrome. Am J Respir Crit Care Med. 1995 Feb;151(2 Pt 1):293-301. [PMID: 7842182]

Johnson W, Nguyen ML, Patel R. Hypertension crisis in the emergency department. Cardiol Clin. 2012 Nov;30(4):533-43. [PMID: 23102030]

Kumar G, Falk DM, Bonello RS, Kahn JM, Perencevich E, Cram P. The costs of critical care telemedicine programs: a systematic review and analysis. Chest. 2013 Jan;143(1):19-29. [PMID: 22797291]

Marik PE. Noninvasive cardiac output monitors: a state-of-the-art review. J Cardiothorac Vasc Anesth. 2013 Feb;27(1):121-34. [PMID: 22609340]

McClave SA, Martindale RG, Vanek VW, et al; A.S.P.E.N. Board of Directors; American College of Critical Care Medicine; Society of Critical Care Medicine. Guidelines for the Provision and Assessment of Nutrition Support Therapy in the Adult Critically Ill Patient: Society of Critical Care Medicine (SCCM) and American Society for Parenteral and Enteral Nutrition (A.S.P.E.N.). JPEN J Parenter Enteral Nutr. 2009 May-Jun;33(3):277-316. [PMID: 19398613]

McConville JF, Kress JP. Weaning patients from the ventilator. N Engl J Med. 2012 Dec 6;367(23):2233-9. [PMID: 23215559]

National Heart, Lung, and Blood Institute Acute Respiratory Distress Syndrome (ARDS) Clinical Trials Network, Wiedemann HP, Wheeler AP, Bernard GR, et al. Comparison of two fluid-management strategies in acute lung injury. N Engl J Med. 2006 Jun 15;354(24):2564-75. [PMID: 16714767]

Nava S, Ambrosino N, Clini E, et al. Noninvasive mechanical ventilation in the weaning of patients with respiratory failure due to chronic obstructive pulmonary disease. A randomized, controlled trial. Ann Intern Med. 1998 May 1;128(9):721-8. [PMID: 9556465]

Needham DM, Davidson J, Cohen H, et al. Improving long-term outcomes after discharge from intensive care unit: report from a stakeholders' conference. Crit Care Med. 2012 Feb;40(2):502-9. [PMID: 21946660]

Nielsen N, Wetterslev J, Cronberg T, et al; TTM Trial Investigators. Targeted temperature management at 33°C versus 36°C after cardiac arrest. N Engl J Med. 2013 Dec 5;369(23):2197-206. [PMID: 24237006]

ProCESS Investigators, Yealy DM, Kellum JA, Huang DT, et al. A randomized trial of protocol-based care for early septic shock. N Engl J Med. 2014 May 1;370(18):1683-93. [PMID: 24635773]

Rivers E, Nguyen B, Havstad S, et al; Early Goal-Directed Therapy Collaborative Group. Early goal-directed therapy in the treatment of severe sepsis and septic shock. N Engl J Med. 2001 Nov 8;345(19):1368-77. [PMID: 11794169]

Simons FE, Sheikh A. Anaphylaxis: the acute episode and beyond. BMJ. 2013 Feb 12;346:f602. [PMID: 23403828]

Ventilation with lower tidal volumes as compared with traditional tidal volumes for acute lung injury and the acute respiratory distress syndrome. The Acute Respiratory Distress Syndrome Network. N Engl J Med. 2000 May 4;342(18):1301-8. [PMID: 10793162]

Vincent JL, De Backer D. Circulatory shock. N Engl J Med. 2013 Oct 31;369(18):1726-34. [PMID: 24171518]

Winters BD, Weaver SJ, Pfoh ER, Yang T, Pham JC, Dy SM. Rapid-response systems as a patient safety strategy: a systematic review. Ann Intern Med. 2013 Mar 5;158(5 Pt 2):417-25. [PMID: 23460099]

Pulmonary and Critical Care Medicine Self-Assessment Test

This self-assessment test contains one-best-answer multiple-choice questions. Please read these directions carefully before answering the questions. Answers, critiques, and bibliographies immediately follow these multiple-choice questions. The American College of Physicians is accredited by the Accreditation Council for Continuing Medical Education (ACCME) to provide continuing medical education for physicians.

The American College of Physicians designates MKSAP 17 **Pulmonary and Critical Care Medicine** for a maximum of **19** *AMA PRA Category 1 Credits*™. Physicians should claim only the credit commensurate with the extent of their participation in the activity.

Earn "Instantaneous" CME Credits Online

Print subscribers can enter their answers online to earn CME credits instantaneously. You can submit your answers using online answer sheets that are provided at mksap.acponline.org, where a record of your MKSAP 17 credits will be available. To earn CME credits, you need to answer all of the questions in a test and earn a score of at least 50% correct (number of correct answers divided by the total number of questions). Take any of the following approaches:

➤ Use the printed answer sheet at the back of this book to record your answers. Go to mksap.acponline.org, access the appropriate online answer sheet, transcribe your answers, and submit your test for instantaneous CME credits. There is no additional fee for this service.

➤ Go to mksap.acponline.org, access the appropriate online answer sheet, directly enter your answers, and submit your test for instantaneous CME credits. There is no additional fee for this service.

➤ Pay a $15 processing fee per answer sheet and submit the printed answer sheet at the back of this book by mail or fax, as instructed on the answer sheet. Make sure you calculate your score and fax the answer sheet to 215-351-2799 or mail the answer sheet to Member and Customer Service, American College of Physicians, 190 N. Independence Mall West, Philadelphia, PA 19106-1572, using the courtesy envelope provided in your MKSAP 17 slipcase. You will need your 10-digit order number and 8-digit ACP ID number, which are printed on your packing slip. Please allow 4 to 6 weeks for your score report to be emailed back to you. Be sure to include your email address for a response.

If you do not have a 10-digit order number and 8-digit ACP ID number or if you need help creating a username and password to access the MKSAP 17 online answer sheets, go to mksap.acponline.org or email custserv@acponline.org.

CME credit is available from the publication date of December 31, 2015, until December 31, 2018. You may submit your answer sheets at any time during this period.

Directions

*Each of the numbered items is followed by lettered answers. Select the **ONE** lettered answer that is **BEST** in each case.*

Item 1

A 55-year-old man is evaluated in the emergency department after being rescued from his burning home by firefighters. His medical history is notable for COPD, and his only medication is an albuterol-ipratropium metered-dose inhaler.

On physical examination, he is alert and in pain. Temperature is 37.8 °C (100.0 °F), blood pressure is 124/60 mm Hg, pulse rate is 116/min, and respiration rate is 22/min; BMI is 31. Oxygen saturation is 98% breathing 3 L/min oxygen by nasal cannula. Soot is noted in the nares and throughout the oral pharynx. The oral mucosa is edematous. Burns are noted on the right upper extremity and lower chest. Cardiac examination reveals a regular rhythm. Pulmonary examination reveals a monophonic wheeze over the anterior chest, diffuse expiratory wheezes, and increased work of breathing.

Arterial blood gas studies breathing 30% oxygen reveal a pH of 7.32, a P_{CO_2} of 50 mm Hg (6.7 kPa), and a P_{O_2} of 78 mm Hg (10.4 kPa).

A chest radiograph shows increased lung volumes consistent with hyperinflation but no infiltrates.

Which of the following is the most appropriate next step in treating this patient's respiratory findings?

(A) Administer a helium-oxygen mixture
(B) Administer methylprednisolone
(C) Perform endotracheal intubation
(D) Start nebulized epinephrine
(E) Start noninvasive ventilation

Item 2

A 72-year-old man is admitted to the ICU for severe community-acquired pneumonia. He was admitted to the hospital 2 days ago with cough and dyspnea. Despite appropriate intravenous antibiotics, his respiratory status declined and he was transferred to the ICU, was intubated, and was placed on mechanical ventilation. A vasopressor was needed for persistent hypotension. Since ICU admission 36 hours ago, he has had stable oxygenation and blood pressure and his oxygen and vasopressor dose are being decreased. Medical history is otherwise unremarkable. Medications are ceftriaxone, azithromycin, norepinephrine, and low-molecular-weight heparin prophylaxis.

On physical examination, the patient is intubated but responsive. Temperature is 38.3 °C (100.9 °F), blood pressure is 95/58 mm Hg, and pulse rate is 110/min; BMI is 27. Chest examination shows decreased breath sounds at the left lung base. Cardiac examination reveals a grade 2/6 systolic flow murmur. The remainder of the examination is unremarkable.

Laboratory studies are significant for a leukocyte count of 15,000/µL (15×10^9/L); the complete blood count is otherwise normal. Complete metabolic profile is normal. Blood and sputum cultures are negative since admission.

A chest radiograph is significant for left lower lobe consolidation but is otherwise unremarkable.

Which of the following is most likely to prevent deconditioning in the ICU?

(A) Passive range of motion exercises only while in the ICU
(B) Progressive physical activity as tolerated starting now
(C) Progressive physical activity as tolerated following discontinuation of vasopressors
(D) Progressive physical activity as tolerated following extubation

Item 3

A 58-year-old woman is evaluated for a right pulmonary nodule that was discovered incidentally 3 weeks ago. She is currently asymptomatic and has not had shortness of breath, fever, chills, weight loss, or night sweats. Medical history is otherwise unremarkable, and she takes no medications. She is a life-long nonsmoker.

On physical examination, temperature is 37.1 °C (98.8 °F), blood pressure is 126/82 mm Hg, pulse rate is 68/min, and respiration rate is 10/min; BMI is 30. There is no cervical or supraclavicular lymphadenopathy. The lungs are clear to auscultation. No clubbing is noted.

The 5-mm nodule seen on CT is shown.

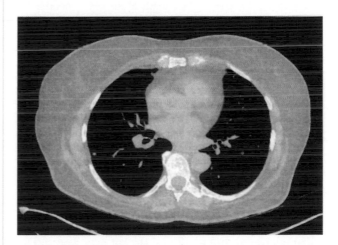

Which of the following is the most appropriate next step in management?

(A) Bronchoalveolar lavage
(B) PET/CT scan
(C) Review any previous chest imaging
(D) Transthoracic needle biopsy

Item 4

A 62-year-old man is evaluated for declining exercise capacity over the past year. He was diagnosed with moderate COPD 3 years ago. His symptoms had previously been well controlled with tiotropium and as-needed albuterol. He has not had any hospitalizations. He is adherent to his medication regimen, and his inhaler technique is good. He quit smoking 2 years ago. All immunizations are up to date, including influenza and pneumococcal vaccination. A chest radiograph performed 3 months ago for increased cough and sputum production was normal. Pulmonary function testing performed 3 years ago showed an FEV_1 of 58% of predicted, an FEV_1/FVC ratio of 60%, and a D_{LCO} of 85% of predicted.

On physical examination, vital signs are normal. Oxygen saturation is 93% breathing ambient air. No jugular venous distention is noted. The lungs are clear. Cardiac examination reveals normal heart sounds. There are no murmurs. No edema is noted.

Which of the following is the most appropriate management?

(A) Add roflumilast
(B) Obtain complete pulmonary function tests
(C) Perform chest CT
(D) Repeat spirometry
(E) Start oxygen therapy

Item 5

A 56-year-old woman is evaluated for a 4-week history of slowly progressive shortness of breath. She has a non-productive cough that started around the same time and did not improve after a course of azithromycin. She has not had fever, chills, chest pain, wheezing, orthopnea, or lower extremity edema. Her medical history is notable for hormone receptor–negative infiltrating ductal carcinoma of the left breast diagnosed 8 months ago and treated with lumpectomy, radiation therapy, and adjuvant chemotherapy. She currently takes no medications.

On physical examination, temperature is 37.1 °C (98.8 °F), blood pressure is 124/76 mm Hg, pulse rate is 110/min, respiration rate is 14/min, and oxygen saturation is 91% breathing ambient air; BMI is 26. Crackles are noted at the left lung base. The left breast shows a well-healed lumpectomy scar and mild radiation skin changes, but no masses. There is no cervical, supraclavicular, or axillary lymphadenopathy. No clubbing is observed.

A complete blood count is normal.

A chest CT with pulmonary embolism protocol was compared with a CT obtained 6 months ago. It shows left hilar and mediastinal lymphadenopathy with new interstitial thickening and beading at the left lung base and no ground-glass opacification. There is no evidence of pulmonary embolism.

Which of the following is the most likely diagnosis?

(A) Atypical pneumonia
(B) Bronchiolitis obliterans organizing pneumonia
(C) Idiopathic pulmonary fibrosis
(D) Lymphangitic carcinomatosis
(E) Radiation fibrosis

Item 6

A 60-year-old woman is evaluated for a 6-month history of worsening dyspnea, especially with exertion. She was diagnosed with COPD 4 years ago, and pulmonary function tests performed 3 months ago showed an FEV_1 of 32% of predicted and an FEV_1/FVC ratio of 55%. She has had three exacerbations in the last year. She completed pulmonary rehabilitation twice within the last 2 years and quit smoking 1 year ago. Medications are combination long-acting β_2-agonist and inhaled glucocorticoid, roflumilast, and albuterol as needed.

On physical examination, she is afebrile. Blood pressure is 120/74 mm Hg, pulse rate is 94/min, and respiration rate is 20/min. BMI is 28. Oxygen saturation breathing ambient air is 89%. There is no jugular venous distention. Pulmonary examination reveals decreased breath sounds. Cardiovascular examination reveals a loud pulmonic component of S_2. Bilateral lower extremity edema is noted to a level above the ankles.

Chest radiograph shows no infiltrate or mass. Arterial P_{O_2} is 57 mm Hg (7.6 kPa) breathing ambient air. Echocardiogram reveals an ejection fraction of 60% and no valvular or wall motion abnormalities. The estimated mean pulmonary artery pressure is 52 mm Hg.

Which of the following is the most appropriate treatment?

(A) Daily prednisone
(B) Long-term oxygen therapy
(C) Overnight pulse oximetry
(D) Repeat pulmonary rehabilitation

Item 7

A 62-year-old man is evaluated for 2-year history of increasing shortness of breath. His symptoms are worse when he walks up steps or lifts heavy objects. He also has an occasional nonproductive cough. His medical history is significant for hypertension, and his only medication is chlorthalidone. He is an active smoker with a 56-pack-year smoking history. He is a former construction worker and worked in a steel mill when he was in high school.

On physical examination, the patient is afebrile, blood pressure is 125/78 mm Hg, pulse rate is 90/min, and respiration rate is 18/min; BMI is 31. Oxygen saturation at rest breathing ambient air is 94%. Pulmonary examination reveals a mildly prolonged expiratory phase but is otherwise normal; no wheezes or crackles are noted. The remainder of the examination is unremarkable.

Chest radiograph shows mildly increased lung markings but no focal findings.

Spirometry shows an FEV_1/FVC ratio of 65%, an FEV_1 of 52% of predicted, and an FVC of 80% of predicted. Lung volumes show a total lung capacity of 120% of predicted, a residual volume of 125% of predicted, and a D_{LCO} of 65% of predicted.

Based on this patient's clinical findings, which of the following is the most likely diagnosis?

(A) Bronchiectasis
(B) COPD
(C) Idiopathic pulmonary fibrosis
(D) Obesity hypoventilation syndrome

Item 8

A 57-year-old woman is evaluated in the emergency department for an episode of hematemesis that occurred 1 hour ago. She had previously felt well except for a recent knee injury, for which she has been taking ibuprofen. She currently is experiencing lightheadedness and weakness. Medical history is otherwise unremarkable. She does not smoke or drink alcohol. She takes no other medications.

On physical examination, she appears ill and pale. Temperature is 36.5 °C (97.7 °F). Blood pressure and pulse rate in the supine position are 90/60 mm Hg and 105/min. When sitting, her blood pressure and pulse rate are 70/35 mm Hg and 128/min. Respiration rate is 14/min; BMI is 26. Mild diaphoresis is noted. Abdominal examination reveals no tenderness and no hepatosplenomegaly. No ecchymoses, rashes, or petechiae are noted.

Laboratory studies are pending and blood typing and cross-match are sent.

Which of the following is the most appropriate form of access for this patient?

(A) Intraosseous catheter
(B) Large-caliber peripheral intravenous catheter
(C) Single-lumen peripherally inserted central venous catheter
(D) Triple-lumen internal jugular venous catheter

Item 9

A 62-year-old man is admitted to the hospital for a 6-week history of progressive cough, hemoptysis, and shortness of breath. Prior to the onset of symptoms, he reports feeling well except for some difficulty rising out of a chair and walking up a flight of stairs because of lower extremity weakness. He has a 50-pack-year history of cigarette smoking. He has no other medical problems and takes no medications.

On physical examination, temperature is 37.6 °C (99.7 °F), blood pressure is 140/84 mm Hg, pulse rate is 102/min, respiration rate is 14/min, and oxygen saturation is 90% breathing ambient air; BMI is 30. Cardiovascular and pulmonary examination findings are unremarkable. On neurologic examination, he has symmetric proximal muscle weakness in both his upper and lower extremities. There is no palpable peripheral lymphadenopathy.

Chest radiograph shows a right hilar mass. Chest CT confirms an 8-cm right hilar mass adjacent to the mediastinum with bulky bilateral mediastinal lymphadenopathy.

Which of the following is the most likely diagnosis?

(A) Adenocarcinoma of the lung
(B) Atypical bronchial carcinoid tumor
(C) Small cell lung cancer
(D) Squamous cell carcinoma of the lung

Item 10

A 60-year-old man is evaluated for a history of advanced COPD. He has fatigue and dyspnea with mild exertion, which significantly impairs his ability to perform routine activities. He is adherent to his medication regimen, and his inhaler technique is good. He has a history of multiple exacerbations, which have required hospitalization over the past year. He participated in pulmonary rehabilitation after his last hospitalization. Medical history is otherwise unremarkable. He quit smoking 3 years ago. Medications are roflumilast, tiotropium, mometasone/formoterol, as-needed albuterol, and 2 L of oxygen via nasal cannula.

On physical examination, respiration rate is 22/min; other vital signs are normal. BMI is 20. Pulmonary examination reveals decreased breath sounds bilaterally with no wheezing or crackles. The remainder of the examination is unremarkable.

Chest radiograph shows changes consistent with COPD, and chest CT shows bilateral homogeneous emphysema. Pulmonary function testing shows an FEV_1 of 18% of predicted, an FEV_1/FVC ratio of 33%, and a D_{LCO} of 52% of predicted. Arterial blood gases on 2 L of oxygen reveal a pH of 7.37, a P_{CO_2} of 64 mm Hg (8.5 kPa), a P_{O_2} of 62 mm Hg (8.2 kPa), and an oxygen saturation of 91%.

Which of the following is the most appropriate next step in management?

(A) Daily oral glucocorticoid therapy
(B) Hospice care
(C) Lung transplantation
(D) Lung volume reduction surgery

Item 11

A 64-year-old man is evaluated for a 2-year history of shortness of breath with exertion and a chronic cough. His symptoms began approximately 1 year ago when he began having mild dyspnea with vigorous exercise; he also noted development of a mild, intermittent, nonproductive cough. Since that time he has had worsening shortness of breath with minimal physical activity, and the cough has become more frequent. He otherwise feels well. Medical history is otherwise unremarkable, and he takes no medications. He is a life-long nonsmoker.

On physical examination, temperature is 37.0 °C (98.6 °F), blood pressure is 128/76 mm Hg, pulse rate is 88/min, and respiration rate is 14/min; BMI is 28. Oxygen saturation is 91% breathing ambient air. There is no jugular venous distention or supraclavicular lymphadenopathy. Lung examination reveals dry crackles at the bases bilaterally. Cardiac examination is unremarkable. Mild clubbing of the fingers is noted. There is no peripheral edema.

Results of a basic metabolic panel are normal.

Chest radiograph shows interstitial thickening at the bases bilaterally.

Which of the following is the most appropriate diagnostic test to perform next?

(A) Chest CT with contrast
(B) Chest CT without contrast
(C) CT pulmonary angiography
(D) High-resolution chest CT

Item 12

A 72-year-old man is evaluated for a 1-year history of cough and shortness of breath. He walks approximately 1 mile per day, but it now takes him twice as long as it did last year. He has noted no clear aggravating or ameliorating factors, and he believes his symptoms have steadily increased over the past year. He has not had chest pain, orthopnea, or paroxysmal nocturnal dyspnea.

On physical examination, vital signs are normal; oxygen saturation is 90% breathing ambient air. No jugular venous distention is noted. Pulmonary examination reveals inspiratory crackles at the bases. Cardiac examination is unremarkable.

Chest radiograph is normal. Pulmonary function testing reveals an FEV_1 of 68% of predicted, an FVC of 75% of predicted, an FEV_1/FVC ratio of 82%, and a DLco of 83% of predicted. Total lung capacity is 65% of predicted.

Which of the following is the most appropriate diagnostic test to perform next?

(A) Bronchoscopy, biopsy, and bronchoalveolar lavage
(B) Cardiopulmonary exercise testing
(C) High-resolution chest CT
(D) Ventilation-perfusion lung scan

Item 13

A 61-year-old woman is evaluated for a 4-month history of progressive dyspnea and fatigue without chest pain. Eighteen months ago, she was diagnosed with liver cirrhosis due to nonalcoholic steatohepatitis (NASH). Medical history is also significant for obesity. Medications are propranolol, spironolactone, and lactulose.

On physical examination, temperature is 36.4 °C (97.5 °F), blood pressure is 112/64 mm Hg, pulse rate is 60/min, and respiration rate is 16/min; BMI is 36. Mild scleral icterus is noted. Cardiac examination reveals a prominent S_2. The lungs are clear. Dilated veins are visible on the trunk and abdomen, and there is no appreciable ascites. Trace symmetric ankle edema is noted.

Chest radiograph shows cardiomegaly and clear lung fields. Pulmonary function tests show normal spirometry but reduced diffusing capacity (42% of predicted). A resting echocardiogram shows a left ventricular ejection fraction of 70% and an estimated right ventricular systolic pressure of 58 mm Hg. No shunt is seen with contrast enhancement. A dobutamine stress echocardiogram is negative for ischemia. A ventilation-perfusion scan shows a low probability of pulmonary embolism. Right heart catheterization reveals a mean pulmonary artery pressure of 48 mm Hg and a pulmonary capillary wedge pressure of 12 mm Hg.

Which of the following is the most likely diagnosis?

(A) Chronic thromboembolic pulmonary hypertension
(B) Hepatopulmonary syndrome
(C) Portopulmonary hypertension
(D) Pulmonary veno-occlusive disease

Item 14

A 72-year-old man is evaluated for fever in the hospital after being on mechanical ventilation for 1 week for hypoxic respiratory failure due to influenza. After an initial period of improvement, his level of purulent sputum production has increased over the past 24 hours, and over the previous 48 hours it has been necessary to increase his FIO_2 to maintain his oxygenation. His only medication is oseltamivir delivered by orogastric tube.

On physical examination, temperature is 38.3 °C (100.9 °F), blood pressure is 110/60 mm Hg, pulse rate is 115/min, and respiration rate is 18/min (ventilator set rate is 14/min). Pulmonary examination reveals diffuse crackles.

Laboratory studies reveal a leukocyte count of 18,000/μL (18×10^9/L), increased from 12,500/μL (12.5×10^9/L) 2 days ago.

Chest radiograph shows worsening pulmonary infiltrates.

Which of the following is the most appropriate next step in management?

(A) Begin empiric ceftriaxone and azithromycin
(B) Chest physiotherapy
(C) Deep sampling of the lower respiratory tract
(D) Substitute zanamivir for oseltamivir

Item 15

A 59-year-old man is evaluated in the emergency department for rapidly progressive dyspnea. His medical history is notable for coronary artery disease, chronic heart failure, and chronic atrial fibrillation. His medications are warfarin; aspirin; lisinopril; metoprolol; atorvastatin, and furosemide, 20 mg/d.

On physical examination, he is alert and in moderate respiratory distress. Temperature is 37.0 °C (98.6 °F), blood pressure is 150/94 mm Hg, pulse rate is 63/min and irregular, and respiration rate is 30/min; BMI is 30. Oxygen saturation is 88% breathing ambient air and increases to 93% breathing 4 L/min of oxygen by nasal cannula. Jugular venous distention is present. Cardiac examination reveals an irregular rhythm and a grade 2/6 holosystolic murmur best heard at the cardiac apex. Pulmonary examination reveals crackles bilaterally and basilar dullness.

A chest radiograph is shown (see top of next page).

An intravenous bolus of furosemide, 40 mg, is administered.

Which of the following is the most appropriate management?

(A) Begin intravenous furosemide infusion
(B) Initiate intubation and mechanical ventilation
(C) Initiate noninvasive positive pressure ventilation
(D) Initiate ultrafiltration

Item 16

A 67-year-old woman is evaluated in the emergency department for a 2-day history of fever, dyspnea, and increased cough with production of green sputum. She has severe

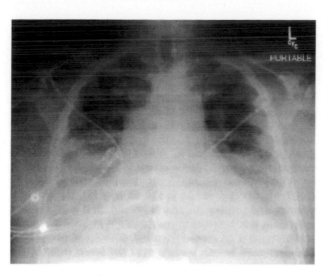

ITEM 15

CONT.

COPD, which was diagnosed 2 years ago. She used albuterol several times yesterday with no relief of dyspnea, and she was unable to sleep last night. Her last spirometry, performed 6 months ago, showed an FEV_1 of 48% of predicted. She is a current smoker with a 24-pack-year history. Medications are tiotropium and as-needed albuterol.

On physical examination, temperature is 38.9 °C (102.0 °F), blood pressure is 124/80 mm Hg, pulse rate is 118/min, and respiration rate is 30/min. Oxygen saturation is 82% breathing ambient air. Pulmonary examination reveals bilateral diffuse expiratory wheezing. After an albuterol nebulizer treatment and breathing 2 L of oxygen by nasal cannula, oxygen saturation is 91%. She remains tachypneic with bilateral expiratory wheezing.

Chest radiograph shows no infiltrate.

In addition to continuing this patient's supplemental oxygen and short-acting bronchodilator, which of the following is the most appropriate treatment?

(A) Azithromycin and prednisone
(B) Clarithromycin and fluticasone
(C) Doxycycline and salmeterol/fluticasone
(D) Erythromycin and roflumilast

Item 17

A 67-year-old man is evaluated for a 6-month history of worsening exertional dyspnea. He has a history of severe COPD diagnosed 4 years ago and previously had minimal exertional symptoms. However, he now notes shortness of breath when walking short distances that is limiting his activity level. He does not have chest pain, gastrointestinal symptoms, or sleep-related symptoms. Medical history is otherwise unremarkable. Medications are a twice-daily fluticasone/salmeterol inhaler and an as-needed albuterol/ipratropium metered-dose inhaler. He has a 55-pack-year smoking history but stopped smoking at the time of his COPD diagnosis.

On physical examination, temperature is 37.0 °C (98.6 °F), blood pressure is 130/84 mm Hg, pulse rate is 82/min, and respiration rate is 16/min; BMI is 24. Oxygen

saturation breathing ambient air is 93%. Jugular venous distention is noted. Pulmonary examination reveals distant breath sounds and no wheezes. Cardiac examination discloses an accentuated S_2 and regular rhythm. Abdominal examination is unremarkable, and there is bilateral lower extremity edema to the level of the ankles.

A chest radiograph shows hyperinflation, prominent central pulmonary arteries, and no infiltrates. A transthoracic echocardiogram shows normal left ventricular size and function with an ejection fraction of 60% and a right ventricular systolic pressure of 52 mm Hg.

Which of the following is the most appropriate diagnostic test to perform next?

(A) High-resolution CT
(B) Oxygen measurement during sleep and exertion
(C) Polysomnography
(D) Right heart catheterization for pressure measurement

Item 18

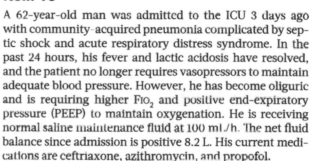

A 62-year-old man was admitted to the ICU 3 days ago with community-acquired pneumonia complicated by septic shock and acute respiratory distress syndrome. In the past 24 hours, his fever and lactic acidosis have resolved, and the patient no longer requires vasopressors to maintain adequate blood pressure. However, he has become oliguric and is requiring higher FIO_2 and positive end-expiratory pressure (PEEP) to maintain oxygenation. He is receiving normal saline maintenance fluid at 100 mL/h. The net fluid balance since admission is positive 8.2 L. His current medications are ceftriaxone, azithromycin, and propofol.

On physical examination, temperature is 37.1 °C (98.8 °F), blood pressure is 92/52 mm Hg, pulse rate is 88/min, and respiration rate is 28/min; BMI is 26. Oxygen saturation is 91% on an FIO_2 of 0.8 and a PEEP of 16 cm H_2O. Mentation seems clear, and the skin is warm. Central venous pressure is 17 cm H_2O. Cardiac examination reveals a regular rhythm without gallop or rub. Chest examination reveals diffuse inspiratory crackles with decreased breath sounds at the bases. There is pitting edema present in all extremities.

Laboratory studies:

Creatinine	2.2 mg/dL (194.5 µmol/L) (baseline 1.2 mg/dL [106.1 µmol/L])
Potassium	4 mEq/L (4 mmol/L)
Arterial blood gases:	
pH	7.30
PCO_2	50 mm Hg (6.7 kPa)
PO_2	86 mm Hg (11.4 kPa)

A chest radiograph shows bilateral infiltrates and interval development of small bilateral pleural effusions.

Which of the following is the most appropriate next step in treatment?

(A) Administer 250 mL of 5% albumin every 6 hours
(B) Discontinue intravenous maintenance fluids
(C) Initiate continuous venovenous hemodialysis
(D) Start hydrocortisone

Item 19

A 58-year-old woman is evaluated because of daily wheezing and breathlessness during allergy season. She has a long history of seasonal allergies, and her usual symptoms include itchy eyes and runny nose. However, over the past several years, these symptoms have been periodically accompanied by episodes of wheezing and shortness of breath. These episodes have increased to the point that they limit her activities several times a week. Medical history is otherwise unremarkable. Her medications are as-needed fexofenadine and antihistamine eye drops. She is a never-smoker.

On physical examination, the patient is afebrile, blood pressure is 130/76 mm Hg, pulse rate is 79/min, and respiration rate is 14/min; BMI is 28. Watery eyes and conjunctival irritation are noted. Pulmonary examination reveals expiratory wheezing. Cardiac examination is normal.

A chest radiograph is unremarkable. Spirometry shows an FEV_1 of 74% of predicted, which improves by 18% with a bronchodilator.

In addition to a short-acting β_2-agonist, which of the following is the most appropriate treatment?

(A) Add a leukotriene antagonist

(B) Add a low-dose inhaled glucocorticoid

(C) Add a low-dose inhaled glucocorticoid and long-acting β_2-agonist

(D) Recommend daily oral antihistamine use

Item 20

An 18-year-old woman is evaluated in follow-up after a recent visit to the emergency department for a 12-day history of shortness of breath, wheezing, and cough productive of yellow sputum. She was started on levofloxacin for a diagnosis of community-acquired pneumonia, and her cough and shortness of breath have now resolved. She was diagnosed with asthma 2 years ago and has been treated for pneumonia twice since that time. Her symptoms typically improve with antibiotics; however, symptoms recur shortly after completing the course of antibiotics. She has tried several inhalers, including a combination inhaled glucocorticoid and long-acting bronchodilator, without relief.

On physical examination, she appears comfortable. Temperature is 37.7 °C (99.9 °F), blood pressure is 114/68 mm Hg, pulse rate is 94/min, respiration rate is 12/min, and oxygen saturation by pulse oximetry is 96% breathing ambient air; BMI is 25. There is no cervical or supraclavicular lymphadenopathy. Decreased breath sounds are noted posteriorly one quarter of the way up on the right, with dullness to percussion and increased tactile fremitus. A localized wheeze is noted over the right lower lung field. There is no clubbing.

Laboratory studies, including a complete blood count with differential, are normal.

Posteroanterior and lateral chest radiographs show a right lower lobe infiltrate that has persisted over the last 8 months.

Which of the following is the most likely diagnosis?

(A) Allergic bronchopulmonary aspergillosis

(B) Bronchial carcinoid tumor

(C) Chronic eosinophilic pneumonia

(D) Cystic fibrosis

Item 21

An 81-year-old man is evaluated in follow-up after a recent hospitalization. He was admitted 2 weeks ago for pneumonia and was discharged 12 days ago with a 10-day course of appropriate antibiotics. For the last week, he has had low-grade fever, fatigue, and increased shortness of breath. He currently is taking no medications.

On physical examination, temperature is 38.4 °C (101.1 °F), blood pressure is 120/65 mm Hg, pulse rate is 80/min, and respiration rate is 28/min. BMI is 21. Oxygen saturation is 90% breathing ambient air. Pulmonary examination reveals decreased fremitus, dullness to percussion, and decreased breath sounds over the lower third of the right hemithorax.

Chest radiograph reveals a moderate right-sided pleural effusion and no effusion on the left side. Thoracic ultrasound shows a moderate echogenic pleural effusion with loculations. Thoracentesis is performed.

Pleural fluid analysis:

Leukocyte count	22,000/µL (22×10^9/L)
Glucose	40 mg/dL (2.2 mmol/L)
Lactate dehydrogenase	1256 U/L
pH	7.1
Gram stain	Negative

Which of the following is the most appropriate management?

(A) Begin ceftriaxone and azithromycin

(B) Insert a large-bore pleural drain (>28 Fr [9.3 mm]) and begin levofloxacin

(C) Insert a small-bore pleural drain (<14 Fr [4.7 mm]) and begin piperacillin-tazobactam

(D) Repeat the chest radiograph in 2 weeks

Item 22

An 18-year-old man is evaluated for a 6-month history of significant chest and throat tightness and acute episodes of a barking cough and a prolonged wheeze that occur during his college basketball practice and games. He also notices episodes of these symptoms occasionally when he is not exerting himself. He has a history of moderate persistent asthma, which had been well controlled. He takes an as-needed short-acting β_2-agonist inhaler at the time his symptoms occur, but this does not relieve his symptoms. He otherwise feels well. Medical history is otherwise unremarkable. In addition to his short-acting β_2-agonist, medications are a low-dose inhaled glucocorticoid and a long-acting inhaled β_2-agonist.

On physical examination, vital signs are normal. There is no jugular venous distention. The lungs are clear without wheezing. Cardiac examination shows no murmur. The remainder of the examination is unremarkable.

Chest radiograph is normal. Spirometry shows no evidence of obstruction.

Which of the following is the most appropriate next step in management?

(A) Allergen immunotherapy

(B) Echocardiography

(C) Otolaryngology evaluation

(D) Switch to a medium-dose inhaled glucocorticoid

Item 23

A 24-year-old man is evaluated in the emergency department for sudden onset of shortness of breath and left-sided chest discomfort. There was no preceding trauma. Medical history is negative and he takes no medications. He does not smoke or use alcohol or illicit drugs.

On physical examination, he appears uncomfortable but is not in acute respiratory distress. Temperature is 37.2 °C (99.0 °F), blood pressure is 117/62 mm Hg, pulse rate is 90/min, and respiration rate is 24/min; BMI is 21. Oxygen saturation is 98% breathing ambient air. There is no jugular venous distention. There is no tracheal deviation. There is hyperresonance to percussion and decreased air entry over the left hemithorax. Asymmetric chest expansion is noted. The cardiac examination is normal, and the remainder of the examination is unremarkable.

A chest radiograph demonstrates a left-sided pneumothorax (4 cm from chest wall to hilum) but no evidence of significant parenchymal disease or lymphadenopathy.

In addition to starting high-flow supplemental oxygen, which of the following is the most appropriate management?

(A) Insert a small-bore thoracostomy tube

(B) Perform needle aspiration of the pneumothorax

(C) Start noninvasive positive pressure ventilation

(D) Observe for 3 to 6 hours, then repeat the chest radiograph

Item 24

A 57-year-old woman is evaluated for a 6-month history of exertional dyspnea. Her medical history is notable for long-standing type 2 diabetes mellitus controlled by diet.

On physical examination, temperature is 37.0 °C (98.6 °F), blood pressure is 144/88 mm Hg, pulse rate is 60/min, and respiration rate is 18/min; BMI is 24. Oxygen saturation is 92% breathing ambient air. Pulmonary examination is normal. Cardiac examination shows a prominent S_2.

Laboratory studies reveal normal hemoglobin, serum electrolyte, and serum creatinine levels.

An electrocardiogram shows left ventricular hypertrophy. Chest radiograph reveals increased pulmonary venous markings. Echocardiogram shows a left ventricular ejection fraction of 54%, normal valves, left ventricular hypertrophy, left atrial dilatation, Doppler evidence of diastolic dysfunction, and a right ventricular systolic pressure of 52 mm Hg.

Which of the following is the most appropriate initial management?

(A) Epoprostenol

(B) Lisinopril

(C) Right heart catheterization

(D) Sildenafil

Item 25

A 44-year-old woman is evaluated in follow-up after multiple recent emergency department visits for worsening asthma. She has had asthma since childhood, but her asthma symptoms have progressively worsened recently. Over the past 2 years, she has had twice-yearly visits to the emergency department requiring treatment with prolonged glucocorticoid tapers. She has required hospitalization twice within the last 4 months. She has no symptoms of gastroesophageal reflux, sinus disease, or other symptoms, and she diligently avoids environmental exposures and likely triggers. Medical history is significant for multiple allergies; skin testing has been positive for allergy to dust mites, cats, and ragweed. She is a never-smoker. Medications are a high-dose inhaled glucocorticoid, a long-acting β_2-agonist, a leukotriene antagonist, a long-acting anticholinergic agent, and an as-needed short-acting β_2-agonist.

On physical examination, vital signs are normal. BMI is 26. Slightly puffy facies are noted. The lungs reveal decreased air movement and mild, diffuse wheezes. Skin fragility is observed on the arms. The remainder of the examination is unremarkable.

Laboratory studies show a serum IgE level of 362 U/mL (362 kU/L) and 6% eosinophils on peripheral blood smear.

Which of the following is the most appropriate treatment?

(A) Allergen immunotherapy

(B) Daily prednisone

(C) Infliximab

(D) Omalizumab

Item 26

A 56-year-old woman is evaluated in the ICU for management of acute respiratory distress syndrome (ARDS) after elective revision of a prosthetic knee. The operation was successful with moderate blood loss, some of which was replaced using an autologous transfusion system. She received no other blood products. Her medical history is notable for osteoarthritis. Her only medication is acetaminophen.

Ventilator settings are unchanged from the operating room: volume-controlled continuous mandatory ventilation (assist/control) mode with a respiration rate of 16/min, a tidal volume of 500 mL, an F_{IO_2} of 0.5, and a positive end-expiratory pressure of 10 cm H_2O.

On physical examination, she is afebrile. Blood pressure is 140/88 mm Hg, pulse rate is 90/min, and respiration rate is 16/min. Her height is 152 cm and weight is 75 kg (165 lb); BMI is 32, and her ideal body weight is 48 kg (106 lb). There is no jugular venous distention. Cardiac examination reveals a grade 2/6 early systolic murmur over the aortic area. There is no S_3 or S_4 and no evidence of peripheral edema. Pulmonary examination reveals diffuse inspiratory crackles. Other than postoperative changes, the remainder of the physical examination is normal.

A chest radiograph shows patchy opacification of airspaces involving all lung fields.

Her plateau pressure is 30 cm H_2O at the time of ICU admission and rises to 38 cm H_2O over the next 24 hours. Her oxygen requirement also increases despite diuresis with a negative fluid balance.

Which of the following is the most likely cause of this patient's acute respiratory distress syndrome?

(A) Obesity hypoventilation syndrome
(B) Pulmonary embolism
(C) Transfusion-associated lung injury
(D) Ventilator-induced lung injury

Item 27

A 57-year-old man is evaluated in follow-up for a right-sided pleural effusion. He initially presented with increasing dyspnea and a constant dull ache on his right side. He also has lost 9.1 kg (20.0 lb) over the last 6 months. Medical history is otherwise unremarkable, and he takes no medications. He has never smoked and is employed as an auto mechanic.

Initial chest radiograph showed a moderate-sized, free-flowing pleural effusion on the right; the left lung field was unremarkable. Thoracentesis showed 3500/µL (3.5 × 10^9/L) nucleated cells with 45% lymphocytes and an exudative profile with negative Gram stain, culture, and cytology. Chest CT following thoracentesis showed no parenchymal lesions but several areas of pleural thickening. A repeat thoracentesis performed 2 weeks later showed similar results, also with negative cultures and cytology.

On physical examination, temperature is 36.7 °C (98.1 °F), blood pressure is 128/72 mm Hg, pulse rate is 81/min, and respiration rate is 18/min; BMI is 23. There is no jugular venous distention. Heart sounds are normal with no murmurs. Dullness to percussion and decreased breath sounds are noted over the lower third of the right hemithorax. The left lung is clear to auscultation. No lower extremity edema is noted.

Repeat chest radiograph shows reaccumulation of the right pleural effusion.

Which of the following is the most appropriate diagnostic test to perform next?

(A) Bronchoscopy
(B) Large-volume pleural fluid cytology
(C) PET/CT scanning
(D) Thoracoscopy

 ## Item 28

A 67-year-old man is evaluated in the emergency department for sepsis secondary to pyelonephritis. He takes no medications.

On physical examination, he is diaphoretic. Temperature is 40.0 °C (104.0 °F), blood pressure is 90/55 mm Hg, pulse rate is 119/min, and respiration rate is 33/min. Oxygen saturation is 93% breathing 50% oxygen by face mask. Respiratory efforts are short and shallow, and the lungs are clear to auscultation. There is tenderness to palpation over the right costovertebral angle. The remainder of the examination is unremarkable.

Urinalysis is positive for too numerous to count leukocytes and many gram-negative rods.

Intravenous fluids and empiric antibiotics are begun, but his mental status declines acutely and he is urgently intubated.

Which of the following is the most appropriate mode of ventilation for this patient?

(A) Continuous mandatory ventilation with pressure control
(B) Continuous mandatory ventilation with volume control
(C) Intermittent mandatory ventilation with pressure control
(D) Intermittent mandatory ventilation with volume control

Item 29

A 28-year-old man is evaluated for shortness of breath, fatigue, and nighttime cough. He has been employed in an auto body shop for the past 4 years and notes that his symptoms began about 6 months ago. He believes his symptoms may be associated with his work. He is being evaluated after several days off from work and currently has no symptoms or medical concerns. Medical history is unremarkable and he takes no medications. He is a never-smoker.

On physical examination, vital signs are normal. BMI is 25; his weight has remained the same for 2 years. Oxygen saturation breathing ambient air is 99%. The sinus examination is normal and the lungs are clear, with no wheezing or crackles noted. The remainder of the examination is unremarkable.

A chest radiograph is normal, and spirometry results are normal.

Which of the following is the most appropriate next step in management?

(A) Advise him to switch employment
(B) High-resolution chest CT
(C) Inhaled glucocorticoid daily
(D) Repeat spirometry after workplace exposure

Item 30

A 42-year-old man is evaluated in follow-up after being diagnosed with obstructive sleep apnea (OSA) 6 weeks ago. Polysomnography showed moderate-severity OSA that was adequately controlled with continuous positive airway pressure (CPAP) at 8 cm H_2O. He has noticed improved daytime alertness since starting CPAP, but he finds that the apparatus is very cumbersome to transport on his frequent business trips. Medical history is otherwise unremarkable, and he takes no medications. He works as a national sales representative.

On physical examination, temperature is 37.0 °C (98.6 °F), blood pressure is 132/82 mm Hg, pulse rate is 82/min, and respiration rate is 14/min; BMI is 27. The neck circumference is 43 cm (17 in). Oropharyngeal examination reveals patent nasal airways, a low-lying soft palate, and a slight dental overjet. Cardiopulmonary examination is normal.

Weight loss is recommended.

Which of the following is the most appropriate alternative treatment to continuous positive airway pressure?

(A) Oral mandibular advancement appliance
(B) Supplemental oxygen
(C) Surgical maxillomandibular advancement
(D) Uvulopalatopharyngoplasty

Item 31

A 61-year-old woman is admitted to the hospital for fever, shortness of breath, and weakness. Symptoms began following initiation of her latest round of chemotherapy for treatment of non-Hodgkin lymphoma 1 week ago. Other than lymphoma, her medical history is unremarkable. Subcutaneous low-molecular weight heparin is begun for venous thromboembolism prophylaxis. She is allergic to penicillin, which caused a rash.

Empiric treatment with meropenem and vancomycin is begun. She experiences steady clinical improvement over the next 2 days. All cultures show no growth, and antibiotics are discontinued. On the morning of the third hospital day, she is found unresponsive in her hospital room.

On physical examination, blood pressure is 68/38 mm Hg, pulse rate is 120/min, and respiration rate is 26/min. Oxygen saturation is 88% on a 100% oxygen nonrebreather mask. Jugular venous distention is noted. The lungs are clear bilaterally with normal breath sounds. Heart rate is regular and a prominent P_2 is noted. There is no rash.

Electrocardiogram shows tachycardia and nonspecific ST-T wave changes.

Which of the following is the most likely diagnosis?

(A) Anaphylaxis
(B) Myocardial infarction
(C) Pulmonary embolism
(D) Septic shock

Item 32

A 55-year-old man is evaluated in follow-up for severe COPD, which was diagnosed 2 years ago. He has had two exacerbations in the past year requiring hospitalization, and his baseline exercise tolerance is low. He completed pulmonary rehabilitation 3 months ago without much improvement in exercise capacity. He quit smoking 1 year ago. His medications are tiotropium, fluticasone/salmeterol, daily roflumilast, and albuterol as needed.

On physical examination, vital signs are normal; BMI is 22. Oxygen saturation is 92% breathing ambient air. Scattered wheezing is noted bilaterally.

Chest radiograph and CT scan both show emphysematous changes in the upper lobes. Spirometry shows an FEV_1 of 40% of predicted and a $DLCO$ of 25% of predicted. His 6-minute walking distance is 240 meters (787 feet), consistent with decreased exercise tolerance.

Which of the following is most likely to benefit this patient?

(A) Change fluticasone/salmeterol to fluticasone/ vilanterol
(B) Daily prednisone

(C) Lung transplantation
(D) Lung volume reduction surgery

Item 33

A 47-year-old man is evaluated for a 6-month history of dry cough. His symptoms began 6 months ago when he noted the paroxysmal onset of persistent coughing spells that make it difficult to carry on a conversation. He was initially diagnosed with allergic rhinitis and was started on a glucocorticoid nasal inhaler with some improvement of his rhinitis symptoms but not his cough. He reports no symptoms of gastroesophageal reflux disease. Medical history is otherwise unremarkable except for a history of dust allergies. Medications are a fluticasone nasal inhaler and an over-the-counter antihistamine as needed. Family history is significant for seasonal allergies and asthma in his children. He is a never-smoker. He works as an upholsterer.

On physical examination, vital signs are normal. Oxygen saturation breathing ambient air is 98%. Slight nasal congestion and dry cough are noted during examination, but both are improved from his previous evaluation. No sinus tenderness is noted. Cardiovascular, pulmonary, and abdominal examination findings are unremarkable.

A chest radiograph is normal. Spirometry shows an FEV_1 of 82% of predicted, an FVC in the normal range, and a slightly reduced FEV_1/FVC ratio of 70%. After bronchodilator challenge, the FEV_1 is increased by 3%.

Which of the following is the most appropriate diagnostic test to perform next?

(A) Allergy skin testing
(B) High-resolution chest CT
(C) Measurement of serum IgE levels
(D) Methacholine challenge testing

Item 34

A 63-year-old woman is evaluated in the emergency department following multiple wasp stings that occurred when she was working in her garden. She is in respiratory distress with wheezing and is confused.

On physical examination after receiving a normal saline fluid bolus, temperature is 37.1 °C (98.8 °F), blood pressure is 76/44 mm Hg, pulse rate is 114/min, and respiration rate is 28/min. Oxygen saturation is 93% breathing 3 L of oxygen per minute by nasal cannula. She appears confused and can follow only simple commands. The skin is flushed, and urticaria is noted. Chest examination reveals diffuse bilateral expiratory wheezes. Cardiac examination reveals regular tachycardic rhythm. The extremities are cool to the touch.

Which of the following is the most appropriate next step in treatment?

(A) Diphenhydramine
(B) Epinephrine
(C) Glucagon
(D) Methylprednisolone

Item 35

A 69-year-old man is evaluated to determine the appropriateness of air travel. He has moderate-severity COPD (FEV_1 is 47% of predicted) with stable exertional dyspnea in the setting of previous cigarette smoking. He and his wife are planning a 4-hour flight. He has not flown in 5 years.

His medical history is also notable for coronary artery disease. His medications are a tiotropium inhaler, an albuterol/ipratropium inhaler, aspirin, rosuvastatin, and metoprolol.

On physical examination, temperature is 36.6 °C (97.9 °F), blood pressure is 124/74 mm Hg, pulse rate is 80/min, and respiration rate is 16/min; BMI is 23. Oxygen saturation is 93% at rest breathing ambient air. Pulmonary examination reveals distant breath sounds, resonance to percussion, and no wheeze.

A chest radiograph performed 6 months ago showed a flattened diaphragm.

Which of the following is the most appropriate management?

(A) Arterial blood gas studies
(B) Echocardiographic assessment of pulmonary artery pressures
(C) Hypoxia altitude simulation test
(D) Recommend not flying

Item 36

A 30-year-old woman is evaluated in follow-up for wheezing and cough that started 6 weeks ago after a viral respiratory illness. At that time she had daily wheezing and cough with nocturnal symptoms that would disturb her sleep. An as-needed β_2-agonist was prescribed for symptomatic relief. She reports feeling much better. Her daytime symptoms of wheezing and cough have resolved, but she notes that she awakens from sleep with shortness of breath approximately twice a week. Medical history is notable for mild asthma as a child that was treated for several years; however, she has not required treatment since age 15 years. Her only medication is as-needed inhaled albuterol. She is a never-smoker.

On physical examination, vital signs are normal. No wheezing is noted on pulmonary examination. The remainder of the examination is normal.

Spirometry demonstrates an FEV_1/FVC ratio of 76%, with an improvement of 15% in the FEV_1 following treatment with a bronchodilator.

Which of the following is the most appropriate management?

(A) Add a glucocorticoid inhaler
(B) Continue current therapy and reevaluate in 4 weeks
(C) Discontinue inhaler medication
(D) Switch to a long-acting β_2-agonist inhaler

Item 37

A 73-year-old man is evaluated for sleep difficulties. He notes unrefreshing sleep that is sometimes interrupted by nocturia, and he occasionally experiences episodes of short-ness of breath that awaken him. He thinks he might snore but has no regular bed partner to provide confirmation. His normal sleep schedule is 10:30 PM to 6:30 AM. Most days of the week he feels sleepy during the daytime and naps for 45 minutes. He has a history of chronic atrial fibrillation and heart failure with stable exertional dyspnea. His medications are lisinopril, atorvastatin, warfarin, and metoprolol.

On physical examination, temperature is 36.6 °C (97.9 °F), blood pressure is 118/70 mm Hg, pulse rate is 76/min, and respiration rate is 14/min; BMI is 27. Respiratory examination shows a low-lying soft palate and clear lung fields. Cardiac examination discloses an irregularly irregular rhythm but no murmurs.

Which of the following is the most appropriate next step in management?

(A) Auto-titrating positive airway pressure (APAP)
(B) In-laboratory polysomnography
(C) Out-of-center sleep testing
(D) Overnight pulse oximetry

Item 38

A 74-year-old man is evaluated in follow-up for a diagnosis of silicosis related to his former occupation as a mine worker. Over the past 4 months he has noted a 4.5-kg (10.0-lb) weight loss. He has not had fever, chills, sweats, or change in his baseline cough or dyspnea with exertion. His medical history is otherwise unremarkable. He has a 15-pack-year smoking history but quit 30 years ago. He takes no medications.

On physical examination, temperature and blood pressure are normal, pulse rate is 85/min, and respiration rate is 18/min. Oxygen saturation breathing ambient air is 97%. No jugular venous distention is noted. Pulmonary examination reveals decreased breath sounds but no wheezes. Cardiac examination is normal. There is no peripheral edema.

His last chest CT 1 year ago showed profuse upper lobe scarring and nodularity. A current chest radiograph is consistent with these findings and is unchanged from a study 6 months ago. His tuberculin skin testing has always been negative, with the last test performed 6 months ago.

Which of the following is the most appropriate next step in management?

(A) Chest MRI
(B) Isoniazid, rifampin, pyrazinamide, and ethambutol
(C) Prednisone
(D) Repeat chest CT

Item 39

A 58-year-old man is evaluated for chronic cough, occasional wheezing, and shortness of breath associated with frequent stops to catch his breath when walking one to two blocks on level ground. His medical history is notable for an episode of bronchitis, for which he underwent outpatient treatment 6 months ago. He is a current smoker with a 30-pack-year smoking history.

On physical examination, vital signs are normal. Examination of the lungs shows mildly decreased breath sounds throughout both lung fields and occasional scattered expiratory wheezes. The remainder of the physical examination is normal. Spirometry shows an FEV_1 of 70% of predicted and a postbronchodilator FEV_1/FVC ratio of 62%. His modified Medical Research Council (mMRC) symptom score is 2.

In addition to smoking cessation, which of the following is the most appropriate treatment?

(A) Combination inhaled glucocorticoid and a long-acting bronchodilator

(B) Phosphodiesterase-4 inhibitor and combination inhaled glucocorticoid and long-acting bronchodilator

(C) Short-acting bronchodilator as needed, a long-acting bronchodilator, and pulmonary rehabilitation

(D) Short-acting bronchodilator as needed and an inhaled glucocorticoid

Item 40

A 55-year-old woman is evaluated in follow-up for a 1-year history of chronic, nonproductive cough. She was recently diagnosed with cough-variant asthma after a methacholine challenge test. She was started on inhaled fluticasone and as-needed albuterol 3 months ago. Her cough initially improved; however, her symptoms have not fully resolved and are worsened at times, most notably when she lies down. She also notes that mild hoarseness occasionally accompanies her cough. She uses alcohol socially, and she works long hours as an attorney.

On physical examination, the patient is afebrile, blood pressure is 132/75 mm Hg, and pulse rate is 82/min; BMI is 28. Dry cough with frequent throat clearing is noted. The chest is clear with no wheezing. The remainder of the examination is unremarkable.

Which of the following is the most appropriate management?

(A) Add a long-acting β_2-agonist

(B) Add a proton pump inhibitor

(C) Repeat methacholine challenge testing

(D) Start nocturnal antitussive therapy

Item 41

A 44-year-old woman is evaluated for a 1-year history of fatigue. She has been on disability owing to chronic low back pain following a motor vehicle accident 18 months ago. She typically goes to bed between midnight and 1 AM. She awakens intermittently overnight because of musculoskeletal aches but usually returns to sleep without much difficulty. She spontaneously awakens between 8 AM and 9 AM and feels unrefreshed. She sometimes naps during the day if she is bored or tired. She does not experience drowsiness when driving. She has no regular bed partner to provide a collateral history. Medications are sustained-release oxycodone twice daily and immediate-release oxycodone/acetaminophen every 6 hours as needed.

On physical examination, temperature is 36.6 °C (97.9 °F), blood pressure is 122/68 mm Hg, pulse rate is 90/min, and respiration rate is 12/min; BMI is 24. The

oropharyngeal airway is patent, and the nasal examination is normal. Cardiopulmonary examination is unremarkable. Trunk flexion is limited owing to pain. There is no peripheral edema.

In-laboratory polysomnography shows central sleep apnea.

Which of the following is the most appropriate next step in management for this patient's sleep apnea?

(A) Adaptive servoventilation

(B) Continuous positive airway pressure

(C) Modafinil

(D) Reduce opioid use

Item 42

A 35-year-old woman is evaluated in follow-up for worsening asthma. Medical history is significant for environmental and food allergies, allergic rhinitis, and asthma diagnosed at age 10 years. Although her asthma had been previously well controlled, her symptoms have worsened over the past year with increased wheezing and a cough productive of dark-colored mucus. She was admitted to the hospital 2 weeks ago for her asthma symptoms and was diagnosed with pneumonia. She was treated with antibiotics and a tapering course of glucocorticoids. Her respiratory symptoms have recurred following completion of therapy. Medical history is otherwise unremarkable. Medications are fluticasone/salmeterol and as-needed albuterol metered-dose inhalers. She works as a school teacher.

On physical examination, temperature is 37.1 °C (98.7 °F), blood pressure is 110/70 mm Hg, pulse rate is 92/min, and respiration rate is 16/min; BMI is 23. Diffuse wheezing is noted on expiration with diminished airflow across the upper right lung field. The remainder of the examination is unremarkable.

Laboratory studies show a leukocyte count of $10,500/\mu L$ (10.5×10^9/L) with 15% eosinophils. Chest radiograph shows a right upper lobe infiltrate and diffusely increased lung markings.

Which of the following is the most likely diagnosis?

(A) Allergic bronchopulmonary aspergillosis

(B) Cystic fibrosis

(C) Eosinophilic granulomatosis with polyangiitis (Churg-Strauss syndrome)

(D) Hypersensitivity pneumonitis

Item 43

A 58-year-old woman was hospitalized 1 week ago for acute-on-chronic kidney injury. Since her hospitalization, she has been receiving hemodialysis through a temporary femoral vein catheter. Last night, she developed a fever of 38.7 °C (101.7 °F).

On physical examination today, she is confused. Blood pressure is 76/40 mm Hg and pulse rate is 108/min. Weight is 60 kg (132 lb). She has adequate peripheral venous access and is given a 1000-mL bolus of intravenous normal saline over 30 minutes. After receiving the fluid bolus, blood

CONT.

pressure is 78/44 mm Hg. Oxygen saturation is 96% breathing ambient air. Cardiac examination reveals an S_1 and S_2 with regular tachycardic rhythm. There is no jugular venous distention, murmur, or gallop. The chest is clear to auscultation. Erythema without purulent discharge is noted at the femoral catheter site. The extremities are warm with bounding pulses and without edema.

Laboratory studies:

Hemoglobin	9.8 g/dL (98 g/L) (baseline 10 g/dL [100 g/L])
Leukocyte count	16,000/μL (16 × 10⁹/L)
Creatinine	2.6 mg/dL (229.8 μmol/L)
Potassium	5.6 mEq/L (5.6 mmol/L)

A blood culture obtained yesterday is growing gram-positive cocci.

A chest radiograph is normal. Electrocardiogram shows sinus tachycardia and no acute ischemic changes.

In addition to replacing the hemodialysis catheter, which of the following is the most appropriate next step in treatment?

(A) Administer another 1000-mL normal saline fluid bolus

(B) Initiate dobutamine infusion

(C) Insert a central venous catheter

(D) Transfuse one unit of packed red blood cells

Item 44

A 75-year-old man is evaluated in the hospital after being admitted 1 week ago for a 2-week history of increased shortness of breath. He was diagnosed with idiopathic pulmonary fibrosis 5 years ago and has had progressive decline in pulmonary function and functional status since then. Two months ago he began requiring 5 L/min of supplemental oxygen at rest. During his hospitalization he has received a 7-day course of meropenem, levofloxacin, and linezolid. He also received a 5-day course of high-dose intravenous methylprednisolone. Diagnostic evaluation in the hospital ruled out pulmonary embolism and infection. He also has hypertension and type 2 diabetes mellitus, for which he takes lisinopril, chlorthalidone, and metformin.

On physical examination, the patient is afebrile, blood pressure is normal, pulse rate is 118/min, and respiration rate is 42/min. Jugular venous distention is present. Pulmonary examination reveals diffuse crackles. The pulmonic component of S_2 is increased. He has peripheral edema and clubbing.

Arterial blood gas studies on 15 L of oxygen via nonrebreathing mask show a pH of 7.32, a P_{CO_2} of 55 mm Hg (7.3 kPa), and a P_{O_2} of 50 mm Hg (6.7 kPa). High-resolution CT scan shows progression of fibrosis without evidence of superimposed ground-glass opacity.

Which of the following is the most appropriate treatment?

(A) Additional intravenous methylprednisolone

(B) Hospice care

(C) Intubation and mechanical ventilation

(D) Lung transplantation

Item 45

An 18-year-old man is evaluated in the emergency department after being found somnolent in a wooded area close to his home. His shirt is covered with emesis. He was last seen in his normal state of health 3 hours ago. His medical history is notable for anxiety, and his only medication is sertraline.

On physical examination, temperature is 38.5 °C (101.3 °F), blood pressure is 98/58 mm Hg, pulse rate is 108/min, and respiration rate is 12/min; BMI is 26. Oxygen saturation is 85% breathing ambient air. The skin is warm. Neurologic examination reveals obtundation and semipurposeful movement of all extremities with painful stimulation. Normal muscle tone is noted, but reflexes are difficult to elicit. Pulmonary examination reveals shallow inspiration with rhonchi in the right lower lung field. Cardiac examination reveals a regular rhythm. The abdomen is soft and nondistended with no overt tenderness.

Laboratory studies:

Blood urea nitrogen	14 mg/dL (5.0 mmol/L)
Electrolytes:	
Sodium	140 mEq/L (140 mmol/L)
Potassium	3.2 mEq/L (3.2 mmol/L)
Chloride	104 mEq/L (104 mmol/L)
Bicarbonate	6 mEq/L (6 mmol/L)
Glucose	180 mg/dL (10 mmol/L)
Lactate	2.8 mEq/L (2.8 mmol/L)
Plasma osmolality	325 mOsm/kg H_2O
Blood ethanol	Absent
Arterial blood gases (breathing 50% oxygen by mask):	
pH	7.17
P_{CO_2}	17 mm Hg (2.3 kPa)
P_{O_2}	120 mm Hg (16.0 kPa)

Which of the following is the most likely diagnosis?

(A) Isopropyl alcohol poisoning

(B) Methanol poisoning

(C) Salicylate poisoning

(D) Serotonin syndrome

Item 46

A 38-year-old woman is evaluated for a 2-week history of fever, right-sided chest pain, cough, and occasional night sweats. Her chest discomfort is sharp and stabbing, and the cough is not productive. Medical history is significant for tuberculosis treated with 6 months of antimicrobial therapy 10 years ago when she lived in Africa; she immigrated to the United States 6 years ago. Medical history is otherwise unremarkable and she takes no medications.

On physical examination, temperature is 36.5 °C (97.7 °F), blood pressure is 132/83 mm Hg, pulse rate is 80/min, and respiration rate is 20/min; BMI is 30. Dullness to percussion and decreased breath sounds are noted over the lower third of the right hemithorax. A pleural rub is noted over the midlateral right lung field.

Chest radiograph shows a moderate right-sided pleural effusion with no infiltrate.

Thoracentesis is performed, and 500 mL of straw-colored fluid is removed.

Laboratory studies:

Serum lactate dehydrogenase	90 U/L
Serum total protein	7.2 g/dL (72 g/L)
Pleural fluid lactate dehydrogenase	600 U/L
Pleural fluid pH	7.30
Pleural fluid total protein	5.6 g/dL (56 g/L)
Pleural fluid total nucleated cell count	5700/µL (5.7×10⁹/L), with 15% neutrophils, 71% lymphocytes, 12% monocytes, and 2% eosinophils

Which of the following tests is most likely to lead to a diagnosis?

(A) Induced sputum culture and stain for acid-fast bacilli

(B) Pleural fluid adenosine deaminase measurement

(C) Pleural fluid culture for acid-fast bacilli

(D) Pleural fluid stain for acid-fast bacilli

Item 47

A 23-year-old man is evaluated in the emergency department for a worsening asthma exacerbation that began 2 days ago following an upper respiratory infection. He has been using an albuterol inhaler at home without improvement. He has a history of poorly controlled asthma and has been hospitalized once a year for the past 4 years; he required intubation 2 years ago. Medical history is otherwise unremarkable. Medications are a long-acting glucocorticoid and an as-needed albuterol inhaler. He is a never-smoker.

On physical examination, he is in moderate discomfort. Temperature is 37.3 °C (99.1 °F), blood pressure is 138/85 mm Hg, pulse rate is 124/min, and respiration rate is 20/min. Audible wheezing is heard, and pulmonary examination reveals diffuse expiratory wheezes. Except for tachycardia, the remainder of the examination is normal.

Chest radiograph shows hyperinflated lungs but is otherwise normal. Arterial blood gas studies breathing ambient air show a pH of 7.48, a P_{CO_2} of 30 mm Hg (4.0 kPa), and P_{O_2} of 85 mm Hg (11.3 kPa).

Systemic glucocorticoids and frequent β_2-agonist nebulizer treatments are administered. After 1 hour, he notes that he feels better. He appears tired, is not speaking in full sentences, and is using accessory muscles of breathing. Pulse rate is now 119/min, respiration rate is 19/min, and repeat arterial blood gas studies breathing ambient air show a pH of 7.38, a P_{CO_2} of 43 mm Hg (5.7 kPa), and a P_{O_2} of 80 mm Hg (10.6 kPa).

Which of the following is the most appropriate management?

(A) Admit to the general medical floor

(B) Admit to the ICU

(C) Continue current treatment and reassess in 2 hours

(D) Discharge home with next-day follow-up

Item 48

A 72-year-old man is evaluated for a 2-year history of cough and a 1-year history of increasing dyspnea. He describes the cough as nonproductive, and his shortness of breath is worse with exertion. He does not have chest pain, orthopnea, paroxysmal nocturnal dyspnea, or any other symptoms. Medical history is otherwise unremarkable. He has a 15-pack-year smoking history but quit 40 years ago. He worked as a construction worker for 40 years. He takes no medications.

On physical examination, temperature, blood pressure, and pulse rate are normal; respiration rate is 18/min. Oxygen saturation breathing ambient air is 96%. BMI is 24. Pulmonary examination reveals inspiratory crackles at the bases bilaterally. Cardiac examination is normal. The remainder of the physical examination is unremarkable.

Chest radiograph shows increased interstitial markings at the bases; calcified parietal pleural plaques are noted bilaterally. High-resolution CT shows bilateral peripheral- and basal-predominant septal line thickening with evidence of honeycomb change at the bases. Pulmonary function tests reveal an FEV_1 of 70% of predicted, an FVC of 75% of predicted, an FEV_1/FVC ratio of 85%, and a D_{LCO} of 65% of predicted.

Which of the following is the most likely diagnosis?

(A) Asbestosis

(B) COPD

(C) Hypersensitivity pneumonitis

(D) Idiopathic pulmonary fibrosis

Item 49

A 52-year-old man is evaluated in follow-up after being diagnosed with severe obstructive sleep apnea 8 weeks ago. Continuous positive airway pressure (CPAP) was prescribed based on a titration during in-laboratory polysomnography. He notes some improvement in his sleep with CPAP, but he still feels drowsy during the day. He does not have problems with nasal congestion. Medical history is otherwise negative and he takes no medications.

On physical examination, temperature is 37.2 °C (99.0 °F), blood pressure is 138/86 mm Hg, pulse rate is 72/min, and respiration rate is 12/min; BMI is 32. A low-lying soft palate and patent nasal airways are noted. The cardiopulmonary examination is unremarkable, and the neurologic examination is normal.

Which of the following is the most appropriate next step in management to address this patient's continued drowsiness?

(A) Prescribe eszopiclone

(B) Prescribe modafinil

(C) Review data from the patient's continuous positive airway pressure device

(D) Switch to a bilevel positive airway pressure device

Item 50

A 30-year-old woman is admitted to the ICU for management of respiratory failure due to influenza A infection.

She is intubated and mechanically ventilated. Ventilator settings are in the volume-controlled continuous mandatory ventilation (assist/control) mode with a respiration rate of 18/min, a tidal volume of 360 mL (6 mL/kg of ideal body weight), an FIO_2 of 0.9, and a positive end-expiratory pressure (PEEP) of 14 cm H_2O. Her plateau pressure is 28 cm H_2O. Because of difficulty with oxygenation, she was paralyzed and is being appropriately monitored for depth of sedation and depth of paralysis. Her medical history is otherwise unremarkable. In addition to her sedative and paralyzing agents, her only medication is oseltamivir.

On physical examination, temperature is 38.8 °C (101.8 °F), blood pressure is 112/64 mm Hg, pulse rate is 85/min, and respiration rate is 18/min; BMI is 29. There is no jugular venous distention. Coarse breath sounds are auscultated throughout both lung fields. Cardiac examination is normal, and there are no other significant findings on her general medical examination.

A chest radiograph shows an appropriately placed endotracheal tube. Diffuse, patchy infiltrates are seen throughout both lung fields, consistent with acute respiratory distress syndrome. Arterial blood gas studies show a pH of 7.41, a PCO_2 of 38 mm Hg (5.0 kPa), and a PO_2 of 57 mm Hg (7.6 kPa).

Which of the following is the most appropriate next step in management?

(A) Aerosolized surfactant
(B) Inhaled nitric oxide
(C) Prone positioning
(D) Systemic glucocorticoids

Item 51

A 66-year-old woman is evaluated for a 6-week history of increasing dyspnea. She has also has right-sided pleuritic chest pain when lying down and an occasional cough. She has lost 9.1 kg (20.0 lb) in the last 3 months. She has no other medical problems and takes no medications.

On physical examination, temperature is 36.4 °C (97.5 °F), blood pressure is 119/63 mm Hg, pulse rate is 77/min, and respiration rate is 20/min; oxygen saturation is 92% breathing ambient air. BMI is 21. There is no jugular venous distention. Heart sounds are normal with no murmurs. Pulmonary examination reveals dullness to percussion and decreased breath sounds over both lower lung zones. A 4-cm right breast mass is palpated.

Chest radiograph demonstrates bilateral pleural effusions but no evidence of infiltrate or pulmonary vascular congestion.

Thoracentesis is performed, and 500 mL of serosanguineous fluid is removed.

Laboratory studies:

Serum lactate dehydrogenase	124 U/L
Serum total protein	6.2 g/dL (62 g/L)
Pleural fluid lactate dehydrogenase	320 U/L
Pleural fluid total protein	4 g/dL (40 g/L)
Pleural fluid glucose	55 mg/dL (3.1 mmol/L)
Pleural fluid total nucleated cells	3500/µL (3.5×10^9/L) (15% lymphocytes)

Pleural fluid Gram stain is negative. Cytology is negative for malignancy.

In addition to evaluation of the breast mass, which of the following is the most appropriate management?

(A) Closed pleural biopsy
(B) Pleural fluid flow cytometry
(C) Repeat thoracentesis and pleural fluid cytology
(D) Thoracoscopic pleural biopsy

Item 52

A 53-year-old woman is evaluated for a 3-month history of progressively worsening exertional dyspnea and chest pressure. She has not had fever, cough, sputum production, or weight loss. Four months ago she underwent left shoulder arthroplasty. Eighteen months ago she had a right lower extremity deep venous thrombosis attributed to hormone replacement therapy. Hormones were discontinued, and she completed a 6-month course of warfarin. She takes no medications at this time.

On physical examination, temperature is 36.0 °C (96.8 °F), blood pressure is 130/74 mm Hg, pulse rate is 90/min, and respiration rate is 18/min; BMI is 26. Oxygen saturation is 89% breathing ambient air. Pulmonary examination reveals clear lung fields. Cardiac examination reveals a single loud S_2. There is no peripheral edema.

Laboratory studies, including a complete blood count and electrolyte measurement, are normal.

Chest radiograph shows no cardiopulmonary abnormalities. Transthoracic echocardiogram shows normal left ventricular and right ventricular function, normal valves, and a right ventricular systolic pressure of 52 mm Hg. Pulmonary function testing reveals an isolated reduction in diffusing capacity. Bilateral lower extremity venous ultrasound shows no evidence of recurrent deep venous thrombosis.

Which of the following is the most appropriate diagnostic test to perform next?

(A) CT angiography of the chest
(B) Polysomnography
(C) Pulmonary angiography
(D) Ventilation-perfusion scan

Item 53

A 66-year-old man is evaluated in the emergency department following a fall 3 days ago, when he struck the right side of his chest against a table. Since that time he has experienced right-sided pleuritic chest pain and difficulty taking a deep breath. His only other medical problem is chronic atrial fibrillation, for which he takes warfarin.

On physical examination, temperature is 37.3 °C (99.1 °F), blood pressure is 132/80 mm Hg, pulse rate is 75/min and irregular, and respiration rate is 15/min with significant left-side splinting; BMI is 26. Oxygen saturation is 85% breathing ambient air. The right side of his chest shows extensive bruising. There is no jugular venous distention and, other than an irregularly irregular rhythm, the cardiac examination is unremarkable. There are diminished breath sounds over the right lower chest with occasional crackles.

CONT. Oxygen saturation does not improve with increasing flow rates of supplemental oxygen delivered by nasal cannula. Oxygen saturation of 90% is achieved with 80% supplemental oxygen delivered by mask.

Laboratory studies reveal a hemoglobin level of 11.8 g/dL (118 g/L) and an INR of 2.5.

Chest radiograph is shown.

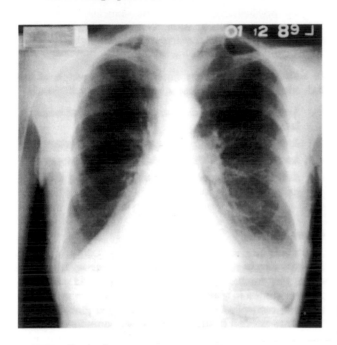

Which of the following is the most likely diagnosis?

(A) Hepatopulmonary syndrome

(B) Intracardiac shunt

(C) Intrapulmonary shunt

(D) Pulmonary arteriovenous malformation

Item 54

A 35-year-old woman is evaluated for a 6-month history of exertional dyspnea. She becomes dyspneic after climbing a flight of stairs or walking two blocks. Her medical history is unremarkable, and she takes no medications.

On physical examination, temperature is 37.4 °C (99.3 °F), blood pressure is 134/86 mm Hg, pulse rate is 84/min, and respiration rate is 18/min; BMI is 26. The lungs are clear. Cardiac examination reveals a prominent S_2. Skin examination is normal. Trace bilateral ankle edema is noted.

Laboratory studies, including serum electrolytes, liver chemistry studies, and serum creatinine, are normal. Antinuclear antibody testing is negative.

Echocardiogram reveals normal left ventricular size and function; the valves are normal. Chest radiograph shows enlarged pulmonary arteries. Pulmonary function tests show an isolated reduction in diffusing capacity (40% of predicted). Ventilation-perfusion scan shows no evidence of venous thromboembolism, and a CT scan of the chest reveals normal lung parenchyma. Right heart catheterization reveals a mean pulmonary artery pressure of 35 mm Hg and a pulmonary capillary wedge pressure of 10 mm Hg.

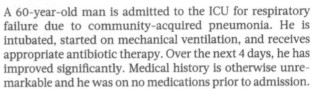
During vasoreactivity testing using inhaled nitric oxide, the mean pulmonary artery pressure remained unchanged.

Which of the following is the most appropriate management?

(A) Epoprostenol

(B) Nifedipine

(C) Restriction of physical activity

(D) Sildenafil

Item 55

A 60-year-old man is admitted to the ICU for respiratory failure due to community-acquired pneumonia. He is intubated, started on mechanical ventilation, and receives appropriate antibiotic therapy. Over the next 4 days, he has improved significantly. Medical history is otherwise unremarkable and he was on no medications prior to admission.

Current physical examination findings include temperature of 37.0 °C (98.6 °F), blood pressure of 120/80 mm Hg, pulse rate of 85/min, and respiration rate of 12/min. Scattered coarse breath sounds are noted throughout both lung fields. The remainder of the examination is normal.

After 30 minutes of a spontaneous breathing trial (SBT), blood pressure is 135/90 mm Hg, pulse rate is 100/min, respiration rate is 28/min, and oxygen saturation is 92% on an FIO_2 of 0.35. He tolerated the SBT without evident onset of arrhythmia, respiratory distress, diaphoresis, or anxiety.

Chest radiograph shows clearing of diffuse infiltrates.

Which of the following is the most appropriate management?

(A) Arterial blood gas studies

(B) Continue mechanical ventilation for 24 hours and reassess

(C) Extubate and discontinue mechanical ventilation

(D) Extubate and initiate noninvasive positive pressure mechanical ventilation

Item 56

A 38-year-old woman is evaluated for exertional dyspnea and fatigue. Her symptoms began 4 months ago and have been steadily worsening. On two recent occasions, she experienced near-syncope walking up two flights of stairs. She notes no shortness of breath at rest or other respiratory symptoms. Medical history is significant for limited cutaneous systemic sclerosis. Her only medication is lansoprazole.

On physical examination, temperature is 36.8 °C (98.2 °F), blood pressure is 122/72 mm Hg, pulse rate is 88/min, and respiration rate is 16/min; BMI is 26. Oxygen saturation breathing ambient air is 94%. Pulmonary examination reveals clear lung fields. Cardiac examination discloses a prominent S_2. Sclerotic changes are noted in the bilateral hands and forearms.

Chest radiograph is normal. Pulmonary function testing shows normal spirometry findings and a DLCO of 48% of predicted. CT angiography shows no evidence of pulmonary embolism. Transthoracic echocardiography shows normal left ventricular function, an enlarged right ventricle, and an estimated pulmonary artery pressure of 52 mm Hg.

Which of the following is the most appropriate diagnostic test to perform next?

(A) 6-Minute walk test

(B) Overnight pulse oximetry

(C) Polysomnography

(D) Right heart catheterization

Item 57

A 66-year-old man is evaluated for a 4-month history of dyspnea on exertion. His symptoms are progressive, and he currently becomes short of breath when getting dressed in the morning. He has not had fever or chills but has lost 9 kg (20 lb) over the past 3 months. His medical history is otherwise unremarkable. He is an active smoker with a 46-pack-year smoking history. He is a retired plumber. He takes no medications.

On physical examination, temperature is 37.2 °C (99.0 °F), blood pressure is 146/82 mm Hg, pulse rate is 90/min, and respiration rate is 16/min; BMI is 27. Oxygen saturation is 92% breathing ambient air. There is no jugular venous distention. There are no palpable cervical or supra-clavicular lymph nodes. Decreased breath sounds are noted on the right, halfway up the hemithorax. There is dullness to percussion and decreased tactile fremitus but no egophony. No pedal edema is noted.

A low-dose chest CT, performed 5 months ago for lung cancer screening, is shown.

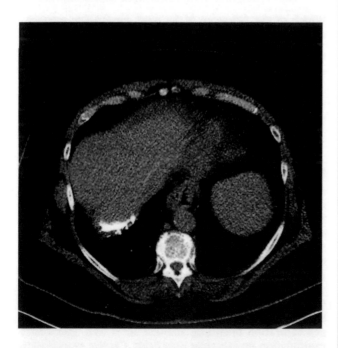

Current laboratory and imaging studies are pending.

Which of the following is the most likely diagnosis?

(A) Heart failure

(B) Lymphoma

(C) Mesothelioma

(D) Pneumonia

Item 58

A 32-year-old woman is evaluated for a 3-month history of dyspnea on exertion and intermittent dry cough. She continues to jog 3 miles per day but notes that it takes her longer than it used to because of increased dyspnea on exertion. She has no other symptoms and takes no medications.

On physical examination, vital signs are normal. The lungs are clear to auscultation. Skin thickening is noted on the backs of the hands, forearms, face, and thighs.

A chest radiograph is normal.

In addition to pulmonary function testing, which of the following will be most helpful in establishing a diagnosis?

(A) Anti–PM-Scl antibody testing and bronchoalveolar lavage

(B) Anti–Scl-70 antibody testing and high-resolution CT

(C) Anticentromere antibody testing and lung biopsy

(D) Antineutrophil cytoplasmic antibody testing and gallium-67 lung scanning

Item 59

A 30-year-old woman is evaluated in follow-up after recently discovering she is 6 weeks pregnant with her first child. Her medical history is notable for mild persistent asthma related to seasonal ragweed allergy. Her symptoms are well controlled on a low-dose inhaled glucocorticoid and an as-needed β_2-agonist. However, symptoms usually flare in fall and winter and with moderate exertion, and she treats these symptoms with an add-on oral leukotriene inhibitor. She currently has no asthma symptoms. Medications are budesonide and albuterol inhalers and montelukast when needed.

On physical examination, vital signs are normal. The lungs show good air movement and no wheezes. The remainder of the physical examination is unremarkable.

The patient's spirometry at the time of diagnosis showed an FEV_1 of 85% of predicted without a significant bronchodilator response. Her last routine spirometry 6 months ago demonstrated normal values with an FEV_1 of 93% of predicted.

Which of the following is the most appropriate treatment?

(A) Continue montelukast and albuterol but stop budesonide

(B) Continue the current drug regimen

(C) Increase budesonide to high dose

(D) Switch to as-needed albuterol therapy only

Item 60

A 70-year-old man is evaluated in follow-up for COPD, which was diagnosed 1 year ago. He has had two exacerbations in the last year, with the second exacerbation 1 month ago. He has also had baseline chronic cough with mucoid sputum consistently for the last 3 years. Sputum culture 6 months ago grew *Haemophilus influenzae* and *Mycobacterium avium-intracellulare*. He has to stop to catch his breath after walking 100 meters (328 feet). His inhaler technique is good. He quit smoking 2 years ago and completed a pulmonary rehabilitation program 4 months ago. His medications are tiotropium, fluticasone/salmeterol, and as-needed albuterol. Spirometry performed 3 months ago showed an FEV_1 of 32% of predicted and an FEV_1/FVC ratio of 50%. Chest radiograph performed last month showed no infiltrate, mass, or increased vascular congestion.

On physical examination, vital signs are normal. Oxygen saturation is 92% breathing ambient air. Pulmonary examination reveals diminished breath sounds.

Which of the following is the most appropriate long-term COPD treatment?

(A) Daily azithromycin
(B) Daily prednisone
(C) Roflumilast
(D) Simvastatin

Item 61

A 76-year-old man is evaluated in the emergency department after being found by his daughter lethargic and confused lying in bed in his apartment. He felt warm to the touch. Emergency medical services personnel noted that the apartment felt warm, with closed windows despite warm weather. He was given 1.5 L of normal saline on the way to the hospital. His medical history is notable for heart failure and depression. His medications are metoprolol, furosemide, lisinopril, and sertraline.

On physical examination, he is arousable only with physical stimulation. Temperature is 41.4 °C (106.5 °F), blood pressure is 98/74 mm Hg, pulse rate is 118/min, and respiration rate is 20/min. Oxygen saturation is 96% breathing ambient air. The mucous membranes and axillae are dry. Normal muscle tone and reflexes are noted.

Which of the following is the most appropriate next step in treatment?

(A) Administer dantrolene
(B) Perform external evaporative cooling
(C) Start cyproheptadine
(D) Start N-acetylcysteine

Item 62

A 50-year-old man is evaluated for a 2-year history of intermittent, nonproductive, chronic cough, as well as mild dyspnea with exertion. He has not had fever, chest pain, heartburn, loss of appetite, or weight loss. He has a 20-pack-year history of smoking and is a current smoker. His medical history is otherwise unremarkable and he takes no medications.

On physical examination, blood pressure is 125/76 mm Hg, pulse rate is 78/min, and respiration rate is 15/min; oxygen saturation is 98% breathing ambient air. BMI is 25. He appears comfortable. There is no jugular venous distention. Heart sounds are normal, and there is no murmur. The lungs are clear. No edema is noted. The remainder of the examination is normal.

A chest radiograph and electrocardiogram are normal.

Which of the following is the most appropriate next step in management?

(A) CT of the chest
(B) Polysomnography
(C) Spirometry
(D) Trial of a proton pump inhibitor

Item 63

A 29-year-old man is being discharged from the hospital following treatment of pneumonia. His medical history is notable for myotonic dystrophy with progressive muscle wasting and increasing dyspnea over the last 12 months. He sleeps in a seated to semirecumbent position and has difficulty breathing on his own when lying flat. He is being treated with cough assistance maneuvers and has not had difficulty in handling his secretions. He has no known underlying lung disease and responded well to antibiotic therapy.

On physical examination, temperature is 37.2 °C (99.0 °F), blood pressure is 128/78 mm Hg, pulse rate is 88/min, and respiration rate is 16/min. Chest examination is significant for mild crackles heard over the right lower lung field. The remainder of the examination is normal except for diffuse wasting of all major muscle groups.

Chest radiograph shows hypoinflation and an improving infiltrate in the upper portion of the right lower lobe. Forced vital capacity is 40% of predicted. Daytime arterial blood gas studies breathing ambient air show a pH of 7.35, a P_{CO_2} of 55 mm Hg (7.3 kPa), and a P_{O_2} of 86 mm Hg (11.4 kPa).

Which of the following is the most appropriate respiratory management for this patient?

(A) Continuous positive airway pressure
(B) Nocturnal noninvasive positive pressure ventilation
(C) Nocturnal supplemental oxygen by nasal cannula
(D) Tracheostomy and continuous mechanical ventilation

Item 64

A 53-year-old woman is evaluated in the emergency department for progressive somnolence. Her neighbors called emergency medical services because she sounded confused on the phone and would not come to her door. On arrival to the hospital, she experienced a generalized tonic-clonic seizure and was subsequently intubated for airway protection; she was admitted to the medical ICU. Her medical history is notable for hypertension, depression, and chronic pain. Her medications are amlodipine, ibuprofen, and amitriptyline.

On physical examination, temperature is 38.5 °C (101.3 °F), blood pressure is 78/46 mm Hg, pulse rate is 108/min, and respiration rate is 16/min; BMI is 26. Oxygen saturation is 96% on an FIO_2 of 0.4. Neurologic examination reveals pupils that are dilated and minimally reactive to light. Muscle tone and reflexes are normal. Cardiovascular examination reveals a regular tachycardic rhythm. Bowel sounds are scarce, and the abdomen is slightly distended.

Laboratory studies:

Creatinine	1.2 mg/dL (106.1 µmol/L)
Electrolytes:	
Sodium	140 mEq/L (140 mmol/L)
Potassium	4.1 mEq/L (4.1 mmol/L)
Chloride	102 mEq/L (102 mmol/L)
Bicarbonate	26 mEq/L (26 mmol/L)
Glucose	90 mg/dL (5.0 mmol/L)
Ethanol	Negative
Plasma osmolality	295 mOsm/kg H_2O
Arterial blood gases	
(performed 2 hours after	
intubation, on F_{IO_2} of 0.4):	
pH	7.43
P_{CO_2}	30 mm Hg (4.0 kPa)
P_{O_2}	130 mm Hg (17.3 kPa)

Urine toxicology studies are pending.

Electrocardiogram shows sinus tachycardia with a PR interval of 180 ms, a QRS interval of 125 ms, and a QTc interval of 420 ms. No ischemic changes are noted.

Which of the following is the most appropriate treatment for this patient?

(A) Calcium gluconate
(B) Fomepizole
(C) Physostigmine
(D) Sodium bicarbonate

Item 65

A 68-year-old man is evaluated in follow-up for a 6-mm solitary pulmonary nodule, which was incidentally discovered on imaging for abdominal pain 3 years ago. The nodule was located at the right lung base and had no associated ground-glass opacification. Follow-up chest CT was obtained at 1- and 2-year intervals, and the pulmonary nodule appears unchanged. He feels well and does not have any respiratory or constitutional symptoms. He has a 23-pack-year smoking history, but he quit smoking 20 years ago.

On physical examination, vital signs and cardiopulmonary examination findings are normal.

Which of the following is the most appropriate management?

(A) Obtain PET/CT now
(B) Perform chest radiograph in 1 year
(C) Repeat chest CT in 1 year
(D) Repeat chest CT in 2 years
(E) No further imaging is necessary

Item 66

A 62-year-old woman is evaluated in the hospital after being admitted 4 days ago for an acute exacerbation of COPD. She has responded well to treatment and is ready to be discharged today. Her medical history is notable for moderate-severity COPD, heart failure, depression, osteoporosis, hypertension, and hyperlipidemia. Her discharge medications are lisinopril, carvedilol, simvastatin,

sertraline, alendronate, vitamin D, calcium, tiotropium, levofloxacin, prednisone, and albuterol.

On physical examination, temperature is normal, blood pressure is 120/84 mm Hg, pulse rate is normal, and respiration rate is 18/min. Oxygen saturation is 93% breathing ambient air. No jugular venous distention is noted. Pulmonary examination reveals a few scattered wheezes and a few basal crackles. She is not using accessory muscles of breathing. Trace pedal edema is noted. She ambulates well without oxygen.

Which of the following factors increases this patient's risk for early hospital readmission for COPD?

(A) Adequacy of discharge medications for COPD
(B) Female gender
(C) Length of hospitalization
(D) Multiple comorbid conditions

Item 67

A 45-year-old woman is evaluated for a history of recurrent bouts of bronchitis that have required treatment with antibiotics. She has had a mild, chronic cough productive of mucopurulent sputum over the past 20 years that has been present between her episodes of acute bronchitis. She does not have shortness of breath with routine activities. She has not had fever, loss of appetite, or weight loss. Medical history is significant for pertussis as a child but is otherwise unremarkable. She takes no medications, and she is a never-smoker.

On physical examination, vital signs are normal. Chest auscultation reveals wheezing over the right lower lung base but is otherwise normal. The remainder of the physical examination is unremarkable.

Chest radiograph shows increased bronchovascular markings in the right lower lobe. Pulmonary function tests show an FEV_1/FVC ratio of 72% and no change after administration of a bronchodilator.

Which of the following is the most appropriate diagnostic test to perform next?

(A) Bronchoscopy
(B) Chest MRI
(C) High-resolution chest CT
(D) Repeat chest radiograph in 8 weeks

Item 68

A 55-year-old woman is evaluated in the emergency department for respiratory failure due to an acute exacerbation of COPD. She is confused and her mental status is rapidly worsening. She is intubated and placed on mechanical ventilation with propofol for sedation. The initial peak inspiratory pressure is 30 cm H_2O and plateau pressure is 15 cm H_2O. Oxygen saturation is 98% on an F_{IO_2} of 0.6. Thirty minutes later, the peak inspiratory pressure is 42 cm H_2O and the plateau pressure is 30 cm H_2O. Oxygen saturation is 92% on an F_{IO_2} of 0.6.

On physical examination, she is afebrile, blood pressure is now 100/60 mm Hg (150/80 mm Hg on admission), pulse rate is 110/min (90/min on admission), and respiration

CONT. rate is 30/min. There is jugular venous distention. Heart sounds are faint. Trachea is midline, and breath sounds are distant but equal bilaterally.

Which of the following is most likely responsible for this patient's change in airway pressures?

(A) Auto–positive end-expiratory pressure
(B) Endotracheal mucus plug
(C) Excessive sedation
(D) Kinked endotracheal tube

Item 69

A 75-year-old man is seen for routine follow-up for very severe COPD. He has constant dyspnea and air hunger and spends most of the day in a chair. He has had no change in baseline cough and sputum production. He has had multiple COPD exacerbations that required ICU admission and intubation. He has not benefited from pulmonary rehabilitation in the past. He quit smoking 3 years ago. His medical history is also notable for hypertension, type 2 diabetes mellitus, and a myocardial infarction 3 years ago. His medications are lisinopril, insulin glargine, budesonide/formoterol, tiotropium, roflumilast, as-needed albuterol, and 2 L of oxygen by nasal cannula. Spirometry performed 1 year ago showed an FEV_1 of 21% of predicted and a DL_{CO} of 35% of predicted. Residual volume/total lung capacity is 105% of predicted.

On physical examination, the patient is very thin and demonstrates a significantly increased work of breathing. He is afebrile, blood pressure is 125/80 mm Hg, pulse rate is normal, and respiration rate is 32/min; BMI is 17. Oxygen saturation is 90% breathing 2 L of oxygen. Pulmonary examination reveals significantly decreased breath sounds, with no crackles or wheezing, and the remainder of the examination is unremarkable.

Laboratory studies reveal a serum albumin level of 2.3 g/dL (23 g/L).

Arterial blood gas studies reveal a P_{CO_2} of 55 mm Hg (7.3 kPa). Chest radiograph shows no acute changes. Echocardiogram shows normal left ventricular function; the estimated pulmonary artery pressure is elevated, suggesting cor pulmonale. CT scan shows diffuse emphysema.

Which of the following is the most appropriate management?

(A) Hospice referral
(B) Lung transplantation
(C) Lung volume reduction surgery
(D) Repeat pulmonary rehabilitation

Item 70

A 75-year-old woman is hospitalized, intubated, and mechanically ventilated for hypoxic respiratory failure due to community-acquired pneumonia. She is empirically started on ceftriaxone and azithromycin.

On physical examination, temperature is 37.8 °C (100.0 °F), blood pressure is 110/65 mm Hg, pulse rate is 110/min, respiration rate is 14/min (ventilator is set at 14/min); BMI is 28. She appears anxious and uncomfortable with pleuritic chest pain, and she has become increasingly anxious with each painful breath. Pulmonary examination reveals diffuse crackles but no wheezing. The remainder of the physical examination is normal.

Chest radiograph shows multifocal infiltrates.

Which of the following is the most appropriate sedation and analgesia protocol for this patient?

(A) Continuous benzodiazepine infusion
(B) Interrupted benzodiazepine infusion
(C) Interrupted opioid infusion
(D) Neuromuscular blockade

Item 71

A 72-year-old woman is evaluated in the emergency department for severe, sharp, substernal chest pain that radiates to her back. Her medical history is notable for hypertension and a 50-pack-year smoking history. Her only medication is hydrochlorothiazide.

On physical examination, temperature is 36.6 °C (97.9 °F), blood pressure is 165/76 mm Hg, pulse rate is 90/min, and respiration rate is 14/min; BMI is 26. Oxygen saturation is 96% breathing ambient air.

Laboratory studies reveal normal serum electrolyte and plasma glucose levels and a serum creatinine level of 1.9 mg/dL (168.0 µmol/L). Arterial blood gas studies on 10 L/min of oxygen by face mask show a pH of 7.52, a P_{CO_2} of 25 mm Hg (3.3 kPa), and a P_{O_2} of 186 mm Hg (24.7 kPa).

A chest radiograph shows a right lower lobe infiltrate. A chest CT with intravenous contrast shows an aortic dissection extending from the descending aorta immediately distal to the left subclavian artery and extending distally into the left renal artery.

She is admitted to the ICU.

Which of the following is the most appropriate next step in treatment?

(A) Intravenous esmolol
(B) Intravenous fenoldopam
(C) Intravenous hydralazine
(D) Intravenous nitroglycerin

Item 72

A 25-year-old man is evaluated to establish care. His medical history is significant for asthma diagnosed as a child. He has a chronic productive cough but no dyspnea. He has also had recurrent sinus infections treated periodically with antibiotics. Medical history is otherwise unremarkable. He is a never smoker. Medications are a beclomethasone metered-dose inhaler and as-needed albuterol.

On physical examination, vital signs are normal; BMI is 20. Oxygen saturation breathing ambient air is 97%. Examination of the nasal passages shows multiple small polyps. Lung examination shows coarse breath sounds throughout both lung fields with occasional diffuse expiratory wheezes. The cardiac and abdominal examinations are unremarkable.

Chest radiograph is shown (see top of next page).

Spirometry shows an FEV_1/FVC ratio of 68%, with 8% improvement after administration of a bronchodilator. Laboratory studies show a normal complete blood count

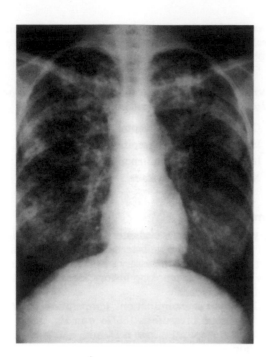

and leukocyte differential, and a normal metabolic profile including kidney function and liver chemistry tests. Urinalysis is normal.

Which of the following is the most appropriate diagnostic test to perform next?

(A) α_1-Antitrypsin measurement
(B) Antineutrophil cytoplasmic antibody assay
(C) Sinus radiographs
(D) Sweat chloride testing

Item 73

A 56-year-old man is evaluated in the emergency department for an episode of coughing up blood. He has had an intermittent nonproductive cough for the past several weeks but has otherwise felt well. Three hours ago he coughed up approximately a half-cup of bright-red blood. Since that episode, he has had several episodes of cough productive of blood-tinged sputum, but he has not had further episodes of frank hemoptysis. Medical history is significant for COPD. His only medications are tiotropium and as-needed albuterol metered-dose inhalers. He has a 55-pack-year smoking history and continues to smoke.

On physical examination, temperature is 37.2 °C (99.0 °F), blood pressure is 130/68 mm Hg, pulse rate is 88/min, and respiration rate is 12/min; BMI is 24. Oxygen saturation is 96% breathing ambient air. There are diffuse, mild expiratory wheezes noted on lung auscultation, but no focal findings. The remainder of the examination is unremarkable.

Laboratory studies reveal a leukocyte count of 9800/µL (9.8×10^9/L), a hemoglobin level of 14.5 g/dL (145 g/L), a normal platelet count, and normal kidney function.

Chest radiograph shows mild hyperinflation and a hazy infiltrate in the right lower lobe. A pulmonary embolism–protocol chest CT shows no evidence of pulmonary embolism; patchy ground-glass opacification is noted in the right lower lobe.

Which of the following is the most appropriate next step in management?

(A) Bronchoscopy
(B) Ceftriaxone and azithromycin
(C) High-resolution chest CT
(D) Upper endoscopy

Item 74

A 63-year-old woman is evaluated for a 2-week history of progressive dry cough and shortness of breath on exertion. She finished combined gemcitabine and radiation therapy 3 months ago for non–small cell lung cancer. Her medical history is otherwise notable for moderate COPD. Medications are a salmeterol inhaler and an ipratropium inhaler.

On physical examination, temperature is 37.2 °C (99.0 °F), blood pressure is 100/60 mm Hg, pulse rate is 94/min, and respiration rate is 24/min. Oxygen saturation is 91% breathing ambient air. Pulmonary examination reveals inspiratory crackles over the left lung anteriorly; the lungs are otherwise clear to auscultation.

Chest radiograph shows increased interstitial markings in both the right and left mid- and upper lung lobes. A representative CT image is shown.

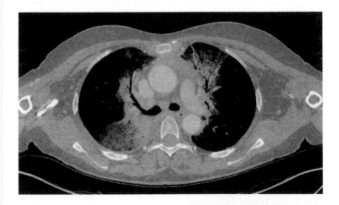

Which of the following is the most likely diagnosis?

(A) Progression of lung cancer
(B) Radiation fibrosis
(C) Radiation pneumonitis
(D) Viral pneumonia

Item 75

A 47-year-old man is evaluated in the emergency department after being found rain-soaked, unresponsive, and pulseless in a local city park by his wife. She had last seen him the previous night when he appeared in his normal state of health. Medical history is notable for alcohol dependence. When emergency medical services personnel arrived, his initial cardiac rhythm was pulseless electrical activity. He was endotracheally intubated and received cardiopulmonary resuscitation (CPR) during transport to the emergency department. Despite ongoing standard advanced cardiac life support, pulseless electrical activity persists. Rectal temperature is 26.0 °C (78.8 °F). His wet clothing is removed and warm blankets are placed over him. After 70 minutes of CPR, his cardiac rhythm converts to sinus bradycardia, but he requires high-dose norepinephrine to maintain a mean arterial blood pressure greater than 60 mm Hg.

On physical examination, temperature is 28.1 °C (82.6 °F), blood pressure is 88/52 mm Hg, pulse rate is 46/min with frequent premature ventricular complexes, and respiration rate is 16/min. Oxygen saturation is 96% on an FIO_2 of 0.5 and a positive end-expiratory pressure of 8 cm H_2O. Neurologic examination reveals mid-sized pupils without light reflex. Corneal reflex is negative. There is no response to verbal or painful stimulation. Muscle tone is normal. No other reflexes can be elicited. He has received no sedation.

Electrocardiogram shows sinus bradycardia, frequent premature ventricular complexes and couplets, and a J-wave in the precordial leads.

Which of the following is the most appropriate next step in management?

(A) Administer 1 L of normal saline warmed to 42.0 °C (107.6 °F)

(B) Administer a lidocaine loading dose followed by infusion

(C) Place on cardiopulmonary bypass for rewarming

(D) Recommend no further cardiopulmonary resuscitation if perfusing rhythm is lost

Item 76

A 58-year-old man is evaluated in follow-up for idiopathic pulmonary fibrosis (IPF), which was diagnosed 2 years ago. He has cough and shortness of breath and now requires supplemental oxygen at rest. Previous evaluations have not identified any cause for his symptoms other than progressive IPF. He has participated in pulmonary rehabilitation and continues in a maintenance program. He is a lifelong nonsmoker. His medical history is otherwise unremarkable, and he takes no medications.

On physical examination, the patient is afebrile, blood pressure is normal, pulse rate is 96/min, and respiration rate is 26/min; BMI is 27. Oxygen saturation is 92% breathing 4 L of oxygen by nasal cannula. Pulmonary examination reveals inspiratory crackles at the bases bilaterally. Results of a 6-minute walk test are 335 meters (1100 feet) (declined from 457 meters [1500 feet] 6 months ago).

Which of the following is the most appropriate management?

(A) Azathioprine

(B) Daily prednisone

(C) Etanercept

(D) Lung transplantation

Item 77

A 22-year-old woman is evaluated for a 3-day history of orthopnea and a 1-month history of progressively worsening dyspnea on exertion. She can no longer participate in lacrosse practice owing to dyspnea. She has generally felt well and has not had fever, chills, weight loss, or night sweats. Medical history is otherwise unremarkable, and she takes no medications.

On physical examination, temperature is 37.1 °C (98.8 °F), blood pressure is 118/64 mm Hg, pulse rate is 110/min, and respiration rate is 12/min; BMI is 22. Cardiac examination reveals a regular rhythm. The lungs are clear bilaterally.

A chest radiograph is shown.

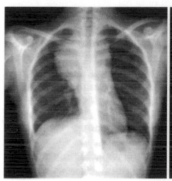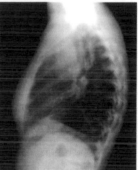

Which of the following is the most likely diagnosis?

(A) Bronchogenic cyst

(B) Hodgkin lymphoma

(C) Neuroblastoma

(D) Schwannoma

Item 78

A 60-year-old woman is evaluated in the emergency department after an aspiration event. Her medical history is notable for multiple sclerosis with a history of infrequent aspiration episodes that occur when she is tired, but is otherwise negative. She is intubated for respiratory distress in the emergency department. She is initially hypotensive. A 3 L intravenous fluid bolus is given, a central venous catheter is placed, and vasopressor medication is started. She is transferred to the ICU 2 hours after intubation. Over the next 12 hours, her blood pressure improves and the day after admission her vasopressor is stopped.

On physical examination, the skin is warm and dry without any signs of underperfusion. Temperature is 37.0 °C (98.6 °F), blood pressure is 128/70 mm Hg, pulse rate is 88/min, and respiration rate is 24/min (set rate on the ventilator is 18/min); BMI is 27. On chest auscultation, diffuse crackles are heard bilaterally. The cardiac examination is normal.

CONT.

Chest radiograph and oxygenation findings are consistent with acute respiratory distress syndrome.

Which of the following is the most appropriate fluid management strategy?

(A) Insert a pulmonary artery catheter and titrate fluid volume to a pulmonary artery occlusion pressure of 4 to 9 mm Hg

(B) Insert a pulmonary artery catheter and titrate fluid volume to a pulmonary artery occlusion pressure of 10 to 14 mm Hg

(C) Titrate fluid volume to a central venous pressure of 4 mm Hg

(D) Titrate fluid volume to a central venous pressure of 10 to 12 mm Hg

Item 79

A 24-year-old man is evaluated for shortness of breath with occasional wheeze that occurs several times per week. He develops significant shortness of breath when playing tennis or soccer outdoors, particularly during cool weather. He notes that it takes several minutes to recover his breath when this occurs. He also notes coughing during exercise as well as episodes of cough in the evenings and nighttime, even when not exerting himself. Medical history is significant only for seasonal allergies as a child, although he now rarely experiences allergy symptoms. He takes no medications.

On physical examination, vital signs are normal. Mild nasal congestion is noted. Lung examination reveals normal air movement and no wheezes. Heart examination is unremarkable, and the remainder of the examination is normal.

A chest radiograph is normal. Spirometry findings are within normal parameters.

Which of the following is the most appropriate next step in management?

(A) Methacholine challenge test

(B) Nasal glucocorticoid

(C) Short-acting β_2-agonist inhaler as needed

(D) Clinical observation

Item 80

A 61-year-old man is admitted to the hospital for a COPD exacerbation requiring intubation and mechanical ventilation. He receives intravenous glucocorticoids, antibiotics, and supportive care. He is a former smoker and is moderately deconditioned.

After 5 days of mechanical ventilation, his condition has improved, but a spontaneous ventilation trial fails, with increased respiration rate and work of breathing after 20 minutes.

On physical examination, he is afebrile, blood pressure is 132/85 mm Hg, and pulse rate is 75/min. Breath sounds are decreased throughout both lung fields. At the end of his spontaneous breathing trial he appears fatigued but is awake and alert. The remainder of the examination is unremarkable.

Which of the following is the most appropriate management?

(A) Extubate now and initiate bilevel noninvasive positive pressure ventilation immediately

(B) Extubate now and provide supplemental oxygen via nasal cannula

(C) Recommend tracheostomy placement

(D) Repeat spontaneous breathing trial in 1 hour

Item 81

A 25-year-old woman is evaluated in the ICU for difficulty in weaning from mechanical ventilation. Medical history is significant for type 1 diabetes mellitus, and she was admitted to the ICU 8 days ago with diabetic ketoacidosis secondary to sepsis from a rectal abscess. Her hospital stay has been prolonged and complicated. Her medications are piperacillin/tazobactam and basal and bolus insulin.

On physical examination, vital signs are normal. Neurologic examination reveals a weak hand grip and difficulty raising her arms. Reflexes are present but reduced.

Which of the following is the most likely diagnosis?

(A) Diabetic neuropathy

(B) Guillain-Barré syndrome

(C) ICU-acquired weakness

(D) Vasculitic neuropathy

Item 82

A 32-year-old woman is evaluated for a 2-year history of progressive dyspnea. She notes a mild, nonproductive cough but has no other symptoms. Medical history is significant only for a spontaneous pneumothorax 3 years ago. She is a never-smoker and takes no medications.

On physical examination, vital signs are normal except for a respiration rate of 20/min. BMI is 24. Oxygen saturation is 94% breathing ambient air. There are mildly decreased breath sounds and scattered crackles heard throughout all lung zones. Cardiac examination is normal. There is no digital clubbing or lower extremity edema. The remainder of the examination is unremarkable.

Laboratory studies reveal a normal complete blood count, comprehensive metabolic panel, and thyroid function studies. Chest radiograph reveals mild hyperinflation and nonspecific interstitial changes. High-resolution CT of the chest is shown (see top of next page).

Which of the following is the most likely diagnosis?

(A) Lymphangioleiomyomatosis

(B) Organizing pneumonia

(C) Pulmonary Langerhans cell histiocytosis

(D) Respiratory bronchiolitis–associated interstitial lung disease

Item 83

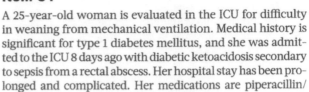

A 38-year-old man is evaluated in the emergency department after being found unresponsive in his closed garage

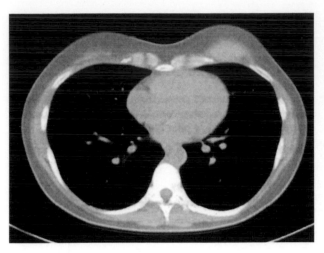

ITEM 82

CONT. with a motor vehicle idling. He was last seen in his usual state of health 2 hours ago. His medical history is notable for epilepsy. His only medication is carbamazepine.

On physical examination, temperature is 37.0 °C (98.6 °F), blood pressure is 106/52 mm Hg, pulse rate is 110/min, and respiration rate is 20/min; BMI is 26. Oxygen saturation is 96% breathing ambient air. He is unresponsive to voice and withdraws all extremities to painful stimulation. No tongue lacerations are noted. The pupils are mid-sized and reactive to light. The chest is clear. Cardiovascular examination reveals a normal S_1 and S_2 with regular tachycardic rhythm and no murmur or gallop.

Laboratory studies reveal a serum troponin I level of 2.4 ng/mL (2.4 µg/L) and a plasma lactate level of 4.2 mEq/L (4.2 mmol/L). Electrocardiogram reveals T-wave inversions involving leads V_2 through V_4. Chest radiograph is normal.

Which of the following tests is most likely to provide the diagnosis?

(A) Carboxyhemoglobin measurement
(B) Cardiac catheterization
(C) Electroencephalography
(D) Urine drug screen

Item 84

A 52-year-old woman is brought to the emergency department after being found walking in the middle of a freeway on-ramp. She was given intramuscular haloperidol by emergency medical personnel for agitation on the way to the hospital. Her medical history is notable for polysubstance use.

On physical examination in the emergency department, she is alert and restless but calms down with verbal reassurance. Blood pressure is 155/90 mm Hg, and pulse rate is 110/min. She is admitted to the observation unit.

One hour later, she becomes severely agitated and tries to leave. Temperature is 38.2 °C (100.8 °F), blood pressure is 210/104 mm Hg, pulse rate is 124/min, and respiration rate is 14/min. Oxygen saturation is 97% breathing ambient air. The pupils are symmetric, dilated, and reactive to light. Slight tremor of the hands is noted. No tongue fasciculations

are observed. The skin is warm and diaphoretic. The chest is clear to auscultation.

Laboratory studies reveal a serum creatine kinase level of 6600 U/L, creatinine level of 1.1 mg/dL (97.2 µmol/L), and a normal troponin level.

An electrocardiogram reveals sinus tachycardia without ischemic changes.

Which of the following is the most appropriate next step in treatment?

(A) Activated charcoal
(B) Lorazepam
(C) Physostigmine
(D) Propranolol

Item 85

A 62-year-old man is evaluated in follow-up after the recent discovery of a 2-cm right apical spiculated pulmonary nodule that in 3 months of follow-up grew 0.5 cm. His medical history is notable for emphysema, but he is otherwise healthy. He uses a tiotropium inhaler daily and an albuterol inhaler as needed.

On physical examination, temperature is 36.6 °C (97.9 °F), blood pressure is 138/74 mm Hg, pulse rate is 82/min, and respiration rate is 12/min; BMI is 30. Pulmonary examination reveals a prolonged expiratory phase, but the lungs are clear to auscultation bilaterally. Clubbing is noted.

Pulmonary function testing shows mild obstruction with a mild diffusion defect. Transthoracic needle aspiration is positive for non–small cell lung cancer (adenocarcinoma of the lung). Hormone receptor testing is negative. PET/CT shows positive uptake in the right apical lung nodule but no other abnormal uptake. MRI of the brain is normal.

Which of the following is the most appropriate treatment?

(A) Airway stent placement
(B) Radiation therapy
(C) Resection
(D) Systemic chemotherapy

Item 86

A 28-year-old man is evaluated for a 6-month history of fatigue, increase in exertional dyspnea, and cough. He has not had weight loss, fever, night sweats, or recent respiratory illness. He lives in the Northeast and has no travel history, occupational exposures, or illness contacts. His medical history is noncontributory and he takes no medications.

On physical examination, vital signs and cardiopulmonary examination are normal. There is no cervical or axillary lymphadenopathy and no skin findings.

Complete blood count and comprehensive metabolic profile are normal. Spirometry testing reveals an FVC of 72% of predicted, an FEV_1 of 75% of predicted, and an FEV_1/FVC ratio of 78%.

Chest radiograph shows bilateral hilar lymphadenopathy and normal lung parenchyma. Chest CT scan with contrast shows bilateral hilar and mediastinal and subcarinal lymphadenopathy, along with bilateral small lung nodules with a perihilar distribution.

Tuberculin skin testing is negative.

Which of the following is the most appropriate next step in management?

(A) Bronchoscopic biopsy

(B) Empiric therapy with prednisone

(C) Interferon-γ release assay

(D) Measurement of angiotensin-converting enzyme level

Item 87

A 63-year-old man is admitted to the ICU for an exacerbation of COPD. He has a 10-year history of COPD with chronic hypercapnia. He recently developed a viral upper respiratory tract infection that worsened his baseline dyspnea, and his family reports increased use of his rescue inhaler. He was brought to the hospital because he became confused. His medical history is otherwise unremarkable. His medications on admission are tiotropium and fluticasone/salmeterol metered-dose inhalers and an as-needed albuterol metered-dose inhaler.

On physical examination, he is responsive but confused and disoriented. Temperature is 36.9 °C (98.4 °F), blood pressure is 117/83 mm Hg, pulse rate is 99/min, and respiration rate is 32/min; BMI is 20. Oxygen saturation is 86% breathing 60% oxygen by Venturi mask. Use of accessory muscles of breathing is present. On oral examination, pooling of secretions in the posterior pharynx and diminished gag reflex are noted. There is no jugular venous distention. Pulmonary examination reveals transmitted upper airway noise and decreased breath sounds with polyphonic end-expiratory wheezing heard throughout both lung fields. There is no clubbing or peripheral edema.

A chest radiograph demonstrates hyperinflation but no infiltrates.

Laboratory studies:

Leukocyte count	11,000/μL (11 × 10⁹/L)
Hematocrit	32.8%
Arterial blood gases (breathing 60% oxygen):	
pH	7.25
P_{CO_2}	72 mm Hg (9.6 kPa)
P_{O_2}	48 mm Hg (6.4 kPa)

Glucocorticoids, antibiotics, and inhaled albuterol by nebulizer are started.

Which of the following is the most appropriate next step in management?

(A) Increase oxygen to 100% by nonrebreather mask

(B) Intubate and start mechanical ventilation

(C) Start noninvasive ventilation with continuous positive airway pressure

(D) Start noninvasive ventilation with inspiratory pressure support and positive end-expiratory pressure

Item 88

A 62-year-old woman is evaluated in follow-up after a 3-mm pulmonary nodule was discovered on chest imaging obtained 1 year ago. She feels well and has not had shortness of breath, cough, hemoptysis, weight loss, or chest pain.

She has a 60-pack-year smoking history and is a current smoker.

On physical examination, vital signs are normal. No cervical or supraclavicular lymphadenopathy is noted. The lungs are clear to auscultation bilaterally. There is no evidence of clubbing.

Her repeat chest CT shows that the nodule has increased in size and now measures 8 mm in diameter. There is no evidence of mediastinal or hilar lymphadenopathy.

Which of the following is the most appropriate management?

(A) Perform bronchoscopy

(B) Perform transthoracic needle aspiration

(C) Refer for thoracic surgery

(D) Repeat chest CT imaging in 3 months

Item 89

A 33-year-old man is evaluated acutely on the inpatient general medicine service for increased heart rate. He was admitted earlier in the day for treatment of neutropenic fever following induction chemotherapy for a recent diagnosis of acute myeloid leukemia after presenting with shaking chills and fever. He was started on broad-spectrum antibiotics and intravenous fluids 8 hours ago.

On physical examination, temperature is 38.6 °C (101.5 °F), blood pressure is 112/60 mm Hg, and respiration rate is 33/min; BMI is 25. Pulse rate was 95/min on admission but has been 150/min for the past hour. Oxygen saturation is 94% breathing ambient air. The skin is very warm and dry. The chest is clear, and the cardiac examination is unremarkable except for tachycardia. The abdomen is soft and nontender. The remainder of the examination is unremarkable.

Laboratory studies on admission were significant for a hemoglobin level of 10 g/dL (100 g/L), a leukocyte count of 10/μL (0.01 × 10⁹/L), and platelet count of 15,000/μL (15 × 10⁹/L). A complete metabolic profile is normal.

Chest radiograph showed no evidence of infiltrates.

Activation of a rapid response team would be expected to decrease which of the following outcomes in a patient such as this?

(A) Chance of cardiopulmonary arrest

(B) ICU utilization

(C) Intubation rate

(D) Length of hospital stay

Item 90

A 28-year-old woman is evaluated for difficulty staying awake during work. She works as a respiratory therapist at a hospital. For the last 9 months, she has been alternating daytime (7 AM to 7 PM) and night shifts (7 PM to 7 AM). When working the night shift, she often feels sleepy by 3 AM and struggles to stay awake. She feels more awake by the time she drives home and then has difficulty falling asleep during the day. Her medical history is unremarkable, and she takes no medications.

On physical examination, vital signs are normal; BMI is 25. The remainder of the examination is normal.

Which of the following is the most appropriate next step in management?

(A) Modafinil
(B) Multiple sleep latency testing
(C) Polysomnography
(D) Sleep hygiene counseling
(E) Zolpidem

Item 91

A 27-year-old man is evaluated for the acute onset of fever, chills, body aches, and dry cough that began last evening after returning home from trimming timber at a saw mill. He has similar symptoms that have been occurring two to three times a month for the past 3 months. These episodes always occur at home and not at the saw mill but never occur on the weekends or when he is away from home on an extended vacation. Two other colleagues who trim timber at work have also reported similar symptoms over the same time period. His medical history is otherwise unremarkable. He takes no medications.

On physical examination, the patient is currently afebrile, blood pressure is normal, pulse rate is 103/min, and respiration rate is 26/min. Pulmonary examination reveals diffuse crackles throughout all lung zones. Cardiac examination is normal except for tachycardia.

Chest radiograph shows ill-defined haziness in the upper lung zones, but no clear infiltrates. CT of the chest shows mid-lobe–predominant changes; representative findings are shown.

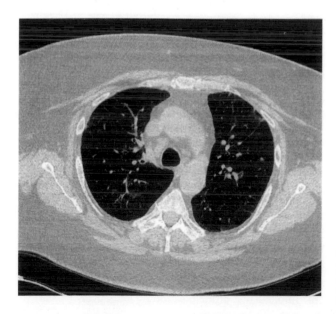

Which of the following is the most likely diagnosis?

(A) Acute hypersensitivity pneumonitis
(B) Acute interstitial pneumonia
(C) Idiopathic pulmonary fibrosis
(D) Nonspecific interstitial pneumonia

Item 92

A 62-year-old woman is evaluated in follow-up after her first hospitalization for an acute exacerbation of COPD. She is currently completing a 5-day course of oral glucocorticoids. She has not had fever, and her cough and sputum production have improved. Although she feels much better, she notes that her exercise capacity has not returned to its preadmission baseline. Medical history is otherwise unremarkable. She has a 30-pack-year history of smoking but stopped smoking 3 years ago. Her medications are tiotropium, mometasone/formoterol, and as-needed albuterol.

On physical examination, vital signs are normal. Oxygen saturation breathing ambient air is 92%. Lung examination shows mildly diminished airflow but is otherwise clear. The remainder of the examination is unremarkable.

Pulmonary function testing performed 5 months ago showed an FEV_1 of 55% of predicted.

Which of the following is the most appropriate treatment?

(A) Add roflumilast
(B) Extend glucocorticoid taper for an additional 5 days
(C) Start 2 L of oxygen by nasal cannula
(D) Start pulmonary rehabilitation

Item 93

A 52-year-old man is hospitalized for a 1- to 2-week history of general malaise and lack of appetite. He has acute-on-chronic kidney injury and has recently been started on dialysis. He has no history of bleeding.

On physical examination, temperature is 36.5 °C (97.7 °F), blood pressure is 80/52 mm Hg, pulse rate is 120/min, and respiration rate is 18/min; BMI is 24. A tunneled dialysis catheter is noted over the left chest wall, and no drainage or redness is noted. The remainder of the physical examination is normal.

After administration of 1 L of fluid, blood pressure is 118/56, pulse rate is 92/min, and respiration rate is 21/min.

Laboratory studies:

Hemoglobin	7.7 g/dL (77 g/L)
Leukocyte count	6750/µL (6.75 × 10⁹/L)
Platelet count	101,000/µL (101 × 10⁹/L), with giant platelets

Blood cultures are positive for methicillin-resistant *Staphylococcus aureus*. Appropriate antibiotics are initiated.

Which of the following is the most appropriate next step in management for this patient's anemia?

(A) Administer epoetin
(B) Transfuse one unit of packed erythrocytes
(C) Transfuse two units of packed erythrocytes
(D) Do not transfuse

Item 94

A 52-year-old man is evaluated in follow-up after undergoing total knee arthroplasty 3 weeks ago. Although the surgical procedure was uncomplicated, he required reintubation in the recovery room owing to persistent hypoxia. He was extubated 24 hours later without difficulty. A postextubation chest radiograph and arterial blood gas study were normal, and the remainder of his hospitalization was unremarkable. Since discharge, he reports normal recovery from surgery and no respiratory problems. Medical history is notable for hypertension, for which he takes lisinopril.

On physical examination, temperature is 36.2 °C (97.2 °F), blood pressure is 128/84 mm Hg, pulse rate is 76/min, and respiration rate is 14/min; BMI is 36. Oxygen saturation breathing ambient air is 97%. Head and neck examination is notable for a low-lying soft palate and thick neck. The lungs are clear, and cardiac examination is normal. His surgical incision is healing well, and the remainder of the examination is unremarkable.

Which of the following is the most appropriate next step in management?

(A) Overnight pulse oximetry
(B) Polysomnography
(C) STOP-Bang questionnaire
(D) No additional testing

Item 95

A 49-year-old woman is evaluated after discharge from the hospital following treatment in the ICU for 6 days for severe sepsis with septic shock requiring aggressive fluid resuscitation and vasopressor support in addition to antibiotic therapy. She feels significantly better since returning home but has had difficulty sleeping. She works as a university professor and has been experiencing anxiety and difficulty with multitasking and other simple cognitive tasks, such as setting up and coordinating meetings with her faculty. She has been able to resume some of her hobbies, including taking short hikes and gardening, but she continues to be limited by fatigue and weakness.

On physical examination, temperature is 37.0 °C (98.6 °F), blood pressure is 115/65 mm Hg, pulse rate is 80/min, and respiration rate is 10/min. BMI is 23, which is an improvement since discharge when BMI was 20. Motor strength is mildly decreased in the major muscle groups and reflexes are normal. Cardiac and pulmonary examinations are unremarkable.

Laboratory studies, including a complete blood count, basic chemistry tests, thyroid-stimulating hormone, and urinalysis, are normal.

Which of the following is the most likely cause of this patient's symptoms?

(A) Critical illness neuromyopathy
(B) Debilitation after prolonged bed rest
(C) Generalized anxiety disorder
(D) Postintensive care syndrome

Item 96

A 67-year-old man is evaluated in the emergency department for the sudden onset of severe periumbilical pain followed by an episode of emesis. His medical history is notable for hypertension, type 2 diabetes mellitus, and chronic

atrial fibrillation. His medications are metformin, metoprolol, glyburide, aspirin, and losartan.

On physical examination, temperature is 38.2 °C (100.8 °F), blood pressure is 92/44 mm Hg, pulse rate is 112/min, and respiration rate is 22/min. Oxygen saturation is 95% breathing ambient air. The chest is clear to auscultation bilaterally. Cardiac examination reveals an irregularly irregular rhythm. The abdomen is nondistended and mildly tender to palpation but without guarding or rebound tenderness. During the examination the patient has a forceful bowel evacuation.

Laboratory studies:

Hemoglobin	14.2 g/dL (142 g/L)
Leukocyte count	18,600/µL (18.6 × 10⁹/L)
Amylase	320 U/L
Lactate	2.2 mEq/L (2.2 mmol/L)

Findings on abdominal radiograph are normal.

Which of the following is the most likely diagnosis?

(A) Acute mesenteric ischemia
(B) Acute pancreatitis
(C) *Campylobacter* enteritis
(D) Colonic ischemia

Item 97

A 63-year-old woman is admitted to the hospital for septic shock secondary to community-acquired pneumonia. After receiving antibiotics, fluids, and vasopressors, her condition stabilizes. However, she subsequently develops respiratory distress and is intubated. Her oxygen requirement increases until she is receiving 100% oxygen. Ventilator settings are in the volume-controlled continuous mandatory ventilation (assist/control) mode with a respiration rate of 15/min, a tidal volume of 330 mL (6 mL/kg of ideal body weight), an F$_{IO_2}$ of 1.0, a positive end-expiratory pressure (PEEP) of 5 cm H$_2$O, a peak inspiratory pressure of 25 cm H$_2$O, and a plateau pressure of 22 cm H$_2$O.

On physical examination, temperature is 38.0 °C (100.4 °F), blood pressure is 115/60 mm Hg, pulse rate is 105/min, and respiration rate is 15/min. The skin is cool. There is no jugular venous distention. Heart sounds are rapid and regular but otherwise unremarkable. Diffuse crackles are heard on pulmonary examination. There is no edema. The remainder of the physical examination is noncontributory.

Arterial blood gas studies show a pH of 7.32, a P$_{CO_2}$ of 50 mm Hg (6.7 kPa), and a P$_{O_2}$ of 54 (7.2 kPa). Chest radiograph shows extensive patchy areas of opacification of the lung fields.

Which of the following is the most appropriate management?

(A) Decrease tidal volume
(B) Implement a prone positioning maneuver
(C) Increase positive end-expiratory pressure
(D) Increase set respiration rate on the ventilator

Item 98

A 59-year-old woman is evaluated in follow-up in November after being diagnosed with moderate COPD 3 months ago.

She has never received the influenza or pneumococcal vaccine. She has no allergies. Her medications are a long-acting inhaled anticholinergic agent and an as-needed short-acting β_2-agonist inhaler.

On physical examination, vital signs and the remainder of the physical examination are normal.

Which of the following vaccinations are recommended for this patient?

(A) Inactivated influenza vaccine and 13-valent pneumococcal conjugate vaccine (PCV13)

(B) Inactivated influenza vaccine and 23-valent polysaccharide pneumococcal vaccine (PPSV23)

(C) Inactivated influenza vaccine, PPSV23, and PCV13

(D) Live attenuated influenza vaccine and PPSV23

(E) Live attenuated influenza vaccine, PPSV23, and PCV13

Item 99

A 20-year-old woman is evaluated in the emergency department for an acute exacerbation of asthma. She has not used her inhalers for several days because she ran out of medications.

On physical examination, she appears to be in respiratory distress. Temperature is 37.1 °C (98.8 °F), blood pressure is 130/75 mm Hg, and pulse rate is 90/min. Oxygen saturation is 96% breathing 4 L/min oxygen by nasal cannula. There is minimal air movement with inspiration and minimal musical wheezing.

Blood gas analysis shows acute respiratory acidosis.

She is intubated. Ventilator settings are in the volume-controlled continuous mandatory ventilation (assist/control) mode with a set respiration rate of 16/min (actual respiration rate is 24/min), a tidal volume of 400 mL, an FIO_2 of 0.4, and a positive end-expiratory pressure of 5 cm H_2O. She is admitted to the ICU. Shortly after arriving in the ICU, peak inspiratory pressure rises to 45 cm H_2O. Blood pressure is now 80/40 mm Hg, pulse rate is 115/min, and oxygen saturation is 80%.

Which of the following is the most appropriate immediate next step in management?

(A) Decrease the set respiration rate to 12/min

(B) Decrease the tidal volume to 300 mL

(C) Increase the inspiratory flow rate

(D) Increase the sedative infusion rate and prepare for therapeutic paralysis

(E) Temporarily disconnect the endotracheal tube from the ventilator

Item 100

An 18-year-old man is evaluated in the emergency department after a near-drowning episode. He was intubated by emergency medical services before arrival at the hospital. He is admitted to the ICU and is mechanically ventilated. The ventilator is set in the volume-controlled continuous mandatory ventilation (assist/control) mode with a respiration rate of 18/min, a tidal volume of 360 mL, an FIO_2 of 0.65,

and a positive end-expiratory pressure (PEEP) of 12 cm H_2O. The ventilator shows a peak inspiratory pressure of 28 cm H_2O and a plateau pressure of 25 cm H_2O.

On physical examination, temperature is 37.5 °C (99.5 °F), blood pressure is 122/68 mm Hg, pulse rate is 75/min, and respiration rate is 18/min. Ideal body weight is 60 kg (132 lb). Crackles are auscultated bilaterally. The remainder of the physical examination is normal.

Arterial blood gas studies show a pH of 7.25, a PCO_2 of 60 mm Hg (8.0 kPa), and a PO_2 of 66 mm Hg (8.8 kPa). Serum bicarbonate level is 26 mEq/L (26 mmol/L). Oxygen saturation is 92%. Chest radiograph shows extensive bilateral opacification.

Which of the following is the most appropriate management?

(A) Decrease tidal volume to 260 mL

(B) Maintain tidal volume at 360 mL

(C) Increase tidal volume to 420 mL

(D) Increase tidal volume to 550 mL

Item 101

A 65-year-old man is evaluated for a 14-month history of progressively worsening cough and shortness of breath, most notable with exertion. His cough is nonproductive and is not associated with fever, chills, or sweats. He has no other symptoms. He is a retired carpenter. He has a 20-pack-year history of smoking but quit 15 years ago. He takes no medications.

On physical examination, respiration rate is 22/min; other vital signs are normal. Oxygen saturation is 95% breathing ambient air. BMI is 27. Pulmonary examination reveals inspiratory dry crackles at the bases bilaterally. Cardiac examination is normal. Mild clubbing is present. There is no lower extremity edema.

Pulmonary function tests reveal an FVC of 60% of predicted, an FEV_1 of 63% of predicted, an FEV_1/FVC ratio of 85%, and a $DLCO$ of 50% of predicted. High-resolution CT shows bilateral peripheral- and basal-predominant septal line thickening with evidence of honeycomb change at the bases. No ground-glass opacities are noted, and there is no mediastinal or hilar lymphadenopathy.

Which of the following is the most likely diagnosis?

(A) COPD

(B) Hypersensitivity pneumonitis

(C) Idiopathic pulmonary fibrosis

(D) Respiratory bronchiolitis–associated interstitial lung disease

Item 102

A 64-year-old man is evaluated for left-sided pleuritic chest pain. The discomfort is localized to the upper left chest and supraclavicular region. He is otherwise asymptomatic. Medical history is unremarkable except for 35-pack-year cigarette use; he continues to smoke. He takes no medications.

On physical examination, blood pressure is 132/72 mm Hg, pulse rate is 68/min, and respiration rate is 12/min.

Multiple firm, nonmobile lymph nodes are present in the left supraclavicular space. The lungs are clear to auscultation bilaterally. The remainder of the examination is normal.

A plain chest radiograph shows a left upper lobe opacity, bilateral hilar lymphadenopathy, and no pleural effusion.

CT of the chest is shown.

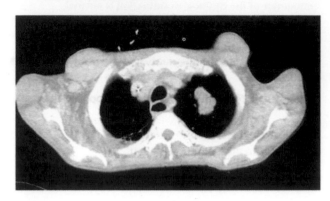

Which of the following is the most appropriate diagnostic test to perform next?

(A) Bronchoscopy with needle aspiration of mediastinal lymph nodes

(B) Bronchoscopy with transbronchial biopsy of the left apical mass

(C) CT-guided biopsy of the left apical mass

(D) Needle aspiration of the left supraclavicular lymph nodes

Item 103

A 29-year-old woman is evaluated for shortness of breath while mountain climbing. She is currently at an elevation of 3200 meters (10,500 feet) and has developed cough and dyspnea, which are present both with exertion and at rest; these symptoms prevent her from continuing the climb. Her medical history is unremarkable, and she takes no medications.

On physical examination, temperature is 36.0 °C (96.8 °F), blood pressure is 154/90 mm Hg, pulse rate is 120/min, and respiration rate is 22/min; BMI is 23. Oxygen saturation is 86% breathing ambient air. She is in moderate respiratory distress. Pulmonary examination reveals a few bibasilar crackles.

Supplemental oxygen is given and arrangements are made for descent from altitude.

Which of the following is the most appropriate adjunctive treatment for this patient?

(A) Acetazolamide

(B) Dexamethasone

(C) Ibuprofen

(D) Nifedipine

Answers and Critiques

Item 1   Answer: C

Educational Objective: Treat thermal upper airway injury with endotracheal intubation.

The most appropriate next step in treating this patient's respiratory findings is to perform endotracheal intubation. This patient sustained significant thermal injury to his upper airway as evidenced by an edematous oropharynx and monophonic wheeze consistent with inspiratory stridor. Intense heat can cause edema and blistering from the mouth to the larynx, and patients with a visibly damaged airway or stridor are at high risk of complete upper airway obstruction due to swelling. It is difficult to predict which patients with acute inhalational injury will develop complete upper airway obstruction, and even patients with minimally apparent inhalational airway injury may develop worsening obstruction associated with intravenous hydration or analgesia needed for burn treatment. Therefore, ensuring upper airway patency is the first priority in patients with significant smoke exposure, and endotracheal intubation is indicated in this patient at high risk of obstruction.

Because helium is less dense than nitrogen, a mixture of helium and oxygen (heliox) may be used in situations in which there is increased airway resistance. The combination of helium and oxygen improves laminar airflow and may decrease the work of breathing in patients with increased airway resistance. However, it would not treat the underlying inhalation-associated airway obstruction.

Methylprednisolone is useful for COPD exacerbations, but systemic glucocorticoids do not have a role in treating upper airway edema or smoke-induced injury of the lower airways.

Nebulized epinephrine can transiently reduce upper airway edema from allergic or anaphylactic reactions, but it does not have a role in the treatment of inhalational injury.

This patient's expiratory wheezes and acute respiratory acidosis suggest the presence of a COPD exacerbation triggered by smoke inhalation, in which case noninvasive ventilation would be appropriate. However, noninvasive ventilation will not prevent this patient from developing complete airway obstruction, and securing the airway with an endotracheal tube while it is still possible takes precedence.

KEY POINT

- In patients with significant smoke inhalation, a visibly damaged airway and stridor are indicators of a high risk for complete upper airway obstruction due to swelling; such patients require immediate endotracheal intubation.

Bibliography

Rex S. Burn injuries. Curr Opin Crit Care. 2012 Dec;18(6):671-6. [PMID: 23037877]

Item 2   Answer: B

Educational Objective: Perform early mobilization in a critically ill patient.

The most appropriate management is early mobilization with progressive physical activity as tolerated starting now. Disabling weakness and motor function impairments are common in ICU survivors and can last up to 5 years following critical illness. Traditionally, patients in the ICU were believed to be too ill to participate in significant physical activity, and any attempt at full mobilization and exercise was reserved until more aggressive therapies were withdrawn or the acute illness had resolved. This was especially true of patients on mechanical ventilation and vasopressors. In many cases, only passive range of motion exercises were provided in the ICU until the patient was believed to be appropriate for mobilization and increased amounts of active physical activity. However, studies have shown that exercise and physical therapy are the only interventions that have a significant effect on decreasing weakness and motor function deficits associated with critical illness. Additionally, it has been demonstrated that patients on ventilators and low-level vasopressors may safely participate in a progressive mobility program once stability is established.

Early mobilization is defined as patient mobilization (such as sitting up in bed and dangling feet over the edge of the bed) within 48 hours of admission to the ICU. Once the patient is awake and interactive, more aggressive bed exercises can be done. If these activities are tolerated without instability, the patient should be assessed for the next level of activity. Early mobilization, along with careful attention to management of pain, agitation, and delirium, has been shown to reduce ICU and hospital length of stay, shorten return to independent functional status, and improve survival. Waiting for discontinuation of vasopressors or extubation is not appropriate because these may not occur for a significant period of time, in which substantial deconditioning may develop.

KEY POINT

- Early mobilization with progressive physical activity, along with careful attention to management of pain, agitation, and delirium, has been shown to reduce ICU and hospital length of stay, shorten return to independent functional status, and improve survival.

Answers and Critiques

Bibliography

Engel HJ, Needham DM, Morris PE, Gropper MA. ICU early mobilization: from recommendation to implementation at three medical centers. Crit Care Med. 2013 Sep;41(9 Suppl 1):S69-80. [PMID: 23989097]

Bibliography

Murrmann GB, van Vollenhoven FH, Moodley L. Approach to a solid solitary pulmonary nodule in two different settings-"Common is common, rare is rare". J Thorac Dis. 2014 Mar;6(3):237-48. [PMID: 24624288]

Item 3   Answer: C

Educational Objective: Evaluate a subcentimeter pulmonary nodule.

The most appropriate next step in management is to review any previous chest imaging the patient may have had. This patient's chest CT shows an incidental finding of a subcentimeter pulmonary nodule. Appropriate evaluation of a subcentimeter pulmonary nodule depends on the patient's risk for lung cancer, which relates to the patient's past or present smoking status and history of other malignancy. Regardless of risk stratification, however, any previous imaging of the chest should be obtained as a comparison. If previous chest imaging confirms stability of the nodule for more than 24 months, further imaging may not be necessary. Previous imaging can also help in determining the best next step in management as well as when to repeat future imaging. For example, if the nodule has been increasing in size, short term follow-up may be indicated whereas documented stability would allow the clinician to extend the time until next imaging. If no previous imaging is available, the clinician should refer to the Fleischner criteria to establish the timing of the next imaging.

Bronchoalveolar lavage provides samples from small bronchi and alveoli and is typically used to diagnose infection or to obtain cell counts in the diagnosis of parenchymal lung disease. It is rarely helpful in determining the cause of a solitary subcentimeter pulmonary nodule. Given the absence of other symptoms to suggest an infection or parenchymal lung disease, bronchoalveolar lavage is not indicated at this time.

Even if previous imaging is not available, a PET/CT would not be indicated at this time. The CT shows a 5-mm nodule, and PET imaging is usually normal in a subcentimeter pulmonary nodule even if the nodule is malignant.

Biopsy of a solitary pulmonary nodule can be obtained by bronchoscopy, CT-guided needle aspiration, or surgical excision. An enlarging pulmonary nodule or a suspicious-appearing nodule warrants more aggressive evaluation with tissue diagnosis or excision depending on the pretest probability of malignancy. This patient, however, has a low pretest probability of cancer because she is a lifetime nonsmoker and has no history of active malignancy. Even if previous imaging is not available, this nodule should be monitored with repeat imaging based on the Fleischner criteria.

KEY POINT

- In patients with a subcentimeter pulmonary nodule, any previous imaging of the chest should be obtained to establish whether the nodule has remained stable or has grown over time.

Item 4   Answer: D

Educational Objective: Evaluate worsening COPD symptoms with repeat spirometry.

The most appropriate management is to repeat spirometry. Lung function can worsen over time in patients with COPD. During each visit, new or worsening symptoms (cough, sputum, dyspnea, fatigue), smoking status, adherence to and effectiveness of the medication regimen, adverse effects of treatment, and inhaler technique should be assessed. The frequency, severity, and causes of exacerbations should be evaluated. Comorbidities should be identified and managed. Spirometry is indicated when patients with COPD experience a change in symptoms. Annual spirometry can help determine which patients have rapid decline in lung function. Because this patient had pulmonary function testing done 3 years ago and has since had a decrease in his exercise capacity, spirometry is indicated. If spirometry shows worsening airflow obstruction in this patient, addition of a long-acting β_2-agonist and an inhaled glucocorticoid may help with symptom control. If spirometry does not show significant worsening of airflow, other comorbidities such as cardiovascular disease should be considered.

Roflumilast is a phosphodiesterase-4 inhibitor that is indicated in patients with severe and very severe COPD with recurrent exacerbations. This patient does not meet these criteria for use of this medication.

Monitoring patients with COPD using complete pulmonary function testing (with lung volumes and diffusing capacity) rather than spirometry is not cost effective and does not change management. Complete pulmonary function testing is not required unless lung volume reduction surgery (LVRS) or lung transplantation is being considered.

CT of the chest is not routinely recommended in the monitoring of COPD. This patient had a recent chest radiograph, which was normal, and there are no symptoms or signs to suggest a tumor that would warrant a CT scan at this time. Chest CT would be useful if this patient was being evaluated for LVRS or lung transplantation.

Oxygen therapy is not indicated because an oxygen saturation greater than 88% is adequate. If oxygen saturation is less than 92%, arterial blood gas studies should be performed.

KEY POINT

- Spirometry is indicated when patients with COPD experience a change in symptoms; annual spirometry can help determine which patients have rapid decline in lung function.

Bibliography

Global Initiative for Chronic Obstructive Lung Disease (GOLD). Global Strategy for the Diagnosis, Management, and Prevention of Chronic Obstructive Pulmonary Disease. www.goldcopd.org/guidelines-global-strategy-for-diagnosis-management.html. Updated 2015. Accessed April 2, 2015.

Item 5   Answer: D

Educational Objective: Diagnose pulmonary lymphangitic spread of metastatic cancer.

The most likely diagnosis is lymphangitic carcinomatosis. Pulmonary metastases most commonly present as multiple, peripheral, or subpleural pulmonary nodules but can also present as solitary pulmonary nodules or lymphangitic spread. Lymphangitic spread of tumor is most commonly associated with adenocarcinoma (lung, breast, and gastrointestinal tract), melanoma, lymphoma, and leukemia; it should be considered if an interstitial abnormality is identified on CT in a patient with one of these malignancies, and is best defined with high-resolution CT if suspected. This patient presents with likely metastatic breast cancer to the mediastinal and hilar lymph nodes with new interstitial changes on chest CT, which raises concern for lymphangitic spread.

Atypical pneumonia can present with interstitial changes. However, this patient has no symptoms to suggest an infection, did not improve with appropriate antibiotic therapy, has had symptoms for 1 month, and has unexplained mediastinal and hilar lymphadenopathy.

Bronchiolitis obliterans organizing pneumonia may be associated with solid-organ malignancies. However, the most common radiographic presentation shows areas of lung consolidation.

The usual CT scan findings associated with idiopathic pulmonary fibrosis are bilateral peripheral and lower lobe-predominant interstitial thickening with honeycombing. Clubbing is present in approximately half of patients. It is not associated with mediastinal and hilar lymphadenopathy.

Patients with radiation pneumonitis present with cough and/or dyspnea approximately 6 weeks after the exposure. CT imaging typically shows hazy opacities with ground-glass attenuation. Affected areas are most commonly found in the field of radiation but can occasionally occur outside the field. The abnormalities in classic radiation pneumonitis typically resolve within 6 months but can progress to a well-demarcated area of fibrosis with volume loss and bronchiectasis. Radiation fibrosis is not consistent with this patient's time course or imaging findings.

KEY POINT

- Lymphangitic spread of tumor to the lungs is most commonly associated with adenocarcinoma (lung, breast, and gastrointestinal tract), melanoma, lymphoma, and leukemia and should be considered if a peripheral interstitial abnormality is identified on CT in a patient with one of these malignancies.

Bibliography

Aquino SL. Imaging of metastatic disease to the thorax. Radiol Clin North Am. 2005 May;43(3):481-95, vii. [PMID: 15847812]

Item 6   Answer: B

Educational Objective: Treat COPD with long-term oxygen therapy.

The most appropriate treatment is to start long-term oxygen therapy (LTOT) for greater than 15 hours per day. The need for oxygen therapy should be evaluated in all stable patients with an FEV_1 less than 35% of predicted or in patients with clinical symptoms or signs suggestive of respiratory failure or right-sided heart failure. LTOT is indicated if patients meet the following criteria: (1) chronic respiratory failure and/or severe resting hypoxemia, defined as an arterial Po_2 less than or equal to 55 mm Hg (7.3 kPa) or oxygen saturation less than or equal to 88% breathing ambient air, with or without hypercapnia; and/or (2) if there is evidence of pulmonary hypertension, peripheral edema suggesting right-sided heart failure, or polycythemia, in combination with an arterial Po_2 less than 60 mm Hg (8.0 kPa) or oxygen saturation less than 88% breathing ambient air. This patient's examination findings (loud pulmonic component of S_2, peripheral edema) and estimated mean pulmonary artery pressure of 52 mm Hg on echocardiography indicate the presence of pulmonary hypertension. Therefore, this patient is an appropriate candidate for LTOT. The resting arterial Po_2 or oxygen saturation values should be repeated and confirmed twice over a 3-week period before a decision about LTOT is made in a stable patient.

A short course of systemic glucocorticoids is recommended in the treatment of acute exacerbations of COPD. However, long-term therapy with systemic glucocorticoids is associated with significant side effects and is not recommended in the management of COPD.

Nocturnal oximetry may be useful in diagnosing hypoxia occurring overnight in patients with COPD that might benefit from oxygen therapy while sleeping. However, this patient's indication for continuous LTOT may be established with available data; therefore, an overnight pulse oximetry study would not be needed to guide therapy.

Although pulmonary rehabilitation is helpful in improving quality of life in patients with advanced COPD, this patient has completed therapy on two occasions, and repeating pulmonary rehabilitation would not address her hypoxemia-associated pulmonary hypertension. However, after LTOT is started, entering a pulmonary rehabilitation program might be appropriate.

KEY POINT

- Long-term oxygen therapy is indicated if patients with COPD meet the following criteria: (1) chronic respiratory failure and/or severe resting hypoxemia, defined as an arterial Po_2 less than or equal to 55 mm Hg (7.3 kPa) or oxygen saturation less than or equal to 88% breathing ambient air, with or without hypercapnia; and/or (2) if there is evidence of pulmonary hypertension, peripheral edema suggesting right-sided heart failure, or polycythemia, in combination with an arterial Po_2 less than 60 mm Hg (8.0 kPa) or oxygen saturation less than 88% breathing ambient air.

Answers and Critiques

Bibliography

Stoller JK, Panos RJ, Krachman S, Doherty DE, Make B; Long-term Oxygen Treatment Trial Research Group. Oxygen therapy for patients with COPD: current evidence and the long-term oxygen treatment trial. Chest. 2010 Jul;138(1):179-87. [PMID: 20605816]

Item 7   Answer: B

Educational Objective: Diagnose COPD using clinical history and pulmonary function testing.

The most likely diagnosis is COPD. The spirometric findings, in conjunction with this patient's clinical history, are most consistent with this diagnosis. His FEV_1/FVC ratio is low, consistent with an obstructive lung defect. The FEV_1/FVC ratio is used to assess for airway obstruction; a value less than 70% (the lower limit of normal) is consistent with airflow obstruction. With evidence of obstruction, the degree of reduction in FEV_1 is then used to characterize the degree of obstruction. An FEV_1 of 50% to 80% of predicted is classified as moderately reduced, 34% to 50% of predicted is severely reduced, and less than 34% of predicted is very severely reduced. This patient's reduction in FEV_1 qualifies as moderately severe. Increased lung volumes with higher than predicted total lung capacity suggests hyperinflation, and high residual volume suggests air trapping from increased lung compliance. The lower than predicted D_{LCO} suggests an effect on the lung parenchyma, which in this patient is most consistent with emphysema. This patient's clinical history demonstrates a progressive course of dyspnea, in contrast to an episodic course with resolution, which would be more compatible with asthma.

Bronchiectasis is a condition that shares features with COPD, including mild to moderate airflow obstruction on pulmonary function testing and an abnormal lung examination with wheezing and crackles. However, patients with bronchiectasis usually have significant coughing with daily sputum (often thick sputum) and airways that are easily inflamed and collapsible. Chest radiographs and CT imaging often show distorted airway architecture. This patient, in contrast, has features of indolent dyspnea, a significant smoking history, and relatively unremarkable chest radiograph, which is more compatible with COPD.

Idiopathic pulmonary fibrosis is a form of diffuse parenchymal lung disease. This condition more typically causes a restrictive pattern on spirometry with parallel decreases in both the FEV_1 and FVC, unlike in this patient who has a decreased FEV_1 but preserved FVC. Additionally, pulmonary fibrosis is more likely to result in decreased lung volumes in contrast to the increased lung volumes seen in this patient.

Obesity hypoventilation syndrome is characterized by fatigue and daytime somnolence in patients who are obese (BMI >30), and the diagnosis is confirmed by arterial blood gas testing showing daytime hypercapnia with an arterial P_{CO_2} greater than 45 mm Hg (6.0 kPa). However, pulmonary function testing typically shows a restrictive pattern without obstruction, with a decreased FEV_1 and FVC but preserved FEV_1/FVC ratio. Although this patient is obese, his clinical symptoms and pulmonary function studies are not consistent with a diagnosis of obesity hypoventilation syndrome.

Bibliography

Pellegrino R, Viegi G, Brusasco V, et al. Interpretative strategies for lung function tests. Eur Respir J. 2005 Nov;26(5):948-68. [PMID: 16264058]

Item 8   Answer: B

Educational Objective: Establish intravenous access in an actively bleeding patient.

Large-caliber peripheral intravenous (IV) access is the preferred route of access in this patient with a hemodynamically significant gastrointestinal bleed. She requires emergent fluid resuscitation because of her bleeding and intravascular volume depletion. When large volumes of crystalloid fluid and blood are needed quickly, large-caliber, shorter catheters allow the highest flow rates to be achieved. Flow of fluid through a catheter is inversely proportional to catheter length and proportional to the fourth radius of the diameter of the catheter. Therefore, the highest flow rates may be achieved through shorter, large-bore catheters. Peripheral IV catheters are typically significantly shorter than either catheters used for central access or peripherally inserted central catheters. Peripheral IV catheters may also be significantly larger than most central catheters, allowing for increased fluid flow. For example, potential flow rates for a 14-gauge (1.73-mm inner diameter) catheter are approximately 3 times greater than an 18-gauge (0.95-mm inner diameter) catheter of equal length. For this reason, use of larger, shorter peripheral catheters is preferred for fluid resuscitation in patients requiring emergent treatment.

Although central access remains a way to administer fluids, it is not recommended for rapid volume infusion. Therefore, a single-lumen peripherally inserted central venous catheter or triple-lumen internal jugular venous catheter would not be appropriate for this patient who requires large fluid volumes quickly. Central access may ultimately be necessary to administer vasopressor therapy, which cannot be given through peripheral access, if this patient does not respond to fluid resuscitation.

Intraosseous infusion is an immediate alternative in medical or trauma resuscitation when other forms of access cannot be rapidly obtained. Sites for intraosseous access in adults include 1 to 2 cm below the tibial tuberosity and the humeral head. Alternative access should replace the intraosseous access catheter within approximately 24 hours of placement to minimize complications.

Bibliography

Lewis GC, Crapo SA, Williams JG. Critical skills and procedures in emergency medicine. vascular access skills and procedures. Emerg Med Clin North Am. 2013 Feb;31(1):59-86. [PMID: 23200329]

Item 9   Answer: C

Educational Objective: Recognize clinical features of small cell lung cancer.

The most likely diagnosis is small cell lung cancer (SCLC). SCLC comprises approximately 15% of all new lung cancer cases diagnosed in the United States and occurs almost exclusively in patients with a history of cigarette smoking. SCLC is the most common pulmonary neuroendocrine tumor in adults. Signs and symptoms of cough, hemoptysis, chest pain, hoarseness, and dyspnea occur frequently. Patients may also present with symptoms related to metastatic disease or to various paraneoplastic syndromes. This patient presents with symptoms of lower extremity weakness with confirmation of upper and lower extremity weakness on neurologic examination. This presentation is consistent with Lambert-Eaton myasthenic syndrome, which has a strong association with SCLC. Because of their rapid growth rate, these tumors are rarely found incidentally. The most common radiographic presentation is a hilar mass with bulky mediastinal lymphadenopathy. It is important to recognize patients with possible SCLC because the cancer is highly aggressive, and most patients start initial chemotherapy during the same hospitalization. SCLC tends to be more aggressive than non–small cell lung cancer (NSCLC); it is usually already disseminated at presentation but is usually more sensitive to chemotherapy and radiation therapy initially.

Most (80%) lung cancers are NSCLC. The most common type is adenocarcinoma of the lung (38% of all lung cancers), followed by squamous cell carcinoma of the lung (20% of all lung cancers). Although NSCLC is still in the differential diagnosis for this patient, the radiographic appearance is classic for SCLC.

Bronchial carcinoid tumors represent only a small percentage of lung cancers and are more common in children and adolescents. Typically, they present with an endobronchial lesion causing proximal airway obstruction.

KEY POINT

- Small cell lung cancer typically presents on imaging as a large hilar mass with bulky mediastinal lymphadenopathy.

Bibliography

Collins LG, Haines C, Perkel R, Enck RE. Lung cancer: diagnosis and management. Am Fam Physician. 2007 Jan 1;75(1):56-63. [PMID: 17225705]

Item 10   Answer: C

Educational Objective: Treat advanced COPD with lung transplantation.

The most appropriate management is to evaluate for lung transplantation. Criteria for referral for lung transplantation include a history of COPD exacerbations associated with acute hypercapnia (arterial P_{CO_2} >50 mm Hg [6.7 kPa]); pulmonary hypertension, cor pulmonale, or both despite oxygen therapy; or FEV$_1$ less than 20% of predicted with DL$_{CO}$ less than 20% of predicted or homogeneous distribution of emphysema. This 60-year-old patient has a history of hospitalization for exacerbations, hypercapnia, an FEV$_1$ of less than 20% of predicted, and bilateral homogeneous distribution of emphysema. Therefore, he is a candidate for lung transplantation. Absolute contraindications to lung transplantation include malignancy within the last 2 years, infection with hepatitis B or C virus with histologic evidence of significant liver damage, active or recent cigarette smoking, drug or alcohol abuse, severe psychiatric illness, documented nonadherence with medical care, and absence of social support. Age greater than 65 years is a relative contraindication, as well as the presence of multiple comorbid conditions, which are not present in this patient.

Short-term use of systemic glucocorticoids is recommended for acute exacerbations of COPD. However, long-term use of oral glucocorticoids has not been shown to improve quality of life or reduce the rate of exacerbations. Because this patient has no evidence of an acute exacerbation, there is no indication for oral glucocorticoid therapy.

Lung volume reduction surgery (LVRS) is indicated in patients with predominantly upper lobe emphysema. Because this patient has homogeneous emphysema, LVRS is not an option. Additionally, LVRS results in higher mortality in patients with an FEV$_1$ less than 20% of predicted.

Hospice is an approach to care in patients with life-limiting illness and focuses on quality of life rather than an attempt at cure of the underlying disease based on the patient's and family's goals and values. Although this patient is significantly limited in his daily activities, it is not clear that he has entered the last months to weeks of life, which is the usual time frame for hospice care (compared with palliative care, which is appropriate for all patients with severe or advanced disease). Additionally, because this patient meets criteria for possible lung transplantation, it is reasonable to offer this as a potential treatment option. Hospice care may be a consideration if he is not a transplant candidate or if he declines further aggressive treatment and his condition progresses.

KEY POINT

- In patients with advanced COPD, criteria for referral for lung transplantation include a history of exacerbations associated with acute hypercapnia (arterial P_{CO_2} >50 mm Hg [6.7 kPa]); pulmonary hypertension, cor pulmonale, or both despite oxygen therapy; or FEV$_1$ less than 20% of predicted with DL$_{CO}$ less than 20% of predicted or homogeneous distribution of emphysema.

Bibliography

Weill D, Benden C, Corris PA, et al. A consensus document for the selection of lung transplant candidates: 2014–an update from the Pulmonary Transplantation Council of the International Society for Heart and Lung Transplantation. J Heart Lung Transplant. 2015 Jan;35(1):1-15. [PMID: 25085497]

Item 11   Answer: D

Educational Objective: Diagnose diffuse parenchymal lung disease.

The most appropriate diagnostic test to perform next is high-resolution chest CT (HRCT). This patient has symptoms (progressive dyspnea on exertion and nonproductive cough), physical examination findings (impaired oxygenation, dry crackles on lung examination, and clubbing), and plain chest radiographic imaging findings (interstitial thickening at the lung bases) consistent with diffuse parenchymal lung disease. HRCT is the most effective CT study for evaluating parenchymal lung disease and is the preferred modality for evaluating patients with possible diffuse parenchymal lung disease. Because of its high resolution, it can help narrow the differential diagnosis based on the distribution of the parenchymal disease and the presence or absence of associated findings such as fibrosis. The HRCT protocol employs very thin image sections that are reconstructed at high resolution to obtain very detailed information about the lung parenchyma. However, these image sections are obtained at relatively wide intervals (typically 1 cm between images); they represent a sampling of the lung parenchyma and do not provide a complete picture of the lungs. Because of this, HRCT should not be performed for suspected localized lung disease (such as pulmonary nodules) as it may miss smaller lesions.

Unenhanced chest CT scanning obtains images at closer intervals and is indicated for evaluation of focal lung lesions, including pulmonary nodules. Contrast may be added to the study when better definition of the mediastinal structures is needed (for example, to assess for lymphadenopathy).

CT pulmonary angiography opacifies the pulmonary arteries and is not designed for detailed definition of the pulmonary parenchyma. It is mainly used in the diagnosis of pulmonary embolism or aortic dissection and would not be an appropriate next diagnostic study in this patient.

KEY POINT

- High-resolution CT is the most effective CT study for evaluating parenchymal lung disease and is the preferred modality for evaluating patients with possible diffuse parenchymal lung disease.

Bibliography
Sundaram B, Chughtai AR, Kazerooni EA. Multidetector high-resolution computed tomography of the lungs: protocols and applications. J Thorac Imaging. 2010 May;25(2):125–41. [PMID: 20463532]

Item 12   Answer: C

Educational Objective: Diagnose diffuse parenchymal lung disease.

High-resolution CT (HRCT) is the gold standard for evaluating parenchymal opacities seen on a plain radiograph. In addition, approximately 20% of patients with diffuse parenchymal lung disease have subtle interstitial abnormalities not detectable on a chest radiograph. For this reason, HRCT should even be considered in symptomatic patients with restrictive physiology on spirometry and a normal chest radiograph, such as this patient. The patterns seen on CT correlate with pathologic findings on an open lung biopsy and are a key diagnostic tool for evaluation of diffuse parenchymal lung disease, as may be present in this patient.

Bronchoscopic lung biopsy can provide enough tissue to demonstrate specific histopathologic features diagnostic of several specific disease processes, including carcinoma, sarcoidosis, and eosinophilic pneumonia. Bronchoalveolar lavage can provide additional diagnostic information, including culture, cytology, and cell differential. However, a lung biopsy and bronchoalveolar lavage would not be indicated until imaging studies confirmed the presence of diffuse parenchymal lung disease.

Cardiopulmonary exercise testing includes assessment of respiratory gas exchange during treadmill or bicycle exercise for a more detailed assessment of functional capacity and differentiation between potential causes of exercise limitation (cardiac, pulmonary, or deconditioning, versus volitional). It would not be the most appropriate next choice in a patient with increasing exercise limitation, pulmonary crackles, and restrictive findings on pulmonary function testing.

A ventilation-perfusion (V/Q) lung scan is the recommended initial test for evaluating chronic thromboembolic pulmonary hypertension (CTEPH). Patients with CTEPH have nonspecific symptoms and the diagnosis is often missed. However, patients with CTEPH typically have a mild restrictive or obstructive defect, although spirometry is often normal. Most patients will have a reduction in the D$_{LCO}$ out of proportion to any abnormalities in spirometry. A V/Q lung scan may be a consideration if this patient's HRCT scan is normal.

KEY POINT

- High-resolution CT (HRCT) is the preferred initial diagnostic study for evaluating diffuse parenchymal lung disease because the pattern and distribution of findings may suggest the underlying disease process, and there is strong correlation of patterns seen on HRCT with findings on an open lung biopsy.

Bibliography
Antoniou KM, Margaritopoulos GA, Tomassetti S, Bonella F, Costabel U, Poletti V. Interstitial lung disease. Eur Respir Rev. 2014 Mar 1;23(131): 40–54. [PMID: 24591661]

Item 13   Answer: C

Educational Objective: Diagnose portopulmonary hypertension.

The most likely diagnosis is portopulmonary hypertension. This diagnosis is suggested by evidence of pulmonary hypertension in the setting of portal hypertension, typically associated with liver cirrhosis. Pulmonary hypertension suggested by echocardiography was confirmed by right heart catheterization. In the classification of pulmonary hypertension, portopulmonary hypertension is part of group 1 (pulmonary arterial hypertension [PAH]). Although the coupling with portal hypertension makes the diagnosis of portopulmonary hypertension most likely, other causes of PAH (such as HIV infection, drug toxicity, connective tissue disease) should be ruled out. However, none of these other causes of PAH are likely in this patient.

This patient has no history of venous thromboembolism; however, some patients with chronic thromboembolic pulmonary hypertension (CTEPH) do not report a history of deep venous thrombosis. This patient's low-probability ventilation-perfusion scan makes CTEPH very unlikely.

Hepatopulmonary syndrome is a disorder caused by dilated small vessels in the pulmonary vasculature resulting in shunting of blood, and it should be considered in a patient with liver disease who is hypoxic. Pulmonary hypertension is not a defining feature. Intrapulmonary shunting is confirmed by the appearance of contrast (bubbles from agitated saline) in the left heart following injection into a peripheral vein. In this patient, the contrast echocardiographic study was normal.

Pulmonary veno-occlusive disease (PVOD) is a rare cause of pulmonary hypertension caused by fibrous occlusion of distal pulmonary veins. Detection in this patient's age group is unusual; most cases are diagnosed in children and young adults. PVOD is confirmed by pathology but can be suggested by radiographic abnormalities such as pleural effusions or a prominent interstitium on chest radiograph and septal thickening on chest CT. This patient had clear lung fields on chest radiograph. PVOD is much less likely than pulmonary hypertension in this patient.

KEY POINT

- The diagnosis of portopulmonary hypertension is suggested by evidence of pulmonary hypertension in the setting of portal hypertension.

Bibliography

Fritz JS, Fallon MB, Kawut SM. Pulmonary vascular complications of liver disease. Am J Respir Crit Care Med. 2013 Jan 15;187(2):133-43. [PMID: 23155142]

Item 14   Answer: C

Educational Objective: Manage ventilator-associated pneumonia.

The most appropriate next step in management is to perform deep sampling of the lower respiratory tract. Ventilator-associated pneumonia (VAP) is a serious, preventable complication of mechanical ventilation. It is defined as pneumonia with onset at least 48 hours after endotracheal intubation. VAP is difficult to diagnose, but potential clues to its presence include temperature greater than 38.0 °C (100.4 °F), leukocytosis or leukopenia, increased purulent secretion, new or progressive pulmonary infiltrates, and worsening ventilation parameters, particularly after a period of improvement.

Patients suspected of having VAP should undergo lower respiratory tract sampling, followed by microscopic analysis and culture of the specimen. Nonbronchoscopic sampling methods are simple suctioning of the endotracheal tube and mini–bronchoalveolar lavage (BAL), which involves use of a telescoping catheter (instead of a bronchoscope) to instill and aspirate physiologic saline for microbiologic analysis. Bronchoscopic methods are standard BAL and protected specimen brush. Deep sampling methods may allow for narrower antibiotic choices and more rapid de-escalation of antibiotics.

While waiting for the microscopic and culture results from the lower respiratory tract sampling, initiating empiric antibiotics is a reasonable option. However, this patient has been in the hospital for 7 days and is at risk for multidrug-resistant organisms, including *Pseudomonas* species. In this situation, an antipseudomonal cephalosporin or carbapenem would be appropriate. Ceftriaxone and azithromycin would be good coverage for community-acquired pneumonia but are inadequate for this patient.

Chest physiotherapy is useful for assisting with the removal of secretions in patients with COPD, cystic fibrosis, and ciliary dyskinesia. In addition to standard chest percussion and drainage, a large number of mechanical devices are now available that help encourage mobilization of secretions with variable results. Although chest physiotherapy will assist with removal of secretions, it will not provide additional information to clarify the diagnosis in this patient. The most appropriate next step in management is a microbiologic diagnosis to guide further therapy.

Switching from oseltamivir to zanamivir is unlikely to help this patient, who demonstrated an initial clinical response to influenza therapy and then declined. VAP is the most likely diagnosis, not influenza resistance to oseltamivir.

KEY POINT

- Patients suspected of having ventilator-associated pneumonia should undergo lower respiratory tract sampling, followed by microscopic analysis and culture of the specimen.

Bibliography

Patel PJ, Leeper KV Jr, McGowan JE Jr. Epidemiology and microbiology of hospital-acquired pneumonia. Semin Respir Crit Care Med. 2002 Oct;23(5):415-25. [PMID: 16088635]

Item 15   Answer: C

Educational Objective: Treat respiratory failure due to heart failure with noninvasive positive pressure ventilation.

The most appropriate management is noninvasive positive pressure ventilation (NPPV) and supplemental oxygen. This patient has developed respiratory insufficiency due to heart failure with pulmonary edema and pleural effusions. His dyspnea and hypoxia are due to fluid in the alveolar space and interstitium of the lungs, as well as to some degree of pulmonary restriction caused by the effusions. NPPV consists of delivery of positive airway pressure breaths without the use of an endotracheal tube; the interface between the patient and NPPV device is a tight-fitting mask. NPPV settings include an inspiratory positive airway pressure (IPAP) and an end-expiratory positive airway pressure (EPAP). The EPAP component of NPPV helps maintain airway patency and recruits atelectatic or flooded alveoli; it also counters the increased workload imposed by high airway resistance. NPPV decreases the need for mechanical ventilation, improves respiratory parameters, and is associated with improved survival, especially in patients with hypercapnia.

The initial dose of loop diuretic should be at least equivalent to, but preferably greater than, the dose of the patient's chronic outpatient diuretic. If response is not adequate, the diuretic dose should be increased, and an additional synergistic diuretic should be added (usually a thiazide). There is no difference in efficacy or safety of furosemide administration for bolus versus continuous infusion, and there is no indication to change this patient's furosemide dosing.

Intubation and mechanical ventilation could be used to deliver positive pressure support, but this process is invasive, requiring intubation and often sedation, and is associated with an increased risk of hospital-acquired pneumonia. Intubation and mechanical ventilation are options if this patient does not respond to NPPV.

Ultrafiltration is an option for fluid removal and can be performed in the setting of diuretic failure before overt need for kidney replacement therapy. Trials of early ultrafiltration for patients hospitalized with acute decompensated heart failure with volume overload did not demonstrate any definitive effects on mortality. This patient has just received a dose of furosemide, and the diagnosis of diuretic failure has not been established.

KEY POINT

- In patients with hypoxemic respiratory failure due to heart failure, noninvasive positive pressure ventilation decreases the need for mechanical ventilation, improves respiratory parameters, and may decrease mortality.

Bibliography

Weng CL, Zhao YT, Liu QH, et al. Meta-analysis: Noninvasive ventilation in acute cardiogenic pulmonary edema. Ann Intern Med. 2010 May 4;152(9):590-600. Erratum in: Ann Intern Med. 2010 Aug 17;153(4):280. Ann Intern Med. 2010 Jul 6;153(1):67. [PMID: 20439577]

Item 16   Answer: A

Educational Objective: Treat an acute exacerbation of COPD with antibiotics and systemic glucocorticoid therapy.

The most appropriate treatment is to start short courses of antibiotics and prednisone. This patient has an acute exacerbation of COPD. In addition to short-acting bronchodilators and supplemental oxygen as needed, antibiotics and systemic glucocorticoids (such as prednisone) are indicated for treatment of acute COPD exacerbations. Acute exacerbations of

COPD are mostly caused by bacterial or viral infections. The combination of cough, dyspnea, and sputum purulence that is increased from baseline generally indicates the need for antibiotics in the treatment of acute COPD exacerbations, especially in patients with severe and very severe COPD. The most common bacterial pathogens that cause exacerbations are *Haemophilus influenzae, Haemophilus parainfluenzae, Streptococcus pneumoniae,* and *Moraxella catarrhalis.* Empiric antibiotic therapy should be chosen on the basis of local bacterial resistance patterns. Commonly used regimens include an advanced macrolide, a cephalosporin, or doxycycline. Systemic glucocorticoids decrease recovery time, improve lung function, improve arterial hypoxemia, and reduce the risk of early relapse. A prednisone dose of 40 mg/d for 5 days is recommended. Earlier studies suggested a 2-week course of prednisone, but a recent study showed that a 5-day course is sufficient. A prompt follow-up visit is necessary after discharge, and pulmonary rehabilitation should be recommended.

The benefits of glucocorticoids in acute COPD exacerbation have been documented with systemic treatment and not with inhaled agents such as fluticasone. Although adding a combination of a long-acting β_2-agonist (LABA) and inhaled glucocorticoid at the time of discharge may be appropriate, treating an acute exacerbation with antibiotics and an inhaled glucocorticoid would not be appropriate.

Short-acting β_2-agonists (albuterol) with or without short-acting anticholinergic agents are preferred for treatment of acute COPD exacerbations. Guidelines suggest adding a LABA or a combination of a LABA and an inhaled glucocorticoid at the time of discharge, in addition to the long-acting anticholinergic agent (tiotropium) that this patient was already taking. However, a combination of a LABA and an inhaled glucocorticoid (such as fluticasone/salmeterol) is not appropriate therapy during an acute COPD exacerbation.

Roflumilast is an oral phosphodiesterase-4 inhibitor that reduces airway inflammation. Roflumilast is indicated for patients with severe or very severe COPD with recurrent exacerbations; it is not indicated for use during acute exacerbations.

KEY POINT

- Antibiotics and systemic glucocorticoids are primary treatments for acute COPD exacerbations in addition to short-acting bronchodilators and as needed oxygen supplementation.

Bibliography

Leuppi JD, Schuetz P, Bingisser R, et al. Short-term vs conventional glucocorticoid therapy in acute exacerbations of chronic obstructive pulmonary disease: the REDUCE randomized clinical trial. JAMA. 2013 Jun 5;309(21):2223-31. [PMID: 23695200]

Item 17   Answer: B

Educational Objective: Diagnose pulmonary hypertension related to lung disease.

The most appropriate diagnostic test to perform next is an oxygen measurement during sleep and exertion. This patient with underlying lung disease has a 6-month history of exertional dyspnea with evidence of pulmonary hypertension (PH) on physical examination and echocardiography. In this setting, PH is most commonly the result of chronic hypoxia causing diffuse pulmonic vasoconstriction; if untreated, this may result in vascular remodeling and sustained PH. Treatment of this form of PH due to underlying lung disease (group 3 classification) focuses on treatment of the underlying lung disease and specifically addressing hypoxia, if present. Although this patient's resting oxygen saturation is within the low-normal range, he may be experiencing sustained hypoxia while asleep or with periods of increased oxygen demand, such as exercise. Therefore, measurement of oxygen saturation with sleep (overnight pulse oximetry) and with exertion (such as with a 6-minute walk test) may determine the need for oxygen therapy in this patient.

High-resolution CT (HRCT) scanning provides detailed information about the lung parenchyma and is particularly valuable for evaluating suspected diffuse parenchymal lung diseases. However, this patient has documented COPD without evidence of another underlying lung process. Therefore, HRCT would not be expected to provide additional useful clinical information in this patient.

There is little evidence in this patient's clinical history to suggest sleep-disordered breathing, and he is not overweight. Therefore, polysomnography is not immediately indicated as a next step in evaluation.

Right heart catheterization is typically used to evaluate PH of unclear cause, and it is generally not necessary when PH is believed to be related to underlying lung disease. In addition, right heart catheterization would not effectively assess the status of the underlying lung disease or the need for supplemental oxygen.

KEY POINT

- Oxygen measurement during sleep (overnight pulse oximetry) and exertion (such as with a 6-minute walk test) may determine the need for oxygen therapy in patients with pulmonary hypertension due to underlying lung disease (group 3 classification).

Bibliography
Galiè N, Hoeper MM, Humbert M, et al; ESC Committee for Practice Guidelines (CPG). Guidelines for the diagnosis and treatment of pulmonary hypertension: the Task Force for the Diagnosis and Treatment of Pulmonary Hypertension of the European Society of Cardiology (ESC) and the European Respiratory Society (ERS), endorsed by the International Society of Heart and Lung Transplantation (ISHLT). Eur Heart J. 2009 Oct;30(20):2493-537. Erratum in: Eur Heart J. 2011 Apr;32(8):926. [PMID: 19713419]

Item 18   Answer: B

Educational Objective: Treat septic shock in a patient developing acute kidney injury.

The most appropriate next step in treatment is to discontinue intravenous maintenance fluids and perhaps start a trial of diuretics. This patient is well past the window (within the first several hours after diagnosis) in which early aggressive fluid resuscitation is known to be beneficial in septic shock. Although individual markers of volume status are imperfect, the combination of a normalized lactic acid level, substantial positive fluid balance, improved blood pressure, and elevated central venous pressure suggest that the patient is euvolemic if not hypervolemic. Additional fluid resuscitation is unlikely to improve kidney function, may make it worse, and could exacerbate this patient's hypoxemia given his acute respiratory distress syndrome and pleural effusions.

Albumin is unlikely to be beneficial and may cause harm in a patient who is in the recovery phase of septic shock and has evidence of intravascular volume overload. Administration of colloids offers no advantage over crystalloids in resuscitating critically ill patients in general; however, sepsis guidelines note that albumin may be advantageous in patients with refractory shock not responding to crystalloids.

Hemodialysis is not clearly indicated at this time. Some concern exists that this patient is developing intravascular volume overload, but reducing intravenous fluids, avoiding nephrotoxins, and perhaps starting a trial of diuretics would be appropriate first steps. This patient does not have other indications for dialysis such as hyperkalemia, uremia, or severe acidosis. His declining kidney function is likely from the residual effect of acute tubular necrosis and may improve in the next few days now that his septic shock is resolving.

Studies of stress-dose glucocorticoids have not consistently shown benefit in patients with septic shock. Their use is generally reserved for patients with persistent shock despite fluid resuscitation and vasopressor support.

KEY POINT

- In patients with septic shock, aggressive fluid resuscitation after the early resuscitation phase (within the first several hours after diagnosis) can be detrimental.

Bibliography
Dellinger RP, Levy MM, Rhodes A, et al; Surviving Sepsis Campaign Guidelines Committee including the Pediatric Subgroup. Surviving sepsis campaign: international guidelines for management of severe sepsis and septic shock: 2012. Crit Care Med. 2013 Feb;41(2):580-637. [PMID: 23353941]

Item 19   Answer: C

Educational Objective: Treat moderate persistent asthma with combination inhaled glucocorticoid and long-acting β₂-agonist therapy.

The most appropriate treatment is the combination of a low-dose inhaled glucocorticoid and long acting β₂-agonist (LABA) in addition to an as-needed short-acting β₂-agonist. Appropriate initial classification of asthma is important in guiding the strength and type of therapy that is likely to be most effective. Underestimating asthma severity may delay resolution of symptoms and may inadequately manage airway inflammation. This patient has newly diagnosed moderate persistent asthma based on her daily symptoms and spirometry showing an FEV₁ of greater than or equal to 60% but less than 80% of predicted that responds to bronchodilator therapy. The preferred regimen for treating moderate persistent asthma is the combination of a low-dose inhaled glucocorticoid and LABA. Adding a LABA to inhaled glucocorticoid therapy has increased synergistic anti-inflammatory properties compared with either agent alone. Additionally, recent data have demonstrated that long-acting anticholinergic therapy may be appropriate as step-up therapy if moderate persistent asthma does not resolve with combination inhaled glucocorticoid and LABA therapy.

A leukotriene agonist or low-dose inhaled glucocorticoid are recommended treatment options for patients with mild persistent asthma, defined as asthma symptoms occurring more than 2 days per week but not daily with an FEV_1 of greater than or equal to 80% of predicted. The addition of either therapy alone may not adequately treat the degree of asthma seen in this patient.

This patient requires anti-inflammatory controller therapy. Recommending daily use of her oral antihistamine would not address her lower airway inflammation and would not be an appropriate intervention to control her asthma symptoms.

KEY POINT

- The most appropriate therapy for moderate persistent asthma is combination low-dose inhaled glucocorticoid and long-acting β_2-agonist therapy.

Bibliography

National Asthma Education and Prevention Program. Expert Panel Report 3 (EPR-3): Guidelines for the Diagnosis and Management of Asthma-Summary Report 2007. J Allergy Clin Immunol. 2007 Nov;120(5 Suppl): S94-138. Erratum in: J Allergy Clin Immunol. 2008 Jun;121(6):1330. [PMID: 17983880]

Item 20   Answer: B

Educational Objective: Diagnose a bronchial carcinoid tumor.

The most likely diagnosis is a bronchial carcinoid tumor. This patient presents with evidence of airway obstruction with a likely postobstructive pneumonia. This should be suspected in patients who have a persistent pulmonary infiltrate and a localized wheeze on examination. Although bronchial carcinoid tumors represent only a small percentage of all lung cancers, they are the most common lung cancer in children and adolescents. Most bronchial carcinoid tumors involve the proximal airways, so patients may present with symptoms related to endobronchial narrowing or obstruction, including postobstructive pneumonia. Only approximately 1% to 5% of patients present with symptoms of carcinoid syndrome. Other endobronchial cancers should be considered in older patients. Foreign body aspiration or airway strictures may also lead to airway obstruction.

Patients with allergic bronchopulmonary aspergillosis can present with recurrent asthma exacerbations in the setting of peripheral eosinophilia, elevated serum IgE levels, and bronchiectasis. Thick sputum can result in airway obstruction with associated atelectasis. However, patients typically respond to systemic glucocorticoids rather than antibiotic treatment, as in this patient. In addition, she has no evidence of peripheral eosinophilia.

Chronic eosinophilic pneumonia is associated with peripheral and upper lobe–predominant areas of consolidation that improve with glucocorticoid therapy. Antibiotics would have no effect on the course of the disease.

Patients with cystic fibrosis can present with recurrent respiratory infections in the setting of bronchiectasis. However, this patient's chest radiograph showed no evidence of bronchiectasis.

KEY POINT

- Most bronchial carcinoid tumors involve the proximal airways, so patients may present with symptoms related to endobronchial narrowing or obstruction, including postobstructive pneumonia.

Bibliography

Travis WD. Advances in neuroendocrine lung tumors. Ann Oncol. 2010 Oct;21 Suppl 7:vii65-71. [PMID: 20943645]

Item 21   Answer: C

Educational Objective: Treat parapneumonic effusion and empyema with thoracostomy drainage and antibiotics.

The most appropriate management is to insert a small-bore pleural drain and begin piperacillin-tazobactam. Complicated parapneumonic effusion and empyema should be suspected in all patients who do not respond to appropriate antibiotic therapy for pneumonia. This patient presented with subacute onset of fever, fatigue, and worsening shortness of breath after antibiotics for pneumonia. Pleural fluid analysis is consistent with a neutrophil-predominant exudate with low pH (<7.2) and negative Gram stain. This defines a complicated parapneumonic effusion that should be drained. If pleural loculations prevent adequate drainage by a single tube, multiple tubes may be needed. Small-bore (10-14 Fr [3.3-4.7 mm]) thoracostomy tubes have been demonstrated to be adequate for most patients with pleural infection and are associated with increased patient comfort.

Large-bore thoracostomy tubes have not demonstrated any advantage over small-bore thoracostomy tubes in the drainage of pleural effusion and are associated with increased patient discomfort.

Some patients with a complicated parapneumonic effusion may respond to appropriate antibiotic therapy alone; however, in most cases simultaneous drainage of the effusion speeds clinical recovery. Empirically selected antibiotics must provide adequate coverage for anaerobic organisms that are common in patients with empyema. Reasonable options include clindamycin, β-lactam plus β-lactamase inhibitors, and carbapenems. Piperacillin-tazobactam is an appropriate antibiotic for this patient, whereas ceftriaxone plus azithromycin and monotherapy with levofloxacin are not appropriate owing to their lack of anaerobic coverage.

Repeating the chest radiograph is not appropriate because this patient requires intervention for his complicated parapneumonic effusion.

- Complicated parapneumonic effusions should be managed with drainage and antibiotics that will treat anaerobic infection.

Bibliography

Rahman NM, Maskell NA, Davies CW, et al. The relationship between chest tube size and clinical outcome in pleural infection. Chest. 2010 Mar;137(3):536-43. [PMID: 19820073]

Item 22   Answer: C

Educational Objective: Diagnose vocal cord dysfunction.

The most appropriate management is otolaryngology evaluation for possible vocal cord dysfunction. Also known as paradoxical vocal fold motion disorder, this condition is characterized by adduction of the vocal cords (instead of abduction) during inspiration. This is an involuntary maneuver that can occur without other chronic conditions, but it can also happen in patients with asthma. Some patients have episodes related to performance (athletes) or exposure to certain irritants such as smoke or perfume. Symptoms include mid-chest tightness, dyspnea, and lack of symptom relief with asthma treatment. Patients may also note cough and dysphonia, and stridor may be present that may be perceived on examination as an inspiratory monophonic wheeze. The gold standard for diagnosis is observation of vocal cord adduction during inspiration with laryngoscopy after provocation with exercise or irritant exposure. Treatment consists of laryngeal control techniques, biofeedback, and relaxation techniques, usually under the direction of a speech pathologist. Management of other potential conditions that might contribute to vocal cord irritation, such as reflux, sinus disease/allergies, and obstructive sleep apnea, can also be very helpful.

Allergen immunotherapy is not indicated in this patient who has no clinical history of allergy symptoms and has normal findings on his upper airway and nasopharyngeal examinations.

Although the patient is experiencing episodes of shortness of breath, mostly with exertion, there is no additional history or findings on physical examination suggestive of heart disease as the cause of his symptoms. Echocardiography is therefore not indicated.

Stepping up asthma therapy by increasing the intensity of inhaled glucocorticoid therapy is not appropriate because this patient's clinical presentation and spirometry results are not consistent with asthma as the cause of his symptoms.

- Vocal cord dysfunction (also known as paradoxical vocal fold motion disorder) is characterized by adduction of the vocal cords during inspiration; symptoms include mid-chest tightness, dyspnea, and lack of symptom relief with asthma treatment.

Bibliography

Matrka L. Paradoxic vocal fold movement disorder. Otolaryngol Clin North Am. 2014 Feb;47(1):135-46. [PMID: 24286687]

Item 23   Answer: B

Educational Objective: Manage a large spontaneous pneumothorax.

The most appropriate management is to perform needle aspiration of the pneumothorax. This patient has a primary spontaneous pneumothorax, because it occurred in the absence of trauma with no clinically apparent lung disease. He is clinically stable but has breathlessness associated with a large pneumothorax (>2 cm from the lung margin to the chest wall at the level of the hilum). High-flow supplemental oxygen is usually given to most patients with pneumothorax to facilitate absorption of the pleural air. Emergent needle thoracostomy followed by thoracostomy tube placement is indicated in patients with a large, hemodynamically significant (tension) pneumothorax. However, in patients such as this one with a large pneumothorax that is symptomatic but stable, it is reasonable to perform needle aspiration of the pneumothorax. If the lung expands after aspiration, the patient may be appropriately observed for several hours with reimaging and discharge if stable. Placement of a one-way (Heimlich) valve is another option with outpatient follow-up.

Insertion of a small-bore thoracostomy tube (<14 Fr [4.7 mm]) is indicated as initial treatment for larger (>2 cm) secondary pneumothoraces in patients who are symptomatic, but it would not be a recommended initial treatment for this patient with a primary pneumothorax.

Noninvasive positive pressure ventilation would not be appropriate, because it does not have an established role in the management of pneumothorax.

Observation alone is not appropriate because this patient is symptomatic, with increased breathlessness, and has a large pneumothorax.

- A large (>2 cm), symptomatic, primary spontaneous pneumothorax may be initially managed with high-flow supplemental oxygen and needle aspiration.

Bibliography

MacDuff A, Arnold A, Harvey J; BTS Pleural Disease Guideline Group. Management of spontaneous pneumothorax: British Thoracic Society Pleural Disease Guideline 2010. Thorax. 2010 Aug;65 Suppl 2:ii18-31. [PMID: 20696690]

Item 24   Answer: B

Educational Objective: Treat pulmonary hypertension due to heart disease.

The most appropriate initial management is treatment of systemic arterial hypertension with lisinopril. This patient has pulmonary hypertension (PH) in the setting of diastolic heart failure (also known as heart failure with preserved ejection fraction [HFpEF]). HFpEF, an increasingly common cause of PH, is often seen in association with systemic hypertension and left ventricular hypertrophy. PH related to left-sided heart disease is classified as group 2, and treatment is directed at the underlying cardiac disease. Therefore, therapy for HFpEF is based on treating the causes and symptoms of the heart failure. Because hypertension is a common cause of HFpEF, aggressive control of the systemic arterial blood pressure is necessary. Because no specific agent has definitively proved to be more effective than another, therapy should follow hypertension treatment guidelines.

Epoprostenol is an advanced therapy; it is an intravenous pulmonary vasodilator reserved for management of group 1 PH (pulmonary arterial hypertension) associated with advanced symptoms and functional limitation.

Right heart catheterization is not an appropriate initial test in the diagnosis or management of patients with PH related to heart failure, although it may be useful later if initial treatments aimed at the underlying condition are not effective in improving symptoms or pulmonary artery pressures.

The pulmonary vasodilator sildenafil is considered advanced therapy, which is directed at PH itself rather than the underlying cause, and is indicated for the treatment of group 1 pulmonary arterial hypertension. Not only is the role of such drugs in the treatment of groups 2 to 5 PH unclear, advanced therapy can alter ventilation-perfusion relationships and be deleterious in these patients.

KEY POINT

- Pulmonary hypertension related to left-sided heart disease is classified as group 2; treatment is directed at the underlying cardiac disease.

Bibliography

McLaughlin VV, Archer SL, Badesch DB, et al; American College of Cardiology Foundation Task Force on Expert Consensus Documents; American Heart Association; American College of Chest Physicians; American Thoracic Society, Inc; Pulmonary Hypertension Association. ACCF/AHA 2009 expert consensus document on pulmonary hypertension a report of the American College of Cardiology Foundation Task Force on Expert Consensus Documents and the American Heart Association developed in collaboration with the American College of Chest Physicians; American Thoracic Society, Inc.; and the Pulmonary Hypertension Association. J Am Coll Cardiol. 2009 Apr 28;53(17):1573-619. [PMID: 19389575]

Item 25   Answer: D

Educational Objective: Treat severe asthma with omalizumab.

The most appropriate treatment is omalizumab. Severe asthma occurs in 10% of patients with asthma and is associated with long-term treatment with high-dose glucocorticoids, frequent exacerbations, and high health care utilization, as in this patient. This patient's asthma has not been controlled despite aggressive nonpharmacologic interventions and treatment with multiple drugs. Omalizumab, a humanized monoclonal antibody directed at IgE, is the first biologic agent approved by the FDA for use in asthma. Administered subcutaneously every 2 to 4 weeks, omalizumab is indicated in patients with moderate to severe persistent asthma with the following characteristics: (1) symptoms inadequately controlled with inhaled glucocorticoids, (2) evidence of allergies to perennial aeroallergens, and (3) serum IgE levels between 30 and 700 U/mL (30-700 kU/L) (normal range, 0-90 U/mL [0-90 kU/L]). Although it is very expensive, omalizumab has been shown to reduce emergency department visits and appears to be cost effective in appropriately selected patients; it is not indicated for use in patients other than those meeting these treatment parameters.

Allergen immunotherapy (allergy shots) can be useful when a single trigger is identified or when a trigger is consistently the source of asthma instability. It is a reasonable longer-term plan in this patient; however, immunotherapy may take 3 to 5 years to achieve a noticeable therapeutic effect. Omalizumab would be expected to provide more immediate control of her asthma than is possible with allergen immunotherapy.

This patient has required frequent and high doses of systemic glucocorticoids and is exhibiting side effects (skin thinning and cushingoid facies). Because of the long-term detrimental effects of prolonged systemic glucocorticoid therapy, particularly in this younger patient, daily glucocorticoid therapy would not be appropriate.

Other forms of immune modulation, such as with tumor necrosis factor-α inhibitors (such as infliximab) or other immunosuppressive agents (such as cyclophosphamide and azathioprine), have not been shown to be effective in controlling severe asthma and are associated with a high level of adverse effects in these patients.

KEY POINT

- Omalizumab is indicated in patients with moderate to severe persistent asthma with the following characteristics: (1) symptoms inadequately controlled with inhaled glucocorticoids, (2) evidence of allergies to perennial aeroallergens, and (3) serum IgE levels between 30 and 700 U/mL (30-700 kU/L) (normal range, 0-90 U/mL [0-90 kU/L]).

Bibliography

Chung KF, Wenzel SE, Brozek JL, et al. International ERS/ATS guidelines on definition, evaluation and treatment of severe asthma. Eur Respir J. 2014 Feb;43(2):343-73. Erratum in: Eur Respir J. 2014 Apr;43(4):1216. [PMID: 24337046]

Item 26   Answer: D

Educational Objective: Diagnose ventilator-induced lung injury.

The most likely diagnosis is ventilator-induced lung injury (VILI), which represents iatrogenic acute respiratory distress syndrome (ARDS) caused by mechanical ventilation. VILI

CONT.

is most likely to occur when tidal volume and/or plateau pressure are too high. It can occur even in patients with no evidence of lung injury at the time of intubation. This patient was ventilated throughout her surgery. Her ideal body weight is 48 kg (106 lb); based on this, the protective tidal volume would be 288 mL (6 mL/kg of ideal body weight). In addition to low tidal volume, protective ventilation also entails keeping the plateau pressure below 30 cm H_2O if possible. An early clue to nonprotective ventilator settings could have been an elevated plateau pressure, as in this patient when she arrived in the ICU.

Obesity hypoventilation syndrome could be seen in a patient with this body habitus and could include low respiratory system compliance, but this condition would not explain the airspace opacification on imaging, poor oxygenation, or worsening compliance over time.

Pulmonary embolism is always a risk postoperatively, especially in those who undergo orthopedic procedures, such as this patient. Pulmonary embolism would certainly worsen ventilation-perfusion matching and oxygenation, but it would not typically worsen lung compliance over the first 24 hours postoperatively.

ARDS can develop in response to transfusion of blood products when antibodies in transfused plasma activate recipient neutrophils; this is known as transfusion-associated lung injury (TRALI). This can occur after transfusion of any blood product, and it appears to be most likely when the volume of transfused plasma is high and comes from a multiparous female donor. TRALI is generally the least severe form of ARDS; however, it can be fatal if not managed appropriately. This patient received an autologous transfusion only and is not at risk for TRALI.

KEY POINT

- Ventilator-induced lung injury is most likely to occur when the tidal volume and/or plateau pressure are too high; tidal volume should be limited to 6 mL/kg of ideal body weight and plateau pressure less than 30 cm H_2O.

Bibliography
Slutsky AS, Ranieri VM. Ventilator-induced lung injury. N Engl J Med. 2013 Nov 28;369(22):2126-36. Erratum in: N Engl J Med. 2014 Apr 24;370(17): 1668-9. [PMID: 24283226]

Item 27   Answer: D

Educational Objective: Diagnose malignant pleural disease.

The most appropriate diagnostic test to perform next is thoracoscopy. This patient has an unexplained unilateral exudative effusion. Owing to his occupation as an auto mechanic, he has a history of potential asbestos exposure (car brakes previously contained asbestos). This potential exposure increases his risk for mesothelioma, which is suggested by his clinical presentation (exudative pleural effusion, chronic chest pain, weight loss) and imaging findings (pleural thickening). Thoracoscopy

allows for the direct visualization of the pleural surface and enables biopsy of pleural sites likely to have a high diagnostic yield. It has a diagnostic sensitivity for malignant disease of greater than 90%. Thoracoscopy is indicated in this patient in whom imaging and thoracentesis have not achieved a diagnosis, which occurs relatively frequently with mesothelioma.

Because endobronchial lesions are rarely seen in mesothelioma, bronchoscopy would not be an appropriate next diagnostic study.

Repeat pleural fluid cytology is not appropriate because this patient has already had two negative studies. The overall mean sensitivity of pleural fluid cytology for identifying malignant disease is approximately 60%. Approximately 65% of positive results are obtained on the initial thoracentesis. The diagnostic yield from sending more than two samples is very low. One study demonstrated an additional yield of 27% on the second sample and only 5% on the third.

PET/CT scanning is a useful tool for staging disease, particularly for identifying extrathoracic disease. However, it is not a preferred initial diagnostic study because both malignant and nonmalignant pleural thickening can be avid for fluorodeoxyglucose and yield a positive finding on this study.

KEY POINT

- If repeat pleural fluid cytology is negative and the suspicion for malignancy is high in an exudative effusion, thoracoscopy is the next step in the evaluation; it has a diagnostic sensitivity for malignant disease of greater than 90%.

Bibliography
Hooper C, Lee YC, Maskell N; BTS Pleural Guideline Group. Investigation of a unilateral pleural effusion in adults: British Thoracic Society Pleural Disease Guideline 2010. Thorax. 2010 Aug;65 Suppl 2:ii4-17. [PMID: 20696692]

Item 28   Answer: B

Educational Objective: Manage initial ventilator settings.

The most appropriate ventilator mode in this patient is volume-controlled continuous mandatory ventilation (VC-CMV). The ventilator mode defines the means by which the ventilator interacts with the patient. Unfortunately, there are numerous mode names (nearly 300 according to a recent review), and the same mode may have different labels depending on the ventilator manufacturer. In an effort to standardize ventilator modes, a taxonomy has been described in an attempt to simplify ordering and understanding the function of the ventilator, although this classification system has not been universally adopted.

Two main variables must be considered when ordering mechanical ventilation. The breath sequence must be determined, with spontaneous and mandatory breaths being the two primary options. Because this patient has respiratory failure and is unable to effectively breathe on his own, a spontaneous breath sequence (in which the patient breathes

CONT.

on his own with no back-up rate) would not be appropriate, and mandatory ventilation is indicated. Mandatory ventilation may be either intermittent or continuous. Intermittent mandatory ventilation allows for spontaneous breaths between or during mandatory breaths; however, this may lead to dyssynchrony, in which the phases of mechanical breaths do not match the phases of patient breaths and is believed to contribute to lung injury. With CMV, all breaths are supported by the ventilator, and the patient may trigger additional supported breaths above the preset frequency; this consistent breath pattern reduces the risk for dyssynchrony. In general, for acutely ill patients who are hemodynamically unstable, supporting all respiratory efforts with CMV is recommended.

The second variable, the breath control method, determines whether breaths are provided based on pressure or volume. Pressure-controlled ventilation, in which a breath is delivered according to a preset inspiratory pressure, has been associated with ventilator-induced lung injury; therefore, volume control, in which tidal volume and inspiratory flow are designated, is the preferred breath control method as the initial strategy for ventilation of critically ill patients.

KEY POINT

- For acutely ill patients who are hemodynamically unstable, supporting all respiratory effort with the volume-controlled continuous mandatory ventilation setting to minimize risk for ventilator-induced lung injury is recommended as the best strategy for initial mechanical ventilation.

Bibliography
Mireles-Cabodevila E, Hatipoğlu U, Chatburn RL. A rational framework for selecting modes of ventilation. Respir Care. 2013 Feb;58(2):348-66. Erratum in: Respir Care. 2013 Apr;58(4):e51. [PMID: 22710796]

Item 29   Answer: D
Educational Objective: Diagnose suspected occupational asthma.

The most appropriate next step in management is to repeat spirometry after workplace exposure. Occupational asthma, related to workplace exposures to agents associated with airway hyperreactivity, should be suspected in all adults with a diagnosis of asthma because it may be a primary target for treatment. It should also be suspected in patients with asthma-like symptoms that vary with exposure to the workplace, as in this patient. This patient has likely been exposed to diisocyanates from spray painting in the auto body shop where he works, which are associated with triggering bronchospasm. Early recognition of an association of asthma symptoms with potential workplace exposure, and testing if indicated, is important for diagnosis and to guide therapy. Serial monitoring of peak flows throughout the workday, with comparison to a baseline time period away from exposures, can be helpful to support the diagnosis. Similarly, spirometry before and after rechallenge with workplace exposures is helpful

to confirm the diagnosis. Because of the possibility that this patient's occupational exposure may be responsible for his asthma symptoms, it is appropriate to perform spirometry before and after exposure to the potential causative agent. If documented, treatment of occupational asthma should follow guidelines for typical asthma, and allergen exposure should be controlled or eliminated if possible. If significant changes in spirometry are not seen post workplace exposure and a suspicion for any underlying asthma remains, a methacholine challenge test may be appropriate.

Advising a change in workplace venue to avoid allergen exposure for occupational asthma would be premature because the diagnosis has not been confirmed.

High-resolution chest CT is indicated for evaluation of suspected parenchymal lung disease. However, this patient's symptoms are most consistent with airways disease, and he has no clinical evidence of a parenchymal process. Therefore, this testing would not be expected to be of benefit.

Empiric therapy for asthma without documentation of the diagnosis or an association of his asthma symptoms with workplace exposure would not be appropriate.

KEY POINT

- Spirometry before and after rechallenge with workplace exposures is helpful to confirm the diagnosis of occupational asthma.

Bibliography
Tarlo SM, Lemiere C. Occupational asthma. N Engl J Med. 2014 Feb 13;370(7): 640-9. [PMID: 24521110]

Item 30   Answer: A
Educational Objective: Treat obstructive sleep apnea with an oral mandibular advancement appliance.

The most appropriate treatment alternative to continuous positive airway pressure (CPAP) in this patient is an oral mandibular advancement appliance. This patient has symptomatic obstructive sleep apnea (OSA) of moderate severity. Although CPAP provided symptomatic improvement and is generally the preferred treatment for OSA, patient preference or intolerance of CPAP should prompt consideration of other treatments. Oral appliances are an alternative to CPAP therapy for mild to moderate OSA. Randomized controlled trials on the use of oral appliances have demonstrated reasonable control of OSA and improvement in symptoms such as daytime sleepiness. In addition, their use as an alternative therapy is consistent with the American College of Physicians Clinical Practice Guideline for Management of Obstructive Sleep Apnea in Adults. These devices act by one of two mechanisms to increase upper airway caliber: (1) advancement of the mandible by traction or (2) preventing posterior displacement of the tongue by suction.

Treatment of OSA should be directed at maintaining upper airway patency. Supplemental oxygen has no effect on the upper airway and is not indicated as primary therapy for OSA.

Evidence supporting surgical procedures as a treatment for OSA is limited. Patient selection is not standardized, and outcomes related to the long-term adverse consequences of OSA are either unknown or inconsistent. Case series have demonstrated significant improvements in the apnea-hypopnea index (AHI) following maxillomandibular advancement; however, in most patients it would not be considered a primary treatment owing to its level of invasiveness. Literature examining uvulopalatopharyngoplasty, a soft-palate procedure, shows limited improvements in the AHI, so it should generally not be recommended for treatment of OSA.

KEY POINT

- Although continuous positive airway pressure (CPAP) is the preferred treatment for obstructive sleep apnea, patient preference or intolerance of CPAP should prompt consideration of other treatments such as oral mandibular advancement appliances.

Bibliography

Phillips CL, Grunstein RR, Darendeliler MA, et al. Health outcomes of continuous positive airway pressure versus oral appliance treatment for obstructive sleep apnea: a randomized controlled trial. Am J Respir Crit Care Med. 2013 Apr 15;187(8):879-87. [PMID: 23413266]

Item 31   Answer: C

Educational Objective: Diagnose acute pulmonary embolism.

This patient most likely has obstructive shock from a hemodynamically significant acute pulmonary embolism (PE). Patients with malignancy are at increased risk of thrombosis and embolic events. Obstructive shock is a subset of cardiogenic shock in which there is mechanical blockage in the central circulation, as can occur with massive PE (as in this patient) or tension pneumothorax. The findings that support obstructive shock due to PE include hypotension, an accentuated P_2, and profound hypoxemia. With hemodynamically significant PE, the electrocardiogram (ECG) may show the classic S1Q3T3 pattern caused by right ventricular strain due to acute obstruction of the pulmonary artery, but this is not a sensitive finding for PE and its absence does not exclude the diagnosis. Thrombolytic therapy or surgical thrombectomy are therapeutic considerations in patients with massive PE causing shock.

Anaphylactic shock is a type of distributive shock, as might occur if a patient with an allergy to penicillin were given either penicillin or a related agent to which she reacted. Anaphylaxis is an IgE-mediated reaction and manifests within minutes to 1 hour after exposure to the implicated antigen. Ninety percent of patients have a cutaneous reaction such as urticaria, angioedema, or flushing. Bronchospasm and wheezing are common. This patient received meropenem 2 days before developing shock and has no evidence of skin changes or wheezing, making anaphylaxis an unlikely diagnosis.

Acute myocardial infarction could lead to sudden deterioration in clinical status based on a rapid decrease in left ventricular output. However, more specific changes associated with significant myocardial ischemia would be expected on the ECG. Additionally, the severe hypoxia in the setting of acute myocardial infarction is usually due to acute PE caused by inadequate cardiac output, and this patient's clear lungs on auscultation are not consistent with this diagnosis. Septic shock is a type of distributive shock and could account for the hypotension seen in this patient, but the sudden appearance of hypotension and hypoxemia in a patient whose clinical condition was improving is not typical of septic shock.

KEY POINT

- Obstructive shock is a subset of cardiogenic shock in which there is mechanical blockage in the central circulation, as can occur with massive pulmonary embolism or tension pneumothorax.

Bibliography

Marshall PS, Mathews KS, Siegel MD. Diagnosis and management of life-threatening pulmonary embolism. J Intensive Care Med. 2011 Sep-Oct;26(5):275-94. [PMID: 21606060]

Item 32   Answer: D

Educational Objective: Treat severe COPD with lung volume reduction surgery.

The most appropriate next step in management is to evaluate for lung volume reduction surgery (LVRS). To be eligible for LVRS, patients must meet the following criteria: (1) severe COPD; (2) symptomatic despite maximal pharmacologic therapy; (3) completed pulmonary rehabilitation; (4) evidence of bilateral predominant upper-lobe emphysema on CT; (5) postbronchodilator total lung capacity greater than 100% and residual lung volume greater than 150% of predicted; (6) maximum FEV_1 greater than 20% and less than or equal to 45% of predicted and D_{LCO} greater than or equal to 20% of predicted; and (7) ambient air arterial P_{CO_2} less than or equal to 60 mm Hg (8.0 kPa) and arterial P_{O_2} greater than or equal to 45 mm Hg (6.0 kPa). In patients with severe COPD and predominantly upper-lobe emphysema and low post-rehabilitation exercise capacity, LVRS results in improved survival compared with medical treatment. However, higher mortality is seen in patients with severe emphysema with an FEV_1 of less than or equal to 20% of predicted and a D_{LCO} less than or equal to 20% of predicted or homogeneous emphysema on high-resolution CT scan. Because of this patient's severe disability associated with his COPD and available parameters suggesting he may be a candidate for LVRS, further evaluation of this option would be appropriate.

This patient is on appropriate medical treatment, and switching from one combination medication to another medication in the same class is not likely to be helpful. Vilanterol is a newer ultra–long-acting β_2-agonist that may be used once daily. Although a once-daily inhaler regimen may be more convenient for some patients than a twice-daily regimen, these formulations tend to be of significantly higher cost, and there are no evidence-based clinical benefits for these newer ultra–long-acting agents. Therefore, making this change in medication would not be expected to have a significant effect in this patient.

Systemic glucocorticoids are recommended for the short-term treatment of acute exacerbations of COPD. However, continuous therapy with systemic glucocorticoids is associated with significant side effects and is not recommended for the chronic management of COPD.

Criteria for referral for lung transplant evaluation include one of the following: pulmonary hypertension, cor pulmonale, or both despite oxygen therapy; history of exacerbation associated with acute hypercapnia; and FEV_1 less than 20% of predicted with D_{LCO} less than 20% of predicted or homogeneous distribution of emphysema. This patient has an FEV_1 greater than 20% of predicted, a D_{LCO} greater than 20% of predicted, and emphysema in the upper lobes; therefore, he is not a candidate for lung transplantation.

KEY POINT

- In patients with severe COPD and predominantly upper-lobe emphysema and low post-rehabilitation exercise capacity, lung volume reduction surgery results in improved survival compared with medical treatment.

Bibliography

Berger RL, Decamp MM, Criner GJ, Celli BR. Lung volume reduction therapies for advanced emphysema: an update. Chest. 2010 Aug;138(2):407-17. [PMID: 20682529]

Item 33   Answer: D

Educational Objective: Evaluate chronic cough with methacholine challenge testing.

The most appropriate diagnostic test to perform next is methacholine challenge testing. This patient has a history of allergies and a family history of asthma, and he is presenting with paroxysms of cough. This presentation is suggestive of possible cough-variant asthma, in which reversible airway obstruction occurs but the primary presenting symptom is a nonproductive cough. Although a classic presentation of asthma on spirometry includes an obstructive pattern and a significant bronchodilator response (200 mL and 12% increase in FEV_1), this finding is not present in all patients with asthma. Asthma is a dynamic airway condition, and obstruction may not be seen at rest or in the absence of an exposure to the asthma trigger. In patients with clinical symptoms suggestive of bronchospastic disease (such as unexplained dyspnea or cough, as in this patient) but with normal spirometry, bronchial challenge testing may be diagnostically helpful. Bronchial challenge testing uses a controlled inhaled stimulus to induce bronchospasm in association with

spirometry; a positive test is indicated by a drop in the measured FEV_1. Methacholine is a commonly used agent that induces cholinergic bronchospasm at low concentrations in patients with asthma.

Although this patient has a history of allergies and allergic rhinitis, it is not clear that the cause of his cough symptoms is associated with an allergic trigger. Allergy testing may be helpful in patients with allergies and asthma in whom treatment for specific triggers would be beneficial and in those whose symptoms are not adequately controlled with usual allergy or asthma therapies.

High-resolution chest CT (HRCT) is used to define the lung parenchyma in great detail and is useful in patients with suspected parenchymal lung disease. However, this patient has no suggestion of an underlying parenchymal disease, and HRCT is therefore not indicated.

Measurement of serum IgE levels may be helpful in diagnosing allergic bronchopulmonary aspergillosis (ABPA), a hypersensitivity reaction of the airways that occurs when bronchi become colonized by *Aspergillus* species. ABPA is characterized by recurrent episodes of fever, bronchial obstruction, and cough productive of brownish mucus plugs. This patient's presentation is not consistent with ABPA; therefore, serum IgE testing is not indicated.

KEY POINT

- In patients with clinical symptoms suggestive of bronchospastic disease (such as cough or unexplained dyspnea) but with normal spirometry, bronchial challenge testing (such as with methacholine) may be helpful to evaluate for asthma.

Bibliography

Katial RK, Covar RA. Bronchoprovocation testing in asthma. Immunol Allergy Clin North Am. 2012 Aug;32(3):413-31. [PMID: 22877619]

Item 34   Answer: B   H

Educational Objective: Treat anaphylaxis with epinephrine.

The most appropriate next step in treatment is to administer epinephrine. This patient's hypotension, bronchospasm, and urticaria are characteristic of a severe anaphylactic reaction. Epinephrine is the drug of choice for anaphylaxis, preferably given as an intramuscular injection because of more rapid and consistent absorption compared with subcutaneous injection. Intravenous delivery may be advantageous in patients with compromised muscle perfusion from shock. Food allergies and insect stings are important anaphylaxis triggers, while a medication is the most likely trigger in a hospitalized patient.

Although antihistamines are the most commonly prescribed drug for anaphylaxis, they do not treat the life-threatening manifestations of anaphylaxis such as bronchospasm and hypotension. It is also likely that epinephrine, rather than antihistamines, is the agent responsible for the resolution of urticaria in these patients.

CONT.

In patients taking β-blocker therapy, glucagon may be an effective treatment for hypotension and bradycardia that is resistant to epinephrine. The inotropic and chronotropic effects of glucagon are not mediated through β-receptors. However, glucagon is a second-line treatment for anaphylaxis, even in patients taking β-blockers.

Methylprednisolone is an adjunctive therapy to prevent delayed or protracted reactions in patients with anaphylaxis. However, the drug takes several hours to take effect and therefore is not useful for rapidly reversing the life-threatening manifestations of anaphylaxis. A recent systematic review did not discover any randomized controlled trials that confirmed the effectiveness of glucocorticoids in the treatment of anaphylaxis.

KEY POINT

- Intramuscular epinephrine is the drug of choice for anaphylaxis; however, intravenous delivery may be advantageous in patients with compromised muscle perfusion from shock.

Bibliography

Simons FE, Sheikh A. Anaphylaxis: the acute episode and beyond. BMJ. 2013 Feb 12;346:f602. [PMID: 23403828]

Item 35   Answer: C

Educational Objective: Manage air travel in a patient with lung disease.

The most appropriate next step is a hypoxia altitude simulation test (HAST). Initial evaluation of patients with lung disease who are not on long-term oxygen therapy and are planning air travel is usually with pulse oximetry at sea level. If the oxygen saturation is greater than 95%, it is unlikely that the patient will have significant desaturation at higher altitudes, and further testing or supplemental oxygen is not usually indicated. For patients with an oxygen saturation of less than 92%, in-flight supplemental oxygen is usually recommended. In patients with sea-level oxygen saturation between 92% and 95%, simulators that mimic altitude hypoxia, available at some centers, can be used to determine the need for oxygen supplementation during flight. Patients at high risk for in-flight hypoxia and its complications are those with COPD with hypercapnia, a recent exacerbation of chronic lung disease, pulmonary hypertension, and restrictive lung disease, in addition to those who have had previous in-flight symptoms. This patient, who has a resting oxyhemoglobin saturation of 93% breathing ambient air, has risk factors for altitude-related hypoxia, which include an FEV_1 less than 50% of predicted and cardiac disease. The HAST predicts the in-flight arterial partial pressure of oxygen and whether supplemental oxygen is needed, accounting for the pressurization of airline cabins that simulate an altitude of less than 2440 meters (8000 feet).

In patients with COPD and a sea-level oxygen saturation between 92% and 95%, an alternative approach in locations where HAST testing is not available is to perform a 6-minute walk test. An oxygen saturation less than 84% suggests likely significant desaturation with altitude, and supplemental oxygen is usually prescribed without additional testing. Those with a walk test saturation greater than or equal to 84% should be referred for HAST testing.

Arterial blood gas studies alone are unlikely to provide important information beyond what is already known about this patient's oxygenation status. It is possible that this patient has chronic hypercapnia due to underlying lung disease, a finding that would support further testing in the form of HAST.

Similarly, echocardiographic evidence of pulmonary hypertension would represent a risk factor for in-flight hypoxia and would require further evaluation, but it does not have adequate predictive value alone in determining the need for in-flight oxygen.

With a proper pre-travel evaluation, it is unlikely that this patient with stable chronic lung disease would have an in-flight problem. Unless the patient declines further testing, recommending against travel is premature.

KEY POINT

- In patients with lung disease and sea-level oxygen saturation between 92% and 95%, hypoxia altitude simulation testing can be used to determine the need for oxygen supplementation during air travel.

Bibliography

British Thoracic Society Standards of Care Committee. Managing passengers with respiratory disease planning air travel: British Thoracic Society recommendations. Thorax. 2002 Apr;57(4):289-304. [PMID: 11923546]

Item 36   Answer: A

Educational Objective: Treat inadequately controlled asthma by stepping up therapy.

The most appropriate management is to step up therapy for this patient's asthma by adding a low-dose glucocorticoid inhaler. This patient has a history of asthma as a child, which has been quiescent for many years and has not required treatment as an adult. She recently experienced a viral respiratory tract infection with associated wheezing and cough. Viral respiratory infections, most commonly with rhinoviruses, may induce bronchospasm in patients without preexisting reactive airways disease and may require acute treatment for symptom relief. However, viral respiratory infections may also exacerbate underlying asthma and require a step-up in treatment. Although this patient has not required therapy for asthma for many years, she remains persistently symptomatic with evidence of ongoing obstruction beyond the time frame when virally induced bronchospasm in patients without asthma typically resolves, which is usually by 6 to 8 weeks after a respiratory infection. Her symptoms and spirometry results are consistent with mild persistent asthma; therefore, the addition of an inhaled glucocorticoid, consistent with guideline-based treatment recommendations, is indicated to control her asthma.

Because this patient remains symptomatic beyond the time frame in which patients without asthma would be expected to have symptom resolution, continuing either an as-needed or long-acting β₂-agonist would not address the underlying mechanism of obstruction and would not provide optimal control of her asthma. Therefore, neither of these interventions is indicated.

Similarly, discontinuing the inhaler medication would not be appropriate in this patient with asthma who remains symptomatic.

KEY POINT

- Viral respiratory infections, frequently due to rhinovirus, may cause airway hyperresponsiveness and obstruction through nonallergic mechanisms in patients without a history of asthma; they may also exacerbate underlying asthma and require step-up therapy.

Bibliography
Irwin RS, Baumann MH, Bolser DC, et al; American College of Chest Physicians (ACCP). Diagnosis and management of cough executive summary: ACCP evidence-based clinical practice guidelines. Chest. 2006 Jan;129(1 Suppl):1S-23S. [PMID: 16428686]

Item 37   Answer: B

Educational Objective: Diagnose suspected obstructive sleep apnea or central sleep apnea.

The most appropriate next step is in-laboratory polysomnography. This patient has risk factors for both obstructive sleep apnea (OSA) (male gender, snoring, overweight) and central sleep apnea (CSA) (heart failure and atrial fibrillation). The lack of history from a bed partner hampers determination of pretest probability. Although out-of-center (performed outside of a sleep laboratory or at home) sleep testing is appropriate for patients with a high pretest probability of uncomplicated moderate to severe OSA, those with heart failure or advanced pulmonary disease or those at risk for CSA should undergo in-laboratory polysomnographic diagnostic testing. In-laboratory polysomnography allows more detailed analysis of the possible underlying disorder than out-of-center methods. Once the type of apnea is clarified during the diagnostic portion of the in-laboratory study, the technician may then utilize the most appropriate mode of positive airway pressure (PAP) therapy and assess the response to treatment. Treatment options include continuous positive airway pressure (CPAP) for OSA, adaptive servoventilation (ASV) for CSA, and the addition of supplemental oxygen, if needed, for gas exchange abnormalities due to chronic heart failure or lung disease.

In this patient, auto-titrating positive airway pressure (APAP) would not be appropriate before diagnostic testing is performed to clarify the predominant type of apnea. APAP is indicated for treatment of OSA but is unlikely to be an effective treatment for CSA or complex sleep apnea, if present.

Out-of-center sleep testing should be used in patients without comorbid cardiopulmonary disease who are likely to have OSA of at least moderate severity, such as in an obese middle-aged man who snores loudly, pauses breathing, and gasps during sleep.

This patient has symptoms of interrupted sleep and daytime sleepiness, which are strong indications for treatment of sleep-disordered breathing. Further screening with overnight pulse oximetry is unlikely to add reliably important diagnostic information, and it will not alter the decision to treat.

KEY POINT

- Although out-of-center sleep testing is appropriate for patients with a high pretest probability of uncomplicated moderate to severe obstructive sleep apnea, those with heart failure or advanced pulmonary disease or those at risk for central sleep apnea should undergo in-laboratory polysomnographic diagnostic testing.

Bibliography
Epstein LJ, Kristo D, Strollo PJ Jr, et al; Adult Obstructive Sleep Apnea Task Force of the American Academy of Sleep Medicine. Clinical guideline for the evaluation, management and long-term care of obstructive sleep apnea in adults. J Clin Sleep Med. 2009 Jun 15;5(3):263-76. [PMID: 19960649]

Item 38   Answer: D

Educational Objective: Evaluate lung cancer risk in a patient with silicosis.

The most appropriate next step in management is to perform repeat CT imaging of the chest. This patient has a history of previously diagnosed silicosis, and silicosis is an independent risk factor for the development of lung cancer. Additionally, this patient also has a smoking history that increases the risk for malignancy. This increased risk, in combination with his history of weight loss, warrant further evaluation for malignancy. Evaluation may be more difficult in patients with silicosis, in whom lung findings tend to be upper lobe predominant, which tends to be the same distribution where lung cancers are more likely to occur. Because of this, plain chest radiography may not define small lesions in the background of nodularity and scarring. Therefore, a more sensitive imaging modality, such as CT, is indicated despite this patient's unchanged plain chest radiograph.

Chest MRI may be useful in evaluating chest wall, pleural, and mediastinal pathology, but it has limited utility in assessing bronchial or parenchymal lesions, primarily due to poorer spatial resolution and longer imaging times required than CT. Therefore, even in the presence of significant lung disease such as in this patient, CT is the preferred imaging modality.

Patients with silicosis are also at increased risk for tuberculosis (TB), which may also cause blood in the sputum and systemic features such as weight loss. This patient's persistently negative tuberculin skin tests and unchanged chest radiograph make this a less likely diagnosis; therefore, empiric treatment for TB would be an inappropriate next step in management. However, further diagnostic evaluation for TB would be reasonable if his evaluation for malignancy is negative.

Although patients with silicosis often have a concomitant smoking exposure and smoking-related lung disease, there is little role for the use of glucocorticoids in treating patients with silicosis who do not have another indication for their use.

KEY POINT

- Silicosis is an independent risk factor for the development of lung cancer.

Bibliography

Liu Y, Steenland K, Rong Y, et al. Exposure-response analysis and risk assessment for lung cancer in relationship to silica exposure: a 44-year cohort study of 34,018 workers. Am J Epidemiol. 2013 Nov 1;178(9):1424-33. [PMID: 24043436]

Item 39   Answer: C

Educational Objective: Treat COPD in a patient with risk category B disease.

The most appropriate treatment for this patient with COPD (Global Initiative for Chronic Obstructive Lung Disease [GOLD] risk category B) is a short-acting bronchodilator as needed, regular use of a long-acting bronchodilator, and pulmonary rehabilitation. The new GOLD risk stratification can be used to classify risk and help make management decisions.

Risk category A COPD is characterized by an FEV_1/FVC ratio less than 70%, an FEV_1 greater than or equal to 50% of predicted, and zero to one exacerbation(s) in the past year. These patients have mild or infrequent symptoms. Symptoms can be objectively quantified using either the Modified Medical Research Council (mMRC) Questionnaire or the COPD Assessment Test (CAT) score. Patients in risk category A have a mMRC score of 0 to 1 or CAT score less than 10. Therapy for category A COPD is an inhaled bronchodilator as needed; a short-acting bronchodilator is preferred.

Patients in risk category B have all the same spirometry measurements and exacerbation frequency as in category A but are more symptomatic, often having to walk slowly or stop owing to breathlessness (mMRC score of ≥2 or CAT score ≥10). These patients are also treated with bronchodilators, typically a short-acting bronchodilator as needed and regular use of a long-acting bronchodilator, as well as with pulmonary rehabilitation. Combinations of a long-acting β_2-agonist (LABA) and long-acting anticholinergic (also known as long-acting muscarinic agent [LAMA]) bronchodilators can be used as alternative therapy.

Risk category C COPD is characterized by an FEV_1/FVC ratio less than 70%, an FEV_1 less than 50% of predicted, or two or more exacerbations per year or one or more hospitalizations

for an exacerbation. Otherwise, patients have mild or infrequent symptoms (mMRC score of 0-1 or CAT score <10). Regular treatment with a combination inhaled glucocorticoid plus a LABA or monotherapy with a LAMA is preferred. Alternatives may include dual combination therapy with a LAMA plus an inhaled glucocorticoid or a LABA, or a phosphodiesterase-4 (PDE-4) inhibitor and a long-acting bronchodilator.

Patients in risk category D have all the same spirometry measurements and exacerbation frequency as category C, but they are more symptomatic (mMRC score of ≥2 or CAT score ≥10). Preferred therapy includes a short-acting bronchodilator as needed and regular use of combination therapy with an inhaled glucocorticoid and a LABA and/or a LAMA, and pulmonary rehabilitation. Alternative therapy includes triple combinations of two long-acting bronchodilators and an inhaled glucocorticoid; an inhaled glucocorticoid plus a LABA and PDE-4 inhibitor; or double combinations of two long-acting bronchodilators, or a LAMA and PDE-4 inhibitor.

KEY POINT

- The recommended therapy for stable patients with symptomatic (Global Initiative for Chronic Obstructive Lung Disease risk category B) COPD consists of a short-acting bronchodilator as needed and regular use of a long-acting bronchodilator, as well as with pulmonary rehabilitation.

Bibliography

Global Initiative for Chronic Obstructive Lung Disease (GOLD). Global Strategy for the Diagnosis, Management, and Prevention of Chronic Obstructive Pulmonary Disease. www.goldcopd.org/guidelines-global-strategy-for-diagnosis-management.html. Updated 2015. Accessed April 2, 2015.

Item 40   Answer: B

Educational Objective: Treat gastroesophageal reflux disease complicating cough-variant asthma.

The most appropriate treatment is to add a proton pump inhibitor to this patient's current asthma treatment regimen. Although she has a clear diagnosis of asthma (based on her methacholine challenge testing results) and her cough has partially responded to asthma therapy, she continues to have symptoms and has additional clinical findings consistent with gastroesophageal reflux disease (GERD) as a potential cause of her persistent cough symptoms. Respiratory symptoms associated with GERD are common, and reflux is frequently a cause of chronic cough. GERD is also extremely common in patients with asthma, with some estimates suggesting some degree of reflux in as many as 90% of patients. GERD can make underlying asthma worse through direct reflux of acidic gastric contents into the respiratory system, resulting in upper airway inflammation or direct airway injury. The reflux of gastric contents into the lower part of the esophagus can also cause reflex bronchoconstriction. There is evidence that treating GERD in patients with asthma improves asthma control. In most patients with asthma and suboptimal control of symptoms, a history consistent with GERD is adequate to justify a trial of empiric antacid therapy without further testing for evidence of reflux. There is no evidence, however, that treating all patients with asthma but without symptoms consistent with GERD is of benefit.

In the setting of asthma treatment, it is necessary to control for confounders such as GERD before escalating the intensity of asthma therapy, such as adding a long-acting β_2-agonist. Stepping up asthma treatment in this patient would be appropriate in the absence of a possible diagnosis of GERD or if her symptoms do not respond to antacid therapy.

Repeating a methacholine challenge test is not indicated if the initial study was adequate for diagnosing asthma and the patient has had a response to treatment. In addition, bronchoprovocation studies carry some risk, making it inappropriate to repeat the study without a clear indication.

Antitussives are frequently used in treating acute cough and may be helpful in patients with chronic cough refractory to other therapies, based on the underlying cause. Treatment with antitussive therapy in this patient with cough-variant asthma and possible comorbid GERD would not be appropriate without further assessing control of these underlying issues.

KEY POINT

- In most patients with asthma and suboptimal control of symptoms, a history consistent with gastroesophageal reflux disease is adequate to justify a trial of empiric antacid therapy without further testing for evidence of reflux.

Bibliography
Hom C, Vaezi MF. Extraesophageal manifestations of gastroesophageal reflux disease. Gastroenterol Clin North Am. 2013 Mar;42(1):71-91. [PMID: 23452632]

Item 41   Answer: D
Educational Objective: Treat opioid-related central sleep apnea.

The most appropriate management is an attempt to reduce this patient's opioid use. A sleep study showed this patient to have central sleep apnea (CSA). Comorbid illnesses that predispose to instability of the ventilatory control system are the most common risk factors for CSA. The most important and prevalent association is between CSA and heart failure, which classically manifests as the Cheyne-Stokes breathing pattern. However, the association between opioid analgesics and CSA is increasingly recognized. Reduction or withdrawal of opioids improves CSA. This patient does not have a history or findings suggestive of heart failure; therefore, opioid analgesics are the most likely cause. The most appropriate next step in management is to seek ways to reduce this patient's opioid intake, possibly through a pain rehabilitation program or in consultation with a pain management specialist.

Adaptive servoventilation (ASV) is a form of positive airway pressure (PAP) therapy sometimes used in patients with CSA. ASV provides a variable amount of pressure during inspiration superimposed on a low level of expiratory PAP, combined with a baseline respiration rate. There is some evidence that ASV may have a positive effect in patients with opioid-induced CSA, but controlled trials showing improvements in important outcomes are lacking. Although a trial of ASV may be warranted in some patients, it should be preceded by an attempt at reduction of opioids.

Continuous positive airway pressure (CPAP) is effective at maintaining upper airway patency in obstructive sleep apnea but is generally ineffective in treating CSA, a disorder of ventilatory control. In fact, CPAP can exacerbate CSA.

Modafinil is used to combat excessive sleepiness associated with the hypersomnia syndromes (such as narcolepsy) and residual sleepiness associated with obstructive sleep apnea despite adequate PAP therapy. There is no role for stimulant medication in the setting of CSA due to opioids.

KEY POINT

- The association between opioid analgesics and central sleep apnea (CSA) is increasingly recognized; reduction or withdrawal of opioids improves CSA.

Bibliography
Rose AR, Catcheside PG, McEvoy RD, et al. Sleep disordered breathing and chronic respiratory failure in patients with chronic pain on long term opioid therapy. J Clin Sleep Med. 2014 Aug 15;10(8):847-52. [PMID: 25126029]

Item 42   Answer: A
Educational Objective: Diagnose allergic bronchopulmonary aspergillosis.

The most likely diagnosis is allergic bronchopulmonary aspergillosis (ABPA). ABPA is a chronic hypersensitivity reaction that occurs in response to colonization of the lower airways with *Aspergillus* species. It occurs most commonly in patients with atopic asthma or cystic fibrosis (CF). The resulting inflammation causes difficult-to-control asthma, impaired mucociliary clearance, destruction of pulmonary parenchyma, and bronchiectasis. Symptoms typically include severe and uncontrolled asthma, cough with expectoration of mucus plugs, and systemic symptoms such as low-grade fever and fatigue. Radiologic findings may be normal or may show recurrent infiltrates or evidence of centrilobular bronchiectasis. Patients will have immediate skin test reactivity to *Aspergillus* antigens; this is often used as an initial diagnostic test. Laboratory studies show peripheral eosinophilia (usually greater than 1000/µL [1×10^9/L]), serum IgE levels greater than 1000 U/mL (1000 kU/L), and precipitating serum antibodies to *Aspergillus*. Treatment consists of standard asthma therapies and the lowest dose of systemic glucocorticoids that effectively controls symptoms. Antifungal agents may be warranted to reduce fungal colonization, and omalizumab may also have a role in therapy.

Cystic fibrosis (CF) is an autosomal recessive disorder causing abnormal chloride transport resulting in thick, viscous secretions in the lungs, pancreas, liver, intestine, and reproductive tract with associated multiorgan dysfunction, with the most prominent disease occurring in the lungs. Although an increasing number of cases of CF are diagnosed in adulthood, this patient has a long history of allergies and asthma, but not chronic respiratory infections or other evidence of multisystem disease suggestive of CF. This lack of consistent symptoms and her older age make CF an unlikely diagnosis in this patient.

Eosinophilic granulomatosis with polyangiitis (formerly known as Churg-Strauss syndrome) is an autoimmune small-vessel vasculitis that presents with peripheral eosinophilia and characteristically involves the lungs as asthma. However, it typically has additional manifestations such as purpura on the hands and legs and sensory or motor neuropathy. This patient does not demonstrate these findings.

Hypersensitivity pneumonitis is an immunologic reaction within the pulmonary parenchyma to a wide variety of inhaled agents. It may be acute, intermittent, or chronic and typically presents with cough, shortness of breath, and fatigue. However, this patient has no clear exposure history, and hypersensitivity pneumonitis is not usually associated with peripheral eosinophilia or wheezing.

KEY POINT

- Allergic bronchopulmonary aspergillosis is a chronic hypersensitivity reaction that occurs in response to colonization of the lower airways with *Aspergillus* species; it occurs most commonly in patients with atopic asthma or cystic fibrosis.

Bibliography

Bains SN, Judson MA. Allergic bronchopulmonary aspergillosis. Clin Chest Med. 2012 Jun;33(2):265-81. [PMID: 22640845]

Item 43   Answer: A

Educational Objective: Treat septic shock with appropriate fluid resuscitation.

The most appropriate next step in treatment is to administer another 1000-mL normal saline fluid bolus. This patient's findings are highly compatible with septic shock from a catheter-related bloodstream infection based on her fever, hypotension, organ failure (encephalopathy), and bacteremia. Aggressive fluid resuscitation and early administration of antibiotics are the highest priorities in managing septic shock. After receiving 1000 mL of fluid, this patient has no evidence of volume overload despite her known kidney injury, and a second bolus of fluid is indicated. Patients with sepsis typically need multiple fluid boluses to achieve adequate intravascular volume repletion.

Dobutamine is not appropriate because this patient's clinical picture is indicative of septic, rather than cardiogenic, shock. There are no changes on electrocardiogram,

she has warm extremities consistent with a low systemic vascular resistance state, and she has signs of infection. Dobutamine is included in early goal-directed therapy protocols, but it is appropriate only after confirming adequate intravascular volume repletion. Also, the recent ProCESS trial calls into question dobutamine use in the absence of confirmed cardiac dysfunction.

The ProCESS trial included 31 emergency departments in the United States that were randomly assigned patients with septic shock to one of three groups for 6 hours of resuscitation: protocol-based early goal-directed therapy (EGDT); protocol-based standard therapy that did not require the placement of a central venous catheter, administration of inotropes, or blood transfusions; or usual care. Protocol-based resuscitation of patients in septic shock did not improve outcomes. In April 2014, the National Quality Forum downgraded use of central venous lines in the resuscitation of patients with septic shock to be at the discretion of clinicians. Because this patient has adequate peripheral venous access, the placement of a central venous catheter is not a priority management step.

Blood transfusion is not appropriate because this patient's stable hemoglobin level and manifestations of sepsis reliably exclude hypovolemic shock from acute blood loss. Crystalloids are the preferred choice for initial resuscitation of patients with sepsis because of their ready access, ease of rapid infusion, safety profile, and low cost. The efficacy of protocol-based blood transfusion as part of early goal-directed therapy is unclear given the results of the ProCESS trial.

KEY POINT

- Aggressive fluid resuscitation and early administration of antibiotics are the highest priorities in managing septic shock; the routine use of central venous catheters, inotropic drugs, and blood transfusion does not improve outcomes in patients with septic shock.

Bibliography

ProCESS Investigators, Yealy DM, Kellum JA, Huang DT, et al. A randomized trial of protocol-based care for early septic shock. N Engl J Med. 2014 May 1;370(18):1683-93. [PMID: 24635773]

Item 44   Answer: B

Educational Objective: Treat advanced idiopathic pulmonary fibrosis with hospice care.

The most appropriate treatment is to recommend hospice care. This patient presents with worsening of his idiopathic pulmonary fibrosis (IPF). The median survival in patients with IPF is 3 to 5 years. IPF has no apparent reversible cause, and patients with IPF have an extremely poor long-term prognosis. This patient has demonstrated significant declines prior to admission with a high supplemental oxygen requirement, and he has now progressed to frank respiratory failure with hypercapnia and hypoxemia refractory to high-flow oxygen. The most common cause of death in IPF is respiratory failure.

CONT.

Although high-dose glucocorticoids are often used for acute exacerbation, their efficacy remains unknown. This patient has already been treated with glucocorticoids without apparent improvement; this indicates that administration of additional glucocorticoids is not likely to be of benefit.

For individuals who develop severe respiratory distress for which there is no underlying reversible cause, intubation and supportive mechanical ventilation is of little long-term benefit. Therefore, the American Thoracic Society recommends palliation of symptoms and consideration of hospice rather than mechanical ventilation for respiratory failure due to progressive IPF.

The only intervention shown to improve survival in selected patients with IPF is lung transplantation. Given the average age of onset of disease and the increased comorbidities associated with increasing age, this intervention is only available to a small portion of patients with IPF. This patient's advanced age, comorbidities, and advanced state of his lung disease (he is likely to die prior to transplantation) make him a poor candidate for lung transplantation.

KEY POINT

- The American Thoracic Society recommends palliation of symptoms rather than intubation and mechanical ventilation for patients with respiratory failure due to progressive idiopathic pulmonary fibrosis.

Bibliography

Raghu G, Collard HR, Egan JJ, et al; ATS/ERS/JRS/ALAT Committee on Idiopathic Pulmonary Fibrosis. An official ATS/ERS/JRS/ALAT statement: idiopathic pulmonary fibrosis: evidence-based guidelines for diagnosis and management. Am J Respir Crit Care Med. 2011 Mar 15;183(6):788-824. [PMID: 21471066]

Item 45   Answer: B

Educational Objective: Diagnose methanol poisoning.

This patient's encephalopathy, high anion gap, and elevated osmolal gap are most consistent with methanol (wood alcohol) or ethylene glycol (antifreeze) ingestion. This patient's anion gap is 30 mEq/L (30 mmol/L), and the upper limit of normal is typically 10 mEq/L (10 mmol/L). The osmolal gap is the difference between calculated and measured plasma osmolality. Plasma osmolality (mOsm/kg H_2O) is calculated as follows:

$$2 \times \text{serum sodium (mEq/L)} + \text{plasma glucose (mg/dL)}/18 + \text{blood urea nitrogen (mg/dL)}/2.8$$

The measured osmolality is 325 mOsm/kg H_2O. The calculated osmolality is 295 mOsm/kg H_2O. The osmolal gap is 30 mOsm/kg, and the normal range is less than 10 mOsm/kg. Methanol is converted to formic acid, which is toxic to the retina of the eye. Ethylene glycol is converted by alcohol dehydrogenase to oxalic acid, which crystalizes in

renal tubules and causes kidney injury. Conversion to toxic metabolites and clearance of these alcohols is greatly diminished by ethanol or intravenous fomepizole. All alcohols can be removed rapidly with dialysis.

Patients with isopropyl alcohol poisoning present with intoxication and an elevated osmolal gap, but they do not have an increased anion gap acidosis as is seen in this patient.

Salicylate toxicity is another cause of increased anion gap acidosis, encephalopathy, and vomiting. However, it does not cause elevation of the osmolal gap, as is seen in this patient.

Serotonin syndrome is a cause of fever and encephalopathy, but it typically manifests with agitation, muscle rigidity, and hyperreflexia, none of which are present in this patient. Serotonin syndrome also would not explain this patient's increased anion gap acidosis and osmolal gap. This patient's fever is most likely related to an aspiration event.

KEY POINT

- Methanol and ethylene glycol ingestion are characterized by encephalopathy, an increased anion gap acidosis, and an elevated osmolal gap.

Bibliography

Kruse JA. Methanol and ethylene glycol intoxication. Crit Care Clin. 2012 Oct;28(4):661-711 [PMID: 22998995]

Item 46   Answer: B

Educational Objective: Diagnose a tuberculous pleural effusion.

The most appropriate next test in this patient is pleural fluid adenosine deaminase (ADA) measurement. This patient likely has a tuberculous pleural effusion from reactivation tuberculosis. She presented with subacute onset of fever, pleuritic chest pain, and nonproductive cough with a history of tuberculosis, and pleural fluid analysis is consistent with a lymphocyte-predominant exudate. All of these features are consistent with a tuberculous pleural effusion. When clinical suspicion is moderate to high, the most appropriate test is pleural fluid ADA measurement. Pleural fluid ADA has been demonstrated to be highly sensitive and specific when levels are greater than 60 U/L (sensitivity 95%, specificity 96%). A level of less than 40 U/L virtually excludes the diagnosis of tuberculosis effusion. In patients with lymphocytic-predominant effusions and elevated ADA levels, empiric therapy for tuberculosis should be initiated and pleural biopsy should be pursued to confirm the diagnosis. In the absence of treatment, patients have a 65% risk of developing pulmonary or extrapulmonary tuberculosis within 5 years.

Sputum culture is more likely to be positive in a patient with concomitant pulmonary parenchymal disease. In the absence of identifiable parenchymal disease, the sensitivity of sputum culture, if present or induced, ranges from 20% to 50%.

Both pleural fluid stain and culture for acid-fast bacilli lack sensitivity to exclude the diagnosis of tuberculosis. In patients without HIV infection, staining is positive in less than 5% of cases, and pleural fluid cultures are positive in only 20% to 30% of cases.

> **KEY POINT**
>
> - When clinical suspicion is moderate to high, the most appropriate test to diagnose a possible tuberculous effusion is pleural fluid adenosine deaminase measurement.

Bibliography

Light RW. Pleural effusions. Med Clin North Am. 2011 Nov;95(6):1055-70. [PMID: 22032427]

Item 47   Answer: B

Educational Objective: Identify the appropriate venue of care for a high-risk asthma exacerbation.

The most appropriate management is to admit the patient to the ICU because of his high-risk asthma and arterial blood gas studies suggesting the possibility of impending respiratory failure. Patients with asthma who are at risk of poorer outcomes include those with limited access to health care or difficulty with medication adherence, poor perception of low lung function (and inability to gauge worsening of airways obstruction), an acute increase in use of short-acting β_2-agonist therapy, and lack of improvement with outpatient treatment. This patient has several of these factors, and he also had severe symptoms before seeking care. His initial blood gas studies showed an acute respiratory alkalosis, which is a typical finding in patients with an acute asthma exacerbation. However, his second blood gas determination after 1 hour of treatment showed a developing respiratory acidosis despite a continued high work of breathing, as reflected by his respiration rate. These changes suggest progressively ineffective ventilation and the possibility of impending respiratory collapse. Therefore, the most appropriate venue for treatment is an ICU setting, in which ventilatory failure could be managed if it occurs.

Admission to a general medical floor would not be appropriate because this patient's clinical indicators suggest the need for more intense monitoring that could not be provided in that setting.

Although ventilatory failure could be managed in an emergency department setting, continued therapy with reassessment in 2 hours would not be appropriate given this patient's changing clinical course.

Discharge with close follow-up would not be appropriate given this patient's current respiratory status and previous issues with poor asthma control.

> **KEY POINT**
>
> - Patients with high-risk asthma exacerbations who are not responding to initial treatment and have persistently high work of breathing are best managed in an ICU.

Bibliography

National Asthma Education and Prevention Program. Expert Panel Report 3 (EPP-3): Guidelines for the Diagnosis and Management of Asthma-Summary Report 2007. J Allergy Clin Immunol. 2007 Nov;120(5 Suppl):S94-138. Erratum in: J Allergy Clin Immunol. 2008 Jun;121(6):1330. [PMID: 17983880]

Item 48   Answer: A

Educational Objective: Diagnose asbestosis.

The most likely diagnosis is asbestosis. The extent of asbestos exposure correlates with risk for disease, with the most common occupational exposures occurring in the construction, automotive servicing, and shipbuilding industries. This patient has a significant exposure history from his construction work for 40 years. History regarding exposure can often be difficult to obtain; however, asking questions regarding limited visibility in the work place due to particulate matter as well as failure to wear protective equipment can suggest an extensive exposure. The latency period between exposure and development of asbestosis is prolonged (15-35 years) and is consistent with this patient's clinical picture. This patient has evidence of fibrosis on lung examination and no evidence to suggest an alternative diagnosis. Pulmonary function testing is consistent with restriction, and chest imaging demonstrates fibrosis and bilateral pleural plaques, which provide evidence of past asbestos exposure. The history, physical examination, and imaging findings are all consistent with diffuse parenchymal lung disease due to asbestosis.

This patient's presentation and laboratory studies are less consistent with COPD. He does not have an extensive tobacco use history, and his physical examination findings are not suggestive of airflow obstruction, which is confirmed by pulmonary function studies. Therefore, COPD is an unlikely cause of this patient's symptoms.

Hypersensitivity pneumonitis in its chronic form may present with indolent symptoms of cough and dyspnea, and it would occur secondary to exposure to an antigen that leads to an immune response. This patient has no exposures other than asbestos. In addition, imaging findings in individuals with hypersensitivity pneumonitis are mid- and upper-lung predominant. Therefore, hypersensitivity pneumonitis is not the most likely diagnosis in this patient.

Idiopathic pulmonary fibrosis (IPF) is the most common form of idiopathic interstitial pneumonia and commonly affects individuals later in life. It is associated with a history of increased dust exposure, and it is also a diagnosis of exclusion. However, this patient has a clear history of asbestos exposure, which is associated with the development of pulmonary fibrosis and precludes a diagnosis of IPF. This is particularly important because the prognosis for patients with asbestosis is better than for those with well-documented IPF.

> **KEY POINT**
>
> - Asbestosis is characterized by slowly progressive pulmonary fibrosis; the presence of pleural plaques confirms asbestos exposure.

Bibliography

Stayner L, Welch LS, Lemen R. The worldwide pandemic of asbestos-related diseases. Annu Rev Public Health. 2013;34:205-16. [PMID: 23297667]

Item 49   Answer: C

Educational Objective: Diagnose nonadherence to continuous positive airway pressure therapy.

The most appropriate next step in management is to review data from the patient's continuous positive airway pressure (CPAP) device to assess adherence to therapy. This patient has severe, symptomatic obstructive sleep apnea (OSA), for which positive airway pressure (PAP) is the preferred therapy. The response to treatment is dependent on adherence, and a substantial proportion of patients, particularly early in the course of therapy, do not wear the PAP device as intended (all night, every night). Downloading and reviewing data from the PAP device yields important information about usage that can be discussed with the patient to explore barriers and formulate a plan to promote compliance.

Despite some limited evidence that the use of hypnotic agents such as eszopiclone may be helpful in promoting CPAP adherence early in therapy, the role of hypnotic agents in promoting CPAP compliance remains controversial. Their use later in the course of PAP, as in this patient, is not established, and the risk of side effects may outweigh the benefit.

Modafinil is a stimulant medication that is approved for use in patients with OSA who are using CPAP optimally and continue to have residual excessive sleepiness. Compliance with CPAP therapy should be established in this patient before prescribing modafinil.

There are few data to support the superiority of a bilevel positive airway pressure (BPAP) device in promoting treatment compliance for OSA. BPAP, which promotes ventilation by delivery of pressure support derived from the gradient between inspiratory and expiratory pressure, is the preferred therapy for hypoventilation syndromes, such as those associated with neuromuscular disease or obesity.

KEY POINT

- The response to obstructive sleep apnea treatment is dependent on adherence to continuous positive airway pressure (CPAP) therapy; the level of adherence to therapy can be established by downloading and reviewing data from the CPAP device.

Bibliography

Epstein LJ, Kristo D, Strollo PJ Jr, et al; Adult Obstructive Sleep Apnea Task Force of the American Academy of Sleep Medicine. Clinical guideline for the evaluation, management and long-term care of obstructive sleep apnea in adults. J Clin Sleep Med. 2009 Jun 15;5(3):263-76. [PMID: 19960649]

Item 50   Answer: C

Educational Objective: Manage acute respiratory distress syndrome using prone positioning.

Prone positioning is most likely to improve this patient's chance of survival. This patient has severe acute respira-

tory distress syndrome (ARDS) due to viral pneumonia, which has significantly impaired oxygenation. A randomized controlled trial has shown that survival was dramatically improved for patients who were placed in the prone position for at least 16 hours per day until their oxygenation improved, compared with patients who were managed identically except for being kept in the supine position. In the study, the 90-day mortality in the group with prone positioning was 23.6%, whereas it was 41% in the supine group. This technique was not associated with increased adverse consequences. The mechanisms by which prone positioning improves oxygenation are likely multifactorial, with optimization of ventilation-perfusion matching likely playing a major role. Therefore, for this patient with severe ARDS, the best option is daily prone positioning based on its demonstrated benefit in improving oxygenation and reducing mortality.

Aerosolized surfactant has been used in infant respiratory distress syndrome, but trials of this therapy in adults have not shown benefit.

Nitric oxide dilates the pulmonary vasculature when administered by inhalation and may have a role in treating patients with pulmonary arterial hypertension. In studies of patients with ARDS, inhaled nitric oxide has been shown to improve oxygenation by temporarily improving ventilation-perfusion mismatch; however, a mortality benefit has not been demonstrated in patients with ARDS. It would therefore not be the most appropriate next step in the management of this patient.

Studies of glucocorticoids in ARDS have shown inconsistent results and have not generally demonstrated improved outcomes. Therefore, systemic glucocorticoids would not be an optimal therapy for treating this patient.

KEY POINT

- Prone positioning is associated with dramatically improved survival for patients with acute respiratory distress syndrome.

Bibliography

Guérin C, Reignier J, Richard JC, et al; PROSEVA Study Group. Prone positioning in severe acute respiratory distress syndrome. N Engl J Med. 2013 Jun 6;368(23):2159-68. [PMID: 23688302]

Item 51   Answer: C

Educational Objective: Diagnose a malignant pleural effusion.

The most appropriate management is repeat thoracentesis and pleural fluid cytology, owing to the increased sensitivity with subsequent samples. If malignancy is suspected, a cytologic analysis is a quick and easy way to obtain a diagnosis. When the suspicion for malignancy is high (breast mass and pleural effusion in this patient), it is appropriate to repeat cytology if the first specimen is negative. The overall mean sensitivity of pleural fluid cytology is 60%. Approximately 65% of positive results are obtained on the initial thoracentesis. The second sample provides an additional 27%, and the third sample provides only 5%.

Closed pleural biopsy is less sensitive than cytology for pleural malignancy and should not be performed.

Flow cytometry is useful with lymphocyte-predominant effusions when lymphoma is a diagnostic consideration. However, this patient's breast mass, weight loss, and bloody effusion suggest otherwise.

Thoracoscopic pleural biopsy is indicated for all undiagnosed exudative pleural effusions following three pleural fluid samplings. Thoracoscopic biopsy is more than 90% sensitive for pleural malignancy. However, this patient has only had one pleural fluid sampling.

KEY POINT

- When suspicion for pleural malignancy is high, it is appropriate to repeat pleural fluid cytology if the first specimen is negative owing to the increased sensitivity with subsequent samples.

Bibliography
Light RW. Clinical practice. Pleural effusion. N Engl J Med. 2002 Jun 20;346(25):1971-7. [PMID: 12075059]

Item 52   Answer: D
Educational Objective: Diagnose chronic thromboembolic pulmonary hypertension.

The most appropriate diagnostic test to perform next is a ventilation-perfusion (V/Q) scan. This patient's presentation strongly suggests chronic thromboembolic pulmonary hypertension (CTEPH), for which V/Q scanning is the preferred and most sensitive diagnostic imaging study. CTEPH usually presents with progressive exertional dyspnea that correlates with the extent of hemodynamic derangement and right ventricular involvement. Patients with CTEPH may have findings of pulmonary hypertension and cor pulmonale and invariably have defects on V/Q scan. This patient's cardiac examination, with an accentuated pulmonic component of S_2, is compatible with pulmonary hypertension, as are the findings on echocardiography. Additionally, her clear lung fields, hypoxia, and findings on pulmonary function testing are consistent with a diffusion defect. If she has an abnormal V/Q scan, right heart catheterization with pulmonary angiography is required to confirm the diagnosis and characterize the degree of thrombosis, which may help guide therapy. The absence of deep venous thrombosis on venous studies of the legs is insufficient to rule out recurrent pulmonary emboli. V/Q scanning can also differentiate CTEPH (group 4 pulmonary hypertension) from pulmonary arterial hypertension (group 1 pulmonary hypertension), which is the other major diagnostic consideration in this patient.

Although CT angiography can identify proximal pulmonary arterial webs and luminal narrowing when present, it is less sensitive than V/Q scanning in detecting CTEPH. Furthermore, in this patient with clear lung fields on chest radiograph, CT scanning is unlikely to provide additional

diagnostically useful information about the pulmonary parenchyma.

Pulmonary hypertension of this severity is typically associated with severe obstructive sleep apnea and marked sleep-related hypoxemia. There is little evidence suggesting sleep-disordered breathing in this nonobese woman; therefore, polysomnography is not indicated at this time.

In operative candidates, CTEPH is best managed surgically with pulmonary thromboendarterectomy. Pulmonary angiography is performed preoperatively to assess the extent and distribution of thrombus. It is not, however, an appropriate test during the initial evaluation.

KEY POINT

- Ventilation-perfusion scanning is the preferred and most sensitive diagnostic imaging study for chronic thromboembolic pulmonary hypertension.

Bibliography
Kim NH, Delcroix M, Jenkins DP, et al. Chronic thromboembolic pulmonary hypertension. J Am Coll Cardiol. 2013 Dec 24;62(25 Suppl):D92-9. [PMID: 24355646]

Item 53   Answer: C
Educational Objective: Diagnose right-to-left intrapulmonary shunt as a cause of hypoxemia.

The most likely diagnosis is intrapulmonary shunt. This patient's profound hypoxia is most likely due to intrapulmonary shunting of blood through his collapsed right lower lobe. Evidence of a collapsed right lower lobe is indicated by the triangular opacity above the diaphragm on the right side on his chest radiograph. Right-to-left intrapulmonary shunts may be anatomical or physiological, but all result in hypoxemia that does not readily correct with supplemental oxygen, as seen in this patient. This patient's physiological shunt results in perfusion of nonventilated alveoli of the collapsed right lower lobe. In most situations, a lobar collapse will not cause such severe shunting because of hypoxic vasoconstriction of arterioles in parts of the lung that are not ventilated; however, in some cases, such as this patient, this compensatory mechanism directing blood flow to other aerated areas of the lung is ineffective.

Hepatopulmonary syndrome, intracardiac shunt, and pulmonary arteriovenous malformation are all examples of anatomic shunts. Although these conditions can be responsible for hypoxemia that is difficult to correct with supplemental oxygen, this patient's trauma, splinting, and abnormal radiographic findings suggest a lower lobe collapse as the most likely diagnosis. In conditions of diagnostic uncertainty, a bubble contrast echocardiogram could be performed. These anatomic shunts are associated with the appearance of left atrial or ventricular bubbles after several cardiac cycles.

Hepatopulmonary syndrome should be suspected in patients with cirrhosis who develop hypoxemia in the absence of other causes. Their shunt worsens with upright posture (orthodeoxia). However, this is not a likely diagnosis in a patient without evidence of cirrhosis.

KEY POINT

- Right-to-left intrapulmonary shunts may be anatomic or physiologic, but all result in hypoxemia that is difficult to correct with supplemental oxygen.

Bibliography

Rodríguez-Roisin R, Roca J. Mechanisms of hypoxemia. Intensive Care Med. 2005 Aug;31(8):1017-9. [PMID: 16052273]

Item 54   Answer: D

Educational Objective: Treat pulmonary arterial hypertension.

The most appropriate management is sildenafil. In patients with pulmonary arterial hypertension (PAH) and respiratory symptoms occurring during exertion but not at rest, oral medications are the preferred initial therapy. Examples of oral agents include phosphodiesterase-5 inhibitors (sildenafil, tadalafil) and endothelin receptor antagonists (bosentan, ambrisentan). Prostanoids are available only as parenteral (epoprostenol) or inhaled (iloprost) forms and are typically reserved for patients with more advanced disease and symptoms and for those in whom disease progresses despite oral therapy. Additional treatments that are provided for most patients with PAH include supplemental oxygen for documented hypoxemia and chronic warfarin therapy. Pregnancy can worsen pulmonary hemodynamics and increase the risk of mortality in patients with PAH, so women of childbearing age should be counseled to avoid pregnancy.

In patients who have a positive response to vasoreactivity testing (a decrease in mean pulmonary artery pressure of at least 10 mm Hg without significant reductions in cardiac output or systemic blood pressure), oral calcium channel blockers such as nifedipine are a reasonable initial therapy. In those with a negative vasoreactivity test, as in this patient, calcium channel blockers are not beneficial.

Recent clinical trials have shown supervised exercise programs to be safe and to improve walking distances and quality of life in patients with PAH. Excessive exertion resulting in respiratory distress should be avoided.

KEY POINT

- In patients with pulmonary arterial hypertension and a negative vasoreactivity test, calcium channel blockers are not beneficial and phosphodiesterase-5 inhibitors (sildenafil, tadalafil) or endothelin receptor antagonists (bosentan, ambrisentan) are preferred.

Bibliography

Galiè N, Corris PA, Frost A, et al. Updated treatment algorithm of pulmonary arterial hypertension. J Am Coll Cardiol. 2013 Dec 24;62(25 Suppl): D60-72. [PMID: 24355643]

Item 55   Answer: C

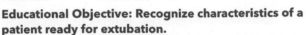

Educational Objective: Recognize characteristics of a patient ready for extubation.

This patient has had a successful spontaneous breathing trial (SBT) and is ready for discontinuation of mechanical ventilation and extubation. The purpose of a SBT is to assess the likelihood that mechanical ventilation can be discontinued successfully. A SBT is performed by placing the patient on a T-piece through which no positive pressure is delivered (only supplemental oxygen) or by adjusting the ventilator so that it applies only enough pressure to overcome the resistance of the endotracheal tube. Criteria that have been suggested for a successful SBT include the ability to tolerate a weaning trial for 30 minutes; maintain a respiration rate of less than 35/min; and maintain an oxygen saturation of at least 90% without arrhythmias, sudden increases in heart rate and blood pressure, or development of respiratory distress, diaphoresis, or anxiety. Because this patient successfully completed a SBT, an attempt at discontinuation of mechanical ventilation and extubation is appropriate.

Arterial blood gas studies are performed when there are concerns about acute or worsening chronic carbon dioxide retention or when exact arterial oxygenation measurement is needed. Even if the carbon dioxide level is elevated, it would not necessarily indicate that the patient is not an appropriate candidate for extubation, especially if the patient is able to perform a SBT and has an otherwise unremarkable examination, as in this patient.

It is unnecessary to continue mechanical ventilation and observe for an additional 24 hours with an endotracheal tube in place. Patients who meet the parameters of success during a SBT can be disconnected from mechanical ventilation and extubated. Continuing mechanical ventilation beyond the time when successful weaning parameters are met adds additional risks to the patient, including ventilator-associated infections or other potential complications of mechanical ventilation.

Direct extubation to noninvasive positive pressure ventilation is effective at weaning patients with obstructive lung disease with ventilatory respiratory failure from mechanical ventilation. However, it is not necessary for patients with primarily hypoxemic respiratory failure such as this patient with pneumonia.

KEY POINT

- Criteria that have been suggested for a successful spontaneous breathing trial in patients requiring intubation and mechanical ventilation include the ability to tolerate a weaning trial for 30 minutes; maintain a respiration rate of less than 35/min; and maintain an oxygen saturation of at least 90% without arrhythmias, sudden increases in heart rate and blood pressure, or development of respiratory distress, diaphoresis, or anxiety.

Bibliography

McConville JF, Kress JP. Weaning patients from the ventilator. N Engl J Med. 2012 Dec 6;267(23):2233-9. [PMID:23215550]

Item 56   Answer: D

Educational Objective: Diagnose pulmonary arterial hypertension.

The most appropriate diagnostic test to perform next is right heart catheterization. This patient has a diagnosis of limited cutaneous systemic sclerosis. Systemic sclerosis, particularly limited cutaneous systemic sclerosis, is associated with pulmonary vascular disease caused by direct proliferative effects on the vascular wall that obliterate pulmonary arterioles and capillaries and lead to fibrosis of the surrounding lung interstitium. These changes result in pulmonary arterial hypertension (PAH, group 1 classification). This patient's symptoms (exertional dyspnea, fatigue), physical examination findings (prominent S_2), and echocardiographic findings (right ventricular enlargement, elevated pulmonary artery pressure) are consistent with PAH. Because echocardiography may underestimate true pulmonary artery pressures, right heart catheterization is required to confirm pulmonary hemodynamics as well as to determine whether there is a specific response to vasodilator infusion, which may help guide therapy. Right heart catheterization should be used to confirm mean pulmonary artery pressures of at least 25 mm Hg, a normal pulmonary capillary wedge pressure, and to determine whether the pulmonary vasculature is vasodilator-responsive to assist defining treatment options.

The 6-minute walk test provides a useful baseline prior to initiation of specific PAH therapy; however, it does not provide the specific diagnostic information obtained by right heart catheterization.

This patient may have gas exchange impairment that causes nocturnal hypoxia, which would be detectable on overnight pulse oximetry. However, this test will not provide specific information about the underlying pulmonary vascular problem and therefore will not be a useful diagnostic study at present.

Polysomnography is useful in diagnosing possible sleep-disordered breathing, such as sleep apnea, as a cause of pulmonary hypertension. However, this patient has no clinical suggestion of sleep apnea, and her clinical presentation is most consistent with PAH associated with her known connective tissue disease. Therefore, polysomnography would not be an appropriate next diagnostic test.

KEY POINT

- In patients with suspected pulmonary arterial hypertension, right heart catheterization is required to confirm pulmonary hemodynamics as well as to determine whether there is a specific response to vasodilator infusion, which may help guide therapy.

Bibliography

Galiè N, Corris PA, Frost A, et al. Updated treatment algorithm of pulmonary arterial hypertension. J Am Coll Cardiol. 2013 Dec 24;62(25 Suppl):D60-72. [PMID: 24355643]

Item 57   Answer: C

Educational Objective: Diagnose mesothelioma.

The most likely diagnosis is mesothelioma. Malignant pleural mesothelioma is a very aggressive tumor that arises from the mesothelial cells of the pleura. Patients most commonly present with symptoms of a slowly enlarging pleural effusion. This patient's physical examination findings (decreased breath sounds, dullness to percussion, decreased tactile fremitus, and no egophony) are consistent with a pleural effusion. The absence of an effusion on this patient's previous screening CT 5 months ago suggests that the effusion developed since then and correlates with development of his symptoms. His previous chest imaging also showed a calcified pleural plaque (*arrows*) that confirms his exposure to asbestos, which likely occurred when he worked as a plumber and is a strong risk factor for mesothelioma. His risk for mesothelioma is further increased by his tobacco use. This combination of history, physical examination, and previous radiographic findings makes mesothelioma the most likely cause of this patient's newly diagnosed pleural effusion.

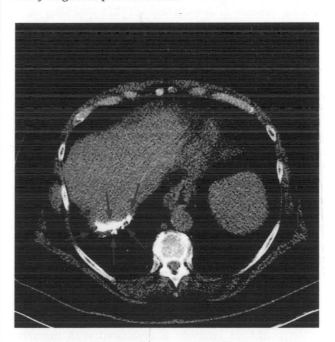

There are many other causes of a pleural effusion, including heart failure. However, this is unlikely in this patient because he has no evidence of volume overload on examination.

Although lymphoma can result in pleural effusions, the patient has no constitutional symptoms or other signs suggestive of lymphoma. Isolated pleural lymphoma is incredibly rare and is much less likely than mesothelioma in this patient.

Both pneumonia (areas of consolidation) and pleural effusion can result in decreased breath sounds and dullness to percussion on physical examination. However, consolidation would cause increased, rather than decreased, tactile fremitus, and egophony would be present.

KEY POINT

- Patients with malignant pleural mesothelioma most commonly present with symptoms of a slowly enlarging pleural effusion.

Bibliography

Wong CL, Holroyd-Leduc J, Straus SE. Does this patient have a pleural effusion? JAMA. 2009 Jan 21;301(3):309-17. [PMID: 19155458]

Item 58   Answer: B

Educational Objective: Diagnose diffuse systemic sclerosis-associated parenchymal lung disease.

In addition to pulmonary function testing, anti–Scl-70 antibody testing and high-resolution CT (HRCT) would be most helpful in establishing a diagnosis. In this particular patient, there are findings of skin thickening in the distal extremities, which suggests diffuse cutaneous systemic sclerosis (dcSSc). Patients with dcSSc are more likely to develop diffuse parenchymal lung disease (DPLD), serositis, and kidney disease (including scleroderma renal crisis). DPLD most commonly occurs in patients with dcSSc and elevated antibody titers to anti–Scl-70. Alveolitis may precede the development of DPLD; presenting manifestations include dyspnea, nonproductive cough, and exercise intolerance. Fine bibasilar Velcro-like inspiratory crackles are frequently present on physical examination. A restrictive impairment with decreased lung volumes and decreased D$_{LCO}$ is typically present on pulmonary function tests. Chest imaging is best performed with HRCT, which is more sensitive than plain radiography in detecting alveolitis and reticular linear opacities present in patients with early stages of lung disease. As a result, anti–Scl-70 antibody testing and HRCT scan are most likely to establish the diagnosis.

Complete pulmonary function testing (spirometry, lung volumes, and diffusing capacity) is an important component of evaluating parenchymal lung disease. It can assess the severity of disease, and the discovery of different patterns can confirm the presence of restrictive lung diseases, such as DPLD, or the presence of obstructive or mixed patterns that can help further focus the differential diagnosis. The finding of a low diffusing capacity that is out of proportion to the decrease in lung volumes suggests the presence of other conditions such as pulmonary hypertension.

Anti–PM-Scl antibody is associated with myositis. Anticentromere antibody is associated with limited cutaneous systemic sclerosis and the risk of developing pulmonary hypertension. Antineutrophil cytoplasmic antibody is associated with granulomatosis with polyangiitis, microscopic polyangiitis, and eosinophilic granulomatosis with polyangiitis (formerly known as Churg-Strauss syndrome); it is not associated with systemic sclerosis.

Bronchoalveolar lavage, lung biopsy, and gallium-67 scanning are generally not helpful in the diagnosis of sys-

temic sclerosis–associated DPLD and would not be performed prior to HRCT scanning.

KEY POINT

- Diffuse parenchymal lung disease most commonly occurs in patients with diffuse cutaneous systemic sclerosis and elevated antibody titers to anti–Scl-70.

Bibliography

Fan MH, Feghali-Bostwick CA, Silver RM. Update on scleroderma-associated interstitial lung disease. Curr Opin Rheumatol. 2014 Nov;26(6):630-6. [PMID: 25191993]

Item 59   Answer: B

Educational Objective: Treat asthma during pregnancy.

The most appropriate management is to continue the current drug regimen. As in all patients with asthma, treatment of asthma during pregnancy should aim for optimal control, and a regimen that adequately controls asthma should be continued. Controlled asthma ensures safety for the fetus as well as the mother and reduces the risk for preeclampsia and preterm birth. Inhaled glucocorticoids are considered safe in pregnancy, and abundant long-term safety evidence exists for budesonide. Short-acting β$_2$-agonists are considered safe in pregnancy, and existing data for long-acting β$_2$-agonists are reassuring that these agents are safe as well. The leukotriene antagonist montelukast is also considered safe in pregnancy. In this patient, who has a history of reduced lung function, it is appropriate to maintain the current regimen that is controlling her asthma because the medications she is taking have evidence of safety in pregnancy. This patient also should have frequent monitoring with regular visits, should be offered a peak flow monitor, and should be counseled regarding the safety of and need for continued asthma medications. The most appropriate management is to continue the current regimen and follow up frequently.

Empirically stepping up asthma therapy in anticipation of worsening asthma symptoms during pregnancy is not warranted. During pregnancy, one third of women have no significant change in their asthma, one third experience worsening of symptoms, and one third experience improvement of symptoms.

Stopping inhaled glucocorticoids and/or montelukast would not be appropriate owing to this patient's likely impairment without controller medications, particularly because these agents are considered safe in pregnancy.

KEY POINT

- Inhaled glucocorticoids, most β$_2$-agonists, and the leukotriene antagonist montelukast are considered safe in pregnancy.

Bibliography

National Asthma Education and Prevention Program. Expert Panel Report 3 (EPR-3): Guidelines for the Diagnosis and Management of Asthma-Summary Report 2007. J Allergy Clin Immunol. 2007 Nov;120 (5 Suppl):S94-138. Erratum in: J Allergy Clin Immunol. 2008 Jun;121(6):1330. [PMID: 17983880]

Item 60   Answer: C

Educational Objective: Treat severe COPD with recurrent exacerbations.

The most appropriate treatment is roflumilast. Roflumilast is a phosphodiesterase-4 (PDE-4) inhibitor that is used as add-on therapy to reduce exacerbations in patients with severe COPD associated with chronic bronchitis and a history of recurrent exacerbations despite other therapies. Inhibition of PDE-4 decreases inflammation, which may be helpful in a limited number of patients with COPD in whom inflammation is a significant factor. Roflumilast has minimal bronchodilator activity; however, small improvements in FEV_1 are seen in patients also treated with a long-acting anticholinergic agent or a long-acting β_2-agonist. Roflumilast should always be used with at least one long-acting bronchodilator. This patent has severe symptomatic COPD (Global Initiative for Chronic Obstructive Lung Disease category D) with recurrent exacerbations, so roflumilast is indicated, along with other agents.

Some studies of macrolide antibiotics suggest that their use reduces exacerbations in a select group of patients with COPD. Macrolides have been shown to reduce exacerbations and improve lung function in patients with cystic fibrosis. However, there is currently insufficient evidence to routinely recommend daily macrolide therapy for the long-term treatment of COPD. There are concerns that long-term azithromycin therapy may be associated with increasing bacterial resistance, especially in patients who previously had *Mycobacterium avium-intracellulare* infection, and an increased risk of QT prolongation.

Oral glucocorticoids should be reserved for limited periodic use to treat acute exacerbations in patients with COPD. Long-term oral glucocorticoid therapy has been shown to have limited, if any, benefits in COPD. In addition, long-term glucocorticoid therapy has a high risk for significant side effects, including diabetes mellitus, muscle weakness, osteoporosis, and decrease in functional status.

The anti-inflammatory effects of simvastatin were previously believed to reduce exacerbations in COPD. However, a large randomized prospective study showed that, in patients at risk for exacerbations, simvastatin along with usual treatment did not reduce exacerbations or the time to first exacerbation. In addition, simvastatin was found to have no effect on lung function, quality of life, rate of severe adverse events, or mortality.

KEY POINT

- Roflumilast is a phosphodiesterase-4 inhibitor that is used as add-on therapy to reduce exacerbations in patients with severe COPD associated with chronic bronchitis and a history of recurrent exacerbations despite other therapies.

Bibliography

Wedzicha JA, Rabe KF, Martinez FJ, et al. Efficacy of roflumilast in the COPD frequent exacerbator phenotype. Chest. 2013 May;143(5):1302-11. [PMID: 23117188]

Item 61   Answer: B

Educational Objective: Treat nonexertional heat stroke with external evaporative cooling.

The most appropriate next step in treatment is external evaporative cooling. Hyperthermia occurs most commonly owing to heat stroke, malignant hyperthermia, and neuroleptic malignant syndrome. A temperature greater than 40.0 °C (104.0 °F) and encephalopathy in the setting of environmental heat exposure are characteristic of heat stroke. The majority of patients with nonexertional heat stroke are older than 70 years or have chronic medical conditions. Medications and recreational drugs with anticholinergic, sympathomimetic, and diuretic effects, including alcohol, pose added risk. This patient's advanced age and diuretic use place him at increased risk for nonexertional heat stroke. External evaporative cooling involves removing all clothing and spraying the patient with a mist of lukewarm water while continuously blowing fans on the patient. Ice water immersion is commonly used for patients with exertional heat stroke, who typically are younger and need less monitoring.

Heat stroke is a cause of rhabdomyolysis, but the combination of fever, encephalopathy, and rhabdomyolysis should also raise the possibility of neuroleptic malignant syndrome (NMS) and serotonin syndrome. NMS can be treated with dantrolene or bromocriptine. However, this patient has no muscle rigidity or medication exposure (antipsychotics in particular), which are characteristic of NMS. Therefore, treatment with dantrolene would not be appropriate.

Cyproheptadine is used to treat serotonin syndrome. Although this patient takes sertraline, serotonin syndrome would not be expected to cause severe hyperthermia. Furthermore, characteristic muscle rigidity and neurologic signs, including tremor, hyperreflexia, and clonus, are absent.

N-acetylcysteine is used to treat acetaminophen toxicity, which is a diagnostic consideration in a patient with encephalopathy and a history of depression and possible suicidality. However, acetaminophen overdose is not associated with severe hyperthermia.

KEY POINT

- Factors that increase risk for nonexertional heat stroke include alcohol use, advanced age, chronic medical conditions, and use of medications or recreational drugs with anticholinergic, sympathomimetic, or diuretic effects.

Bibliography

Atha WF. Heat-related illness. Emerg Med Clin North Am. 2013 Nov;31(4):1097-108. [PMID: 24176481]

Item 62   Answer: C

Educational Objective: Diagnose COPD with spirometry.

The most appropriate next step in management is spirometry. This patient, who is a smoker with intermittent cough and dyspnea, likely has COPD. Although dyspnea, cough, and sputum production are characteristic symptoms of COPD, these symptoms can be variable and the cough can be non-productive. This patient requires spirometry, which measures the FEV_1 and FVC, and the FEV_1/FVC ratio to assess for and quantify any degree of airflow obstruction present. Patients with COPD have a FEV_1/FVC ratio of less than or equal to 70%. Spirometry is reproducible and provides an objective measurement of airflow obstruction. Screening for COPD with spirometry in individuals without respiratory symptoms is not recommended, but it is indicated in this patient with symptoms and a suggestive clinical history for COPD.

CT scanning is used to evaluate parenchymal lung lesions (such as nodules) and other potential chest pathology (such as pleural or mediastinal disease). However, it is not effective in diagnosing COPD, particularly in this patient with a normal plain chest radiograph. In addition, guidelines recommend low-dose CT scanning for current or former smokers aged 55 to 80 years with a smoking history of at least 30-pack-years with no history of lung cancer; this patient does not fit these criteria.

Polysomnography is used for evaluation of suspected sleep-disordered breathing (such as sleep apnea). However, this patient does not have symptoms suggestive of sleep apnea or other sleep or nocturnal breathing disorders. Therefore, polysomnography is not indicated.

Although gastroesophageal reflux disease (GERD) is a common cause of chronic cough, and a trial of an empiric proton pump inhibitor is reasonable in patients with unexplained cough and otherwise negative evaluation, GERD would not account for this patient's dyspnea symptoms. Because his clinical presentation is more consistent with mild COPD, empiric treatment for GERD would not be the preferred next management step.

KEY POINT

- Spirometry should be performed to evaluate for COPD in patients with suggestive symptoms (dyspnea, cough, sputum production) and risk factors such as a history of smoking.

Bibliography

Qaseem A, Wilt TJ, Weinberger SE, et al; American College of Physicians; American College of Chest Physicians; American Thoracic Society; European Respiratory Society. Diagnosis and management of stable chronic obstructive pulmonary disease: a clinical practice guideline update from the American College of Physicians, American College of Chest Physicians, American Thoracic Society, and European Respiratory Society. Ann Intern Med. 2011 Aug 2;155(3):179-91. [PMID: 21810710]

Item 63   Answer: B

Educational Objective: Treat chronic respiratory failure due to muscular weakness.

The most appropriate respiratory management for this patient is nocturnal noninvasive positive pressure ventilation (NPPV). He has chronic respiratory failure due to progressive muscular weakness. Although there are no clear guidelines regarding when to institute respiratory support in patients with progressive muscle weakness, this patient's inability to breathe while lying flat is highly suggestive of diaphragm weakness, and his low vital capacity is below the threshold at which most patients require mechanical support. Frequently used clinical indicators for the need of ventilatory assistance include an FVC less than 50% of predicted, a vital capacity below 60% of predicted (or 1 L), or a maximal inspiratory pressure of less than -30 cm H_2O. In patients requiring ventilator support, NPPV is the usual initial method used, typically on an intermittent, nocturnal basis. NPPV has been shown to improve quality of life and delay the progression of respiratory failure in patients with progressive neuromuscular disease.

Nocturnal continuous positive airway pressure is typically used in patients with upper airway obstruction such as obstructive sleep apnea, but it would not improve this patient's respiratory mechanics and ventilatory impairment.

Nocturnal oxygen therapy is not indicated and would not be expected to be helpful in this patient with adequate arterial oxygenation despite his chronic hypoventilation.

Continuous mechanical ventilation, usually through a tracheostomy, is generally indicated for patients with a contraindication to NPPV or for those requiring continuous mechanical ventilation for an extended period of time. This patient does not have a contraindication to noninvasive ventilation, and his response to a trial of NPPV therapy is not yet known. Therefore, pursuing tracheostomy and continuous mechanical ventilation would be premature in this patient. It should be noted that he will probably eventually require a tracheostomy, and this would be a good time to introduce that idea for ongoing discussion.

KEY POINT

- No clear guidelines exist for when to start mechanical ventilation in patients with chronic respiratory failure due to progressive muscular weakness; however, signs that ventilatory support is required include the inability to breathe while lying flat, low FVC, low vital capacity, and decreased negative inspiratory pressure.

Bibliography

Ambrosino N, Carpenè N, Gherardi M. Chronic respiratory care for neuromuscular diseases in adults. Eur Respir J. 2009 Aug;34(2):444-51. [PMID: 19648521]

Item 64   Answer: D

Educational Objective: Treat tricyclic antidepressant overdose with sodium bicarbonate therapy.

The most appropriate next step in treatment is to begin intravenous sodium bicarbonate therapy. The combination of progressive somnolence, hypotension, widening of the QRS interval, seizure, and anticholinergic signs (fever, tachycardia, mydriasis, reduced bowel sounds) is concerning for severe tricyclic antidepressant overdose. Tricyclic antidepressants inhibit fast sodium channels in the myocardium

CONT.

and conduction system, resulting in decreased ventricular function and increased duration of repolarization that predisposes to ventricular arrhythmias. Electrocardiographic findings in tricyclic overdose include nonspecific changes in QRS morphology and QRS prolongation that predisposes to ventricular arrhythmia; a QRS duration of greater than 100 ms is often used as an indicator of significant tricyclic cardiotoxicity. Sodium bicarbonate increases the serum pH, which inhibits the ionized form of the drug that binds sodium channels, making it less available. Sodium bicarbonate also increases extracellular sodium, which increases the electrochemical gradient across myocardial cell membranes and minimizes the effect of blockade of rapid sodium channels. Clinically, this improves myocardial contractility and results in a reduction in the risk of arrhythmias.

Intravenous calcium gluconate is used in the management of calcium channel blocker overdose, which is a possibility given this patient's baseline use of amlodipine, her hypotension, and the possibility of hypotension-associated encephalopathy. Verapamil and diltiazem poisoning is associated with bradycardia, but this is not typically seen in the case of poisoning with dihydropyridines like amlodipine. Amlodipine poisoning would not explain this patient's anticholinergic signs, widened QRS interval, and seizure.

Fomepizole is an alcohol dehydrogenase inhibitor that prevents the breakdown of methanol and ethylene glycol into toxic metabolites. This patient's somnolence and history of depression raise the possibility of methanol and ethylene glycol poisoning, but the normal osmolal gap, QRS interval widening, and anticholinergic signs would not be expected.

Physostigmine is a potential antidote for anticholinergic toxicity and may be particularly helpful in the management of associated agitated delirium. Although this patient has anticholinergic symptoms, her somnolence, widened QRS interval, and baseline use of amitriptyline are more compatible with tricyclic antidepressant overdose. Physostigmine has reportedly precipitated asystole when used in the setting of tricyclic overdose and should not be given to this patient.

KEY POINT

- The combination of progressive somnolence, hypotension, widening of the QRS interval, seizure, and anticholinergic signs (fever, tachycardia, mydriasis, reduced bowel sounds) is characteristic of severe tricyclic antidepressant overdose.

Bibliography
Body R, Bartram T, Azam F, Mackway-Jones K. Guidelines in Emergency Medicine Network (GEMNet): guideline for the management of tricyclic antidepressant overdose. Emerg Med J. 2011 Apr;28(4):347-68. [PMID: 21436332]

Item 65   Answer: E
Educational Objective: Manage surveillance of a solitary pulmonary nodule.

The most appropriate management is to discontinue further imaging. This patient was found to have a subcentimeter pulmonary nodule. The Fleischner criteria recommend surveillance with repeat chest imaging in a high-risk patient (history of smoking or other risk factors for lung cancer) at intervals based on the size of the nodule. For subcentimeter nodules at 6 mm, the recommendation is initial follow-up CT at 6 to 12 months and then at 18 to 24 months if no change. If imaging demonstrates stability of the nodule (and no other new findings) for 24 months, no further imaging is required.

Given the higher probability of malignancy with ground-glass opacification and partly solid nodules, patients with these types of tumors may warrant longer, if not lifelong, surveillance. Patients with such nodules would benefit from a pulmonary consultation. This patient, however, has no evidence of associated ground-glass opacification and does not currently meet any other criteria for further imaging with a repeat CT, PET/CT, or chest radiograph.

Recent guidelines recommend screening with annual low-dose CT for 3 consecutive years in patients with at least a 30-pack-year history of smoking who are currently smoking or quit within the last 15 years if the patient is between the ages of 55 and 80 years. This patient, however, quit smoking 20 years ago, so he does not meet criteria for screening.

KEY POINT

- If imaging demonstrates stability of a solitary pulmonary nodule (and no other new findings) for 24 months, no further imaging is required.

Bibliography
Murrmann GB, van Vollenhoven FH, Moodley L. Approach to a solid solitary pulmonary nodule in two different settings-"Common is common, rare is rare". J Thorac Dis. 2014 Mar;6(3):237-48. [PMID: 24624288]

Item 66   Answer: D
Educational Objective: Identify risk factors for early readmission in a patient hospitalized for COPD exacerbation.

Comorbidities such as heart failure, lung cancer, anxiety, depression, and osteoporosis are important causes of increased early hospital readmission in patients with COPD exacerbation. The rates of early readmission for COPD exacerbation increase as the number of comorbidities increases. Higher rates of readmissions were noted in patients with COPD and combinations of comorbidities like heart failure and osteoporosis (21%), heart failure and anxiety (18.2%), heart failure and depression (15.9%), and heart failure and alcohol abuse (14.4%).

Inadequate discharge medications for COPD exacerbation were also associated with early readmission rates, specifically the failure to prescribe a short-acting bronchodilator, oral glucocorticoid, and an antibiotic. This patient was discharged on all of these medications; therefore, inadequate discharge medications should not be a cause of early readmission.

Another patient factor associated with early readmission is male gender. Female gender does not increase the risk for early readmission.

Answers and Critiques

CONT.

Patients who were discharged less than 2 days or more than 5 days after admission are at risk for early readmission. This patient's hospital stay was 4 days, so this is unlikely to contribute to her risk of early readmission.

KEY POINT

- The rates of early hospital readmission for COPD exacerbation increase as the number of comorbidities increases.

Bibliography

Sharif R, Parekh TM, Pierson KS, Kuo YF, Sharma G. Predictors of early readmission among patients 40 to 64 years of age hospitalized for chronic obstructive pulmonary disease. Ann Am Thorac Soc. 2014 Jun;11(5):685-94. [PMID: 24784958]

Item 67   Answer: C

Educational Objective: Diagnose bronchiectasis with high-resolution CT.

The most appropriate diagnostic test to perform next is high-resolution CT (HRCT). This patient most likely has bronchiectasis. Symptoms of bronchiectasis include chronic cough with purulent sputum and recurrent pneumonia (in both smokers and nonsmokers). Pulmonary function tests commonly detect mild to moderate airflow obstruction, which may overlap with other disease findings (such as COPD). Physical examination findings may include crackles and/or wheezing on lung auscultation. This patient has a history of pertussis as a child, has a chronic cough with mucopurulent sputum, and has increased bronchovascular markings on chest radiograph. The cause of bronchiectasis in this patient may be lung damage associated with her history of pertussis. In most patients with bronchiectasis, the chest radiograph shows nondiagnostic radiologic findings, including linear atelectasis or dilated and thickened airways ("tram" or "parallel" lines). HRCT is the gold standard diagnostic test for parenchymal lung disease, such as bronchiectasis, and should be performed in this patient. Contrast enhancement is not necessary. Airway dilatation with lack of tapering, bronchial wall thickening, and cysts may be seen on HRCT. After the diagnosis is confirmed, evaluation for underlying causes, such as cystic fibrosis, immunoglobulin deficiencies, and mycobacterial disease, should be performed based on the clinical circumstances of the patient.

Bronchoscopy may be helpful for evaluating a mass or foreign body if identified on CT. However, bronchoscopy is less useful in evaluating bronchiectasis and would not be the next study of choice in this patient.

MRI of the chest has a limited role in evaluating bronchiectasis owing to multiple technical factors. It is an established diagnostic modality for evaluating pleural, hilar, and mediastinal abnormalities. However, it would not be an indicated study in this patient.

Although repeat chest imaging might be helpful to document resolution or progression of a pulmonary finding,

delaying further evaluation in this patient with chronic symptoms would likely not be beneficial.

KEY POINT

- High-resolution CT is the gold standard diagnostic test for bronchiectasis.

Bibliography

McShane PJ, Naureckas ET, Tino G, Strek ME. Non-cystic fibrosis bronchiectasis. Am J Respir Crit Care Med. 2013 Sep 15;188(6):647-56. [PMID: 23898922]

Item 68   Answer: A

Educational Objective: Diagnose auto-positive end-expiratory pressure.

This patient with severe COPD has developed auto-positive end-expiratory pressure (auto-PEEP) on mechanical ventilation. Her obstructive lung disease slows her expiratory flow rate so that she cannot completely exhale before the next breath is initiated by the ventilator (breath stacking). The volume of air that remains in the lungs after each breath builds up, resulting in increased intrathoracic pressure; this can progress to severe consequences such as hypoxemia, cardiovascular collapse (due to decreased venous return and reduced cardiac preload), and barotrauma. When auto-PEEP is diagnosed, the ventilator circuit should be disconnected from the patient's endotracheal tube to allow for a prolonged exhalation which enables trapped intrathoracic air to escape, intrathoracic pressure to drop, and venous return to improve. The ventilator settings should then be adjusted to allow for more effective exhalation to avoid further air trapping. Slowing the respiration rate, decreasing the tidal volume, and increasing the inspiratory flow rate while tolerating respiratory acidosis are ways to increase the exhaled volume with each cycle.

Partial tube obstruction (as with a kink or partially obstructing mucus plug) usually causes a rise in only the peak inspiratory pressure because it affects resistance to flow of air through the tube. Plateau pressure is measured in the absence of flow, so it is unaffected by changes in resistance. Because this patient's plateau pressure increased along with the peak inspiratory pressure, partial tube obstruction is not the most likely cause of her findings.

If a patient has anxiety and triggers breaths more frequently than the set rate, sedation may be required to slow the respiration rate and avoid potential auto-PEEP. This is especially true with hypercapnia, as it is a potent stimulus to increase respiration rate. However, sedation itself is not associated with increased airway and plateau pressures.

KEY POINT

- Patients with obstructive lung disease on mechanical ventilation are susceptible to air trapping due to resistance to expiratory flow, which leads to auto-positive end-expiratory pressure (auto-PEEP) and subsequently to increased intrathoracic pressure.

Bibliography

Marini JJ. Dynamic hyperinflation and auto-positive end-expiratory pressure: lessons learned over 30 years. Am J Resph Crit Care Med. 2011 Oct 1;184(7):756-62. [PMID: 21700908]

Item 69   Answer: A

Educational Objective: Manage advanced COPD with referral to hospice care.

The most appropriate management is to refer this patient for hospice care. Hospice is considered appropriate for patients in whom attempted curative therapy is not likely to be beneficial, and specifically in those who are predicted to have less than 6 months to live. In hospice care, treatment goals are refocused from cure and life-prolonging therapy toward maintaining the highest possible quality of life. In patients with COPD, parameters that portend a poor prognosis and trigger more extensive discussions regarding end-of-life care include an FEV_1 of less than 30% of predicted, oxygen dependence, multiple hospital admissions for COPD exacerbations, significant comorbidities, weight loss and cachexia, decreased functional status, and increasing dependence on others. This patient has very severe COPD, cor pulmonale, decreased functional capacity, constant dyspnea and air hunger, poor nutritional status, and a history of multiple COPD exacerbations on maximal medical therapy and home oxygen. Given these factors and an overall poor prognosis, discussion of a hospice approach to care would be an appropriate next step in management.

In any patient with advancing COPD, it is important to have ongoing discussions regarding the goals of care as the disease progresses so that appropriate management decisions may be made based on anticipated outcomes and patient values and preferences. Involvement of clinicians trained in palliative care may be helpful in these discussions. Palliative care focuses on the many implications of any significant illness with an emphasis on establishing patient-centered goals of care and symptom management. Palliative care does not preclude active treatment of disease and is appropriate regardless of estimated survival time.

Although this patient might meet several of the criteria for possible lung transplantation, most transplant centers use 65 years of age as an arbitrary cutoff, and the presence of other comorbidities such as diabetes mellitus, coronary artery disease, and osteoporosis should also be considered. This patient's age and comorbid conditions likely would preclude lung transplantation.

Lung volume reduction surgery (LVRS) is indicated for patients with severe COPD with predominant upper lobe emphysema who are symptomatic despite optimal medications. Because this patient has diffuse emphysema, he is not a candidate for LVRS.

This patient has completed pulmonary rehabilitation in the past without improvement, and chair-bound patients may not benefit from it; therefore, pulmonary rehabilitation is not an appropriate option for this patient.

KEY POINT

- In patients with COPD, parameters that portend a poor prognosis and trigger more extensive discussions regarding end-of-life care include an FEV_1 of less than 30% of predicted, oxygen dependence, multiple hospital admissions for COPD exacerbations, significant comorbidities, weight loss and cachexia, decreased functional status, and increasing dependence on others.

Bibliography

Curtis JR. Palliative and end-of-life care for patients with severe COPD. Eur Respir J. 2008 Sep;32(3):796-803. [PMID: 17989116]

Item 70   Answer: C

Educational Objective: Manage pain and sedation in a patient with critical illness.

The most appropriate management of this patient's pain and related anxiety is to use an opioid such as fentanyl as an interrupted infusion. Untreated pain increases the risk of posttraumatic stress disorder in patients in the ICU. Although pain assessment is difficult in critically ill patients, it should be monitored with a validated pain scale and not just with vital signs alone; physiologic indicators such as hypertension and tachycardia correlate poorly with valid measures of pain. The 2013 Society of Critical Care Medicine clinical practice guidelines for pain, agitation, and delirium recommend preemptive analgesia and/or nonpharmacologic interventions to alleviate pain. Opioids are considered the drug class of choice for treatment of non–neuropathic pain in critically ill patients, including mechanically ventilated adult patients in the ICU. Therefore, for this patient, an opioid analgesic such as fentanyl should be given as an interrupted infusion. Daily interruption of analgesia and sedation and spontaneous breathing trials should be used as a standard of care for appropriate patients in ICUs. Their use will shorten the need for mechanical ventilation by an average of 1.5 days, dramatically decrease the number of patients who require mechanical ventilation for more than 3 weeks, decrease ICU length of stay, and lower 1-year mortality.

Benzodiazepines, such as lorazepam, given either intermittently or continuously, should generally be avoided or used sparingly because benzodiazepines are a risk factor for delirium in patients in the ICU.

Neuromuscular blocking agents are sometimes used in patients with acute respiratory distress syndrome or in other critical care scenarios where control of carbon dioxide or patients' movements to allow mechanical ventilation are needed. This patient does not have an indication for neuromuscular blockade. Additionally, if needed, neuromuscular blockade should never be used as a single agent. It should only be used when adequate pain control and sedation of the patient are assured prior to its administration.

Answers and Critiques

KEY POINT

- Opioids are the drug class of choice for treatment of non-neuropathic pain in critically ill patients, including mechanically ventilated adult patients in the ICU, and should be given in an interrupted fashion when needed.

Bibliography

Barr J, Fraser GL, Puntillo K, et al; American College of Critical Care Medicine. Clinical practice guidelines for the management of pain, agitation, and delirium in adult patients in the intensive care unit. Crit Care Med. 2013 Jan;41(1):263-306. [PMID: 23269131]

Item 71   Answer: A

Educational Objective: Treat a dissecting aortic aneurysm.

The most appropriate next step in treatment is to start an esmolol infusion. Acute medical therapy is indicated in aortic dissection to lower blood pressure and heart rate, both of which are elevated in this patient. β-Blockers are the drug of choice owing to their antihypertensive and negative chronotropic effects, which lead to reduced shear stress on the aortic wall. Options include propranolol, labetalol, and esmolol. Esmolol is a very short-acting intravenous agent that allows careful titration of blood pressure and heart rate and may be useful in patients with aortic dissection. Nondihydropyridine calcium channel blockers are preferred second-line agents in patients who are unable to tolerate β-blockade. In patients with aortic dissection, the target systolic blood pressure should be 100 to 120 mm Hg, and the target heart rate should be below 65/min.

Fenoldopam is a dopamine agonist that acts as an antihypertensive agent. Because it effectively lowers blood pressure without impairing kidney perfusion, it may be advantageous in patients with hypertensive emergencies accompanied by acute kidney injury. However, unlike β-blockers, it does not reliably lower the heart rate and would not be a preferred treatment for this patient with acute aortic dissection.

Direct vasodilators such as hydralazine increase aortic wall shear stress and are more difficult to use in predictably controlling blood pressure. They are therefore not used in treating acute aortic dissection.

Nitroglycerin produces relatively greater venodilation than arteriolar dilation and would not reliably reduce blood pressure into target range in this patient. A second agent would also be required to lower heart rate, as nitroglycerin does not have chronotropic effects.

KEY POINT

- In patients with aortic dissection, initial medical therapy (preferably with β-blockers) is indicated to lower the blood pressure and heart rate and reduce shear stress on the aortic wall.

Bibliography

Nienaber CA, Clough RE. Management of acute aortic dissection. Lancet. 2015 Feb 28; 385(9970):800-11. [PMID: 25662791]

Item 72   Answer: D

Educational Objective: Diagnose cystic fibrosis.

The most appropriate diagnostic test to perform next is sweat chloride testing. Although traditionally considered a pediatric disease, an increasing number of cases of cystic fibrosis (CF) are diagnosed in adult patients. Conditions suggesting the diagnosis of CF in adults include chronic asthma-like symptoms, chronic sinusitis, nasal polyposis, recurrent pancreatitis, male infertility, nontuberculous mycobacterial infection, allergic bronchopulmonary aspergillosis, bronchiectasis, and positive sputum culture for *Burkholderia cepacia* and/or *Pseudomonas aeruginosa*. This young patient has a history of pulmonary disease since childhood with a chronic productive cough, chronic sinus disease, nasal polyps on physical examination, findings suggestive of CF (such as hyperinflation) on chest radiograph, and pulmonary function tests showing obstruction; therefore, based on this history, he should be evaluated for CF. Diagnosis of CF is based on a combination of CF-compatible clinical findings in conjunction with either biochemical (sweat chloride testing, nasal potential difference) or genetic (*CFTR* mutations) techniques. Sweat chloride testing and *CFTR* analysis are the definitive diagnostic tests.

α_1-Antitrypsin (AAT) is an inhibitor of proteolytic enzymes, with deficiency leading to accelerated emphysema and liver disease. A characteristic radiographic finding of the emphysema associated with AAT is bullous changes most prominent at the bases, which are not present in this patient. Additionally, liver disease is more common in younger patients, which is also not present in this patient; lung disease usually occurs beyond the second and third decades of life. Therefore, AAT testing would not be the most appropriate next diagnostic test in this patient with a clinical history suggestive of possible CF.

Antineutrophil cytoplasmic antibody assays are useful in diagnosing granulomatosis with polyangiitis (GPA), which may present with both upper and lower airway disease as well as kidney involvement. Although this patient has evidence of both upper and lower airway disease, he has no apparent kidney involvement, and his lung imaging is more consistent with bronchiectasis, compared with the common findings in GPA of nodules, diffuse opacities, transient pulmonary infiltrates, and hilar lymphadenopathy. Additionally, GPA tends to affect an older patient population and also has a more acute onset than the symptoms present in this patient, making this a less likely diagnostic consideration. ANCA antibodies are also associated with eosinophilic granulomatosis with polyangiitis (formerly known as Churg-Strauss syndrome). There is no eosinophilia in this patient, and the chronicity since childhood makes this an unlikely diagnosis.

Although imaging of the sinuses may be helpful in defining the extent of polyposis noted on examination, it would not be useful in determining the cause of the polyps or underlying lung disease. Additionally, CT is the preferred imaging modality for sinus disease because of inadequate sensitivity and specificity of plain radiography, making this an inappropriate next diagnostic intervention.

KEY POINT

- Cystic fibrosis should be a diagnostic consideration in young adults presenting with suggestive findings, including chronic asthma-like symptoms, chronic sinusitis, nasal polyposis, recurrent pancreatitis, male infertility, nontuberculous mycobacterial infection, allergic bronchopulmonary aspergillosis, bronchiectasis, and positive sputum culture for *Burkholderia cepacia* and/or *Pseudomonas aeruginosa*.

Bibliography

Smyth AR, Bell SC, Bojcin S, et al; European Cystic Fibrosis Society. European Cystic Fibrosis Society Standards of Care: Best Practice guidelines. J Cyst Fibros. 2014 May;13 Suppl 1:S23-42. [PMID: 24856775]

Item 73   Answer: A

Educational Objective: Evaluate hemoptysis with bronchoscopy.

The most appropriate next step in management is bronchoscopy. Bronchoscopy is generally indicated for evaluation of new respiratory symptoms that may be associated with airway pathology (for example, hemoptysis or stridor). This patient presents with massive hemoptysis, which is generally defined as expectoration of at least 100 mL of blood (one-half U.S. cup equals approximately 120 mL). Chest imaging in this patient showed no evidence of pulmonary embolism but did show ground-glass opacification in the right lower lobe. Although this could represent a source of infection, it more likely represents aspirated blood in this patient without symptoms of an infection. Because of this patient's extensive smoking history, he is at increased risk of lung cancer, which may present as an endobronchial lesion causing hemoptysis. Therefore, he should undergo bronchoscopy with airway inspection to evaluate for an endobronchial lesion; a bronchial wash can also be sent for cytologic and microbiologic studies. Even if there is no endobronchial lesion, bronchoscopy could confirm the source of bleeding if blood is seen originating from the right lower lobe.

Although respiratory infections can lead to hemoptysis, this patient has no symptoms or laboratory studies suggesting an infection such as community-acquired pneumonia or an exacerbation of his COPD, for which antibiotic therapy might be indicated. It is also unusual for pulmonary parenchymal infections to cause massive hemoptysis. Therefore, antibiotic treatment would not be indicated in this patient.

High-resolution CT is used to evaluate the pulmonary parenchyma in greater detail than standard-protocol chest

CT and is the study of choice for evaluating disorders such as interstitial lung disease. However, it would not adequately define endobronchial lesions as a possible cause of hemoptysis and would therefore not be an appropriate next study in this patient.

Some patients may have difficulty distinguishing between hemoptysis and hematemesis, making the history a key component of evaluation to identify the likely source of bleeding. In patients in whom a gastrointestinal cause is suspected, upper endoscopy would be appropriate for further evaluation. However, this patient's presentation is consistent with a pulmonary source of bleeding, and upper endoscopy would not be appropriate before excluding hemoptysis.

KEY POINT

- Bronchoscopy is generally indicated for evaluation of new respiratory symptoms that may be associated with airway pathology (for example, hemoptysis or stridor).

Bibliography

Casal RF, Ost DE, Eapen GA. Flexible bronchoscopy. Clin Chest Med. 2013 Sep;34(3):341-52. [PMID: 23993807]

Item 74   Answer: C

Educational Objective: Diagnose radiation pneumonitis.

The most likely diagnosis is radiation pneumonitis. Patients with radiation pneumonitis present with cough and/or dyspnea approximately 6 to 12 weeks after the exposure. Patients with a high total dose of radiation, preexisting lung disease (especially COPD), and concomitant chemotherapy and radiation therapy are at increased risk. The disease can be severe, with progression over days to weeks leading to acute respiratory failure. Gemcitabine is associated with radiation pneumonitis and drug-induced pneumonitis. The factor that is most pathognomonic of radiation pneumonitis is the imaging finding of a nonanatomic straight line demarcating involved versus uninvolved lung parenchyma as can be seen in this patient's CT scan (*arrows*). However, this finding is no longer an absolute diagnostic criterion owing to differing types of radiation delivery, such as stereotactic

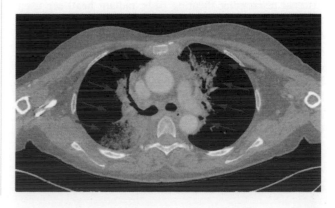

and conformal regimens. The abnormalities in classic radiation pneumonitis typically resolve within 6 months but can progress to a well-demarcated area of fibrosis with volume loss and bronchiectasis.

Although this patient is at risk for progression of her malignancy, the ground-glass and nonanatomic straight line imaging findings are not typical for non–small cell lung cancer recurrence. Additionally, the clinical and radiographic worsening over days to weeks is a helpful clue to distinguish radiation pneumonitis from recurrent local or metastatic cancer.

Radiation fibrosis is clinically distinct from radiation pneumonitis, although the diseases may have overlapping clinical presentations. Radiation fibrosis can occur in patients with or without a history of radiation pneumonitis. Radiation fibrosis occurs 6 to 24 months after radiation therapy and represents a long-term fibrotic sequela of lung damage, most often within the radiation field. Symptoms are uncommon, but patients with previous marginal lung function may have worsening dyspnea. The fibrotic process is irreversible. This patient's symptoms and time course are not compatible with radiation fibrosis.

Viral pneumonia is also part of the differential diagnosis, but the radiographic finding of a straight line of demarcation makes this an unlikely diagnosis.

KEY POINT

- The imaging finding of a nonanatomic straight line demarcating involved versus uninvolved lung parenchyma is pathognomonic of radiation pneumonitis.

Bibliography

Fogh S, Yom SS. Symptom management during the radiation oncology treatment course: a practical guide for the oncology clinician. Semin Oncol. 2014 Dec;41(6):764-75. [PMID: 25499635]

Item 75   Answer: C

Educational Objective: Treat severe hypothermia in a patient with hemodynamic instability.

This patient is hemodynamically unstable as a result of severe accidental hypothermia and should undergo extracorporeal rewarming to maximize the rate of temperature correction. Passive external rewarming (blankets, insulation) and active external rewarming (heating pads, radiant heat) are used for mild or moderate hypothermia. However, this patient has severe hypothermia with hemodynamic instability, and more aggressive warming techniques are indicated. In this case, extracorporeal support, including cardiopulmonary bypass, is recommended because it maximizes the rewarming rate and can also provide hemodynamic support. Cardiopulmonary bypass, most frequently used in cardiac surgical procedures, can provide hemodynamic stabilization and can increase the body temperature by approximately 9.0 °C (16.2 °F) per hour.

Other forms of active internal warming, such as administering warmed intravenous fluids or intraperitoneal and pleural irrigation, are indicated for severe hypothermia, as in this patient. However, these methods do not provide hemodynamic support and do not raise body temperature as rapidly as cardiopulmonary bypass. For example, 1 L of fluid at 42.0 °C (107.6 °F) would raise this patient's core temperature by approximately 0.25 °C (0.45 °F).

This patient is at risk of developing hypothermia-related sustained ventricular tachycardia and fibrillation, but limited data indicate that core temperatures greater than 34.0 °C (93.2 °F) are needed for pharmacologic therapies such as lidocaine to be effective. Additionally, electrical cardioversion is often ineffective in patients with core temperatures less than 30.0 °C (86.0 °F). Rewarming is the surest method of stabilizing this patient, and attempts at treating or preventing arrhythmias should not detract from this.

Although this patient's clinical presentation is concerning for potential severe anoxic encephalopathy, there are numerous reports of survival with good neurologic outcomes in patients with hypothermia requiring prolonged periods of cardiopulmonary resuscitation. The neurologic examination is not reliable in assessing neurologic injury in severe hypothermia. Given the potential for recovery, recommending no CPR in the event of recurrent nonperfusing cardiac rhythm is not the best option for this patient.

KEY POINT

- In patients with severe hypothermia and hemodynamic instability, extracorporeal support, including cardiopulmonary bypass, is recommended because it maximizes the rewarming rate and can provide hemodynamic support.

Bibliography

Brown DJ, Brugger H, Boyd J, Paal P. Accidental hypothermia. N Engl J Med. 2012 Nov 15;367(20):1930-8. Erratum in: N Engl J Med. 2013 Jan 24;368(4):394. [PMID: 23150960]

Item 76   Answer: D

Educational Objective: Manage idiopathic pulmonary fibrosis with evaluation for lung transplantation.

The most appropriate management is referral to a lung transplantation program. Individuals considered for lung transplantation are most often at high risk of death within 2 years due to respiratory failure and also have a high likelihood of long-term survival following the procedure. This patient with idiopathic pulmonary fibrosis (IPF) has a significant oxygen requirement at rest in addition to a documented decline in his 6-minute walk distance. Both of these factors substantially increase his risk for the development of respiratory failure. Furthermore, he has no history of comorbidities that would limit posttransplant survival, and he continues to actively participate in pulmonary rehabilitation. Lung transplantation remains the only intervention with a clear survival benefit for select patients with IPF.

Medical options for treatment of IPF are limited. The immunosuppressant azathioprine, given along with prednisone and N-acetylcysteine, has been studied in patients with IPF. However, this combination therapy was associated with increased mortality and adverse effects. Therefore, azathioprine is not recommended for use in patients with IPF. In related studies, N-acetylcysteine used as single-agent therapy in IPF showed no benefit over placebo; thus, N-acetylcysteine is also no longer considered of value for treatment of IPF.

Although there is some debate as to the benefit of glucocorticoids in the treatment of patients with an acute exacerbation of IPF, there is no benefit to either short- or long-course prednisone in patients with IPF without an exacerbation. IPF is a disease with ongoing fibrosis but with limited inflammation. Consequently, glucocorticoids do little to affect the progressive fibrosis, and their many associated side effects only place the patient at increased risk of complications.

Treatment with tumor necrosis factor-α (TNF-α) inhibitors has been proposed as a method for decreasing the progressive pulmonary fibrosis associated with IPF. However, a trial of the TNF-α inhibitor etanercept failed to show benefit, and its use is not recommended in IPF.

Two new medical therapies have recently been approved for treatment of IPF. These are nintedanib, a tyrosine kinase inhibitor that moderates production of fibrogenic growth factors, and pirfenidone, whose mechanism is unclear but also modulates production of fibrosis. Both agents slow the decline in pulmonary function tests but do not affect quality of life and are not curative. The effect of these agents on disease progression appears to be very similar. To date, these agents have not been studied extensively in patients with acute exacerbation of IPF or severely advanced IPF. Pulmonary subspecialty assessment to confirm IPF and assess risk/benefit for the use of these drugs in selected patients is recommended. Consideration of participation in clinical trials for patients with this progressive disorder remains important for the development of future, more effective, medical therapies.

KEY POINT

- Patients with idiopathic pulmonary fibrosis who have a high risk for the development of respiratory failure and a high likelihood of long-term posttransplant survival should be referred to a lung transplantation program.

Bibliography

Weill D, Benden C, Corris PA, et al. A consensus document for the selection of lung transplant candidates: 2014-An update from the Pulmonary Transplantation Council of the International Society for Heart and Lung Transplantation. J Heart Lung Transplant. 2015 Jan;34(1):1-15. [PMID: 25085497]

Item 77   Answer: B

Educational Objective: Diagnose Hodgkin lymphoma.

The most likely diagnosis in this patient is Hodgkin lymphoma. This patient's chest radiograph shows a mass that originates from the mediastinum, given the convex angles

resulting from the mass impinging on the pleura. The lateral film localizes the mass to the anterior mediastinum. Thymomas are the most common mediastinal lesion in adults and are also located in the anterior mediastinum. However, they occur more commonly in patients between the ages of 40 and 50 years old and can present with paraneoplastic syndromes such as myasthenia gravis. The second most common cause of anterior mediastinal masses is lymphoma; affected patients, such as this one, are typically younger at the time of presentation. Hodgkin lymphoma is the most common lymphoma to involve the mediastinum, followed by lymphoblastic lymphoma and primary mediastinal diffuse large B-cell lymphoma. Other causes of anterior mediastinal masses include germ cell tumors, including teratomas. However, Hodgkin lymphoma is the most common cause of anterior mediastinal masses in patients aged 20 to 30 years, such as this patient.

Bronchogenic cysts are congenital anomalies that develop in the middle mediastinal compartment and most commonly present in the second decade of life. Although they may be found incidentally as rounded lesions on imaging, they may be symptomatic if large owing to compression of normal tissues. Other anomalies such as pericardial cysts and esophageal duplication cysts may also be seen in this compartment. The mass seen on this patient's chest radiograph does not arise from the middle mediastinum compartment.

A mass in the posterior mediastinum is usually a neurogenic tumor. In children, these typically arise from the sympathetic ganglia (for example, neuroblastomas), whereas in adults neurogenic tumors tend to arise from the nerve sheaths (for example, schwannomas). The mass on this patient's chest radiograph is located in the anterior mediastinal compartment.

KEY POINT

- The second most common cause of anterior mediastinal masses is lymphoma; affected patients are typically younger at the time of presentation than are patients with thymomas, which are the most common anterior mediastinal masses.

Bibliography

Takahashi K, Al-Janabi NJ. Computed tomography and magnetic resonance imaging of mediastinal tumors. J Magn Reson Imaging. 2010 Dec; 32(6):1325-39. [PMID: 21105138]

Item 78   Answer: C

Educational Objective: Manage acute respiratory distress syndrome with a conservative fluid strategy.

The most appropriate fluid-management strategy is to titrate this patient's fluid volume to a central venous pressure (CVP) of 4 mm Hg or less. This patient has acute respiratory distress syndrome (ARDS). A large multicenter trial has shown that a conservative fluid strategy leads to discontinuing mechanical ventilation sooner than the traditional or "liberal" fluid strategy. Limiting intravenous fluids and using diuretics to keep CVPs at lower targets has been associated with a more rapid improvement in lung function, shorter duration of mechanical ventilation, and shorter ICU length of stay. However, the study did not show an effect on mortality. The target CVP for the conservative strategy was 4 mm Hg.

A CVP target of 12 mm Hg would be more consistent with the "liberal" fluid management arm of the study, which was associated with longer duration of ventilation and is therefore not recommended.

Traditionally, a pulmonary artery catheter had been used to guide hemodynamic resuscitation; however, at least four international studies have shown that neither pulmonary artery catheters nor specific protocols that incorporate data from such catheters yield superior outcomes in most patients. In addition, these catheters have more risk associated with their use compared with a simple central line.

KEY POINT

- In patients with acute respiratory distress syndrome, a conservative fluid-management strategy is associated with more rapid improvement in lung function, shorter duration of mechanical ventilation, and shorter ICU length of stay.

Bibliography

National Heart, Lung, and Blood Institute Acute Respiratory Distress Syndrome (ARDS) Clinical Trials Network, Wiedemann HP, Wheeler AP, Bernard GR, et al. Comparison of two fluid-management strategies in acute lung injury. N Engl J Med. 2006 Jun 15;354(24):2564-75. [PMID: 16714767]

Item 79   Answer: A

Educational Objective: Diagnose exercise-induced bronchospasm and possible asthma with bronchial challenge testing.

The most appropriate next step in management is a methacholine challenge test. Testing will confirm the degree to which this patient's symptoms are caused by hyperreactivity of the lungs. The frequency and degree of this patient's symptoms are concerning, and he has several risk factors and clinical factors (such as a history of allergies, cough without exercise, and symptoms occurring several times a week) that suggest the possibility of asthma as the underlying diagnosis. Though some patients with asthma wheeze with exercise, it is not a necessary symptom to consider the diagnosis; exercise intolerance, breathlessness, and cough can be the primary symptoms as well. Because of the significant morbidity and mortality associated with undiagnosed and untreated asthma, further evaluation of this possibility is indicated in this patient. Because spirometry results are normal, which can occur in patients with asthma, further confirmatory testing with a bronchial challenge test (such as with methacholine) is warranted to further evaluate for possible asthma.

Managing only this patient's allergic rhinitis with a nasal glucocorticoid would not treat possible underlying asthma adequately to protect him from nighttime cough and shortness of breath during exercise. However, counseling avoidance of exercise in locations with allergens would be appropriate.

Although a therapeutic trial of an as-needed β_2-agonist inhaler may seem reasonable, a more extensive assessment and proper diagnosis of this patient's symptoms concerning for asthma will ensure that adequate medications are prescribed for chronic management.

In patients with asthma, spirometry results between episodes are often normal. Additionally, this patient is experiencing frequent and disruptive symptoms. Therefore, clinical observation without further evaluation would not be appropriate.

KEY POINT

- In patients with symptoms of exercise-induced bronchospasm and/or asthma but normal spirometry findings, bronchial challenge testing is warranted for further evaluation.

Bibliography

Parsons JP, Hallstrand TS, Mastronarde JG, et al; American Thoracic Society Subcommittee on Exercise-induced Bronchoconstriction. An official American Thoracic Society clinical practice guideline: exercise-induced bronchoconstriction. Am J Respir Crit Care Med. 2013 May 1;187(9):1016-27. [PMID: 23634861]

Item 80   Answer: A

Educational Objective: Manage extubation in a patient with hypercapnic COPD using noninvasive positive pressure ventilation.

The most appropriate management is to extubate the patient now and initiate bilevel noninvasive positive pressure ventilation (NPPV). This patient's condition is improving after intubation for a COPD exacerbation with hypercapnic respiratory failure. For most patients on invasive ventilatory support, the use of NPPV after extubation to facilitate weaning has not been shown to have improved outcomes. However, patients such as this one, with COPD and hypercapnia who can be extubated and started on NPPV, are an exception to this general rule. This strategy has been shown in some studies to decrease the ICU length of stay and improve survival, and would be a reasonable next step in this patient who has been steadily improving, is otherwise stable, and has a normal mental status. These patients require careful follow-up and observation for reintubation if they do not remain stable on NPPV.

Extubating this patient without immediate NPPV support could be considered, but there are indications that he may not be ready for unsupported breathing yet.

Tracheostomy is a good option for patients who have been intubated for an extended period of time and likely require continued mechanical ventilation to avoid damage to the vocal cords and subglottic airway. However, this patient's condition is improving and he is unlikely to need mechanical ventilation for an extended period of time; therefore, placing a tracheostomy tube is unnecessary.

CONT.

Continuing spontaneous breathing trials on invasive ventilation would probably lead to gradual improvement and eventual extubation, but the risk of complications from mechanical ventilation increases with longer use, and the opportunity to extubate sooner should be pursued if available.

KEY POINT

- In patients with COPD and hypercapnia, extubation followed by noninvasive positive pressure ventilation support may decrease the ICU length of stay and improve survival.

Bibliography

Burns KE, Meade MO, Premji A, Adhikari NK. Noninvasive positive-pressure ventilation as a weaning strategy for intubated adults with respiratory failure. Cochrane Database Syst Rev. 2013 Dec 9;12:CD004127. [PMID: 24323843]

Item 81   Answer: C

Educational Objective: Diagnose ICU-acquired weakness.

The most likely diagnosis is ICU-acquired weakness. ICU-acquired weakness includes critical illness polyneuropathy (with axonal nerve degeneration) and critical illness myopathy (with muscle myosin loss), resulting in profound weakness. These two conditions are difficult to differentiate and may overlap. Some experts recommend that biopsies and more formal electrophysiologic studies be reserved for patients in whom the diagnosis is more ambiguous and where other diagnoses are more likely to exist. ICU-acquired weakness is associated with long-term functional disability, prolonged ventilation, and in-hospital mortality. Risk factors include female sex, hyperglycemia, sepsis, multiple organ dysfunction and systemic inflammatory response, immobility, and long duration of mechanical ventilation. Strategies to limit or prevent ICU-acquired weakness include sedation limitation, early mobilization, and moderate glucose control. The strategies that have the most impact are not yet known.

Diabetes predisposes to multifactorial nerve injury due to nerve compression, ischemia, inflammation, and metabolic changes. Distal sensorimotor peripheral neuropathy is the most common disorder and presents with numbness, tingling, and burning pain in a stocking-glove distribution. Weakness may occur late in the course of the disease. However, this pattern is not present in this patient and would be unlikely to account for this patient's symmetric muscle weakness.

Guillain-Barré syndrome is the most common cause of acute diffuse neuromuscular paralysis. Affected patients initially experience rapid onset of symmetric weakness of the upper and lower limbs over days to weeks, generally in the setting of a recent infection, trauma, or surgery. The disorder generally progresses over 2 weeks, with 90% patients at their worst by 4 weeks. Although many patients describe paresthesias or neuropathic pain in the hands and feet,

objective sensory loss is usually mild or absent. Neurologic examination reveals weakness and decreased or absent deep tendon reflexes. The time course and absence of paresthesias in this patient make Guillain-Barré syndrome an unlikely diagnosis.

Vasculitic neuropathy is usually found in association with a systemic vasculitis that involves other organs (skin, lungs, kidneys), but it can be found in isolation. Patients most commonly present with both sensory and motor nerve dysfunction that is asymmetric and distal, typically involving the longest nerves of the body first. This patient's painless and symmetric loss of muscle function is not compatible with vasculitis neuropathy.

KEY POINT

- ICU-acquired weakness includes critical illness polyneuropathy (with axonal nerve degeneration) and critical illness myopathy (with muscle myosin loss), resulting in profound weakness; it may impair weaning from the ventilator.

Bibliography

Kress JP, Hall JB. ICU-acquired weakness and recovery from critical illness. N Engl J Med. 2014 Jul 17;371(3):287-8. [PMID: 25014703]

Item 82   Answer: A

Educational Objective: Diagnose lymphangioleiomyomatosis.

The most likely diagnosis is lymphangioleiomyomatosis (LAM). LAM is a very uncommon disorder that occurs in association with the genetic changes found in tuberous sclerosis complex, and a sporadic form that is seen almost exclusively in women during childbearing years. Histopathology shows infiltration of atypical smooth muscle cells into the pulmonary interstitium caused by activation of the mammalian target of rapamycin (mTOR) signaling pathway. This results in the development of thin-walled cysts scattered throughout the pulmonary parenchyma and increases the risk of spontaneous pneumothorax. Diagnosis is based on imaging studies showing the characteristic diffuse cystic changes and elevated levels of vascular endothelial growth factor-D (VEGF-D). Hormonal therapy, which was used in the past, is not effective in altering the disease course. Sirolimus, an mTOR inhibitor, has shown promise in stabilizing pulmonary function in patients with LAM and is increasingly used to treat patients with progressive lung disease.

Organizing pneumonia is a noninfectious diffuse parenchymal lung disease that may occur in association with other underlying conditions (such as collagen vascular diseases or use of certain drugs), but may also occur in the absence of another condition or exposure (cryptogenic organizing pneumonia). Onset is typically over 4 to 6 weeks and symptoms rarely persist for longer than 6 months; its presentation may mimic community-acquired pneumonia. Chest imaging typically shows patchy airspace disease with consolidation and ground-glass opacities but no cystic changes.

This patient's presentation and imaging findings are not consistent with a diagnosis of organizing pneumonia.

Pulmonary Langerhans cell histiocytosis (PLCH), which involves an increased number of Langerhans and inflammatory cells in the lung interstitium, may present with nonspecific respiratory symptoms and a history of spontaneous pneumothorax. Most cases occur in young adults between 20 and 40 years of age. There is also a very strong association with smoking. The duration of symptoms is usually less than 1 year before the diagnosis is made. Although pulmonary cysts are found in PLCH, they tend to be thicker-walled and are accompanied by interstitial thickening and nodularity seen in radiographic findings. This patient's clinical course and imaging studies make a diagnosis of PLCH unlikely.

Respiratory bronchiolitis–associated interstitial lung disease results from inflammation of bronchioles and occurs primarily in smokers. It results in characteristic radiographic findings of centrilobular nodules with air-trapping and scattered ground-glass attenuation. This patient's absence of a smoking history and CT findings do not support this diagnosis.

KEY POINT

- Lymphangioleiomyomatosis is a rare cystic lung disease that occurs sporadically in women of childbearing age or in association with tuberous sclerosis; characteristic findings include diffuse, thin-walled, small cysts on CT.

Bibliography

Meraj R, Wikenheiser-Brokamp KA, Young LR, McCormack FX. Lymphangioleiomyomatosis: new concepts in pathogenesis, diagnosis, and treatment. Semin Respir Crit Care Med. 2012 Oct;33(5):486-97. [PMID: 23001803]

Item 83   Answer: A

Educational Objective: Diagnose carbon monoxide poisoning with carboxyhemoglobin measurement.

The most appropriate diagnostic test is measurement of the carboxyhemoglobin level. The history of exposure to an idling car in an enclosed space is a risk factor for carbon monoxide poisoning. Symptoms of carbon monoxide poisoning vary and include headache, confusion, nausea, vomiting, and, in severe cases, loss of consciousness. Routine pulse oximetry measures and compares the light absorption of oxygenated and deoxygenated hemoglobin to calculate the percentage of hemoglobin saturated with oxygen. However, it is not able to detect the presence of other abnormal hemoglobin moieties, such as methemoglobin or carboxyhemoglobin. Because of this, standard pulse oximetry may not indicate the presence of either of these abnormal hemoglobins, and a normal hemoglobin saturation by pulse oximetry is inadequate to exclude their presence. Therefore, co-oximetry of an arterial blood gas sample, which measures both types of hemoglobin, is indicated if either of these conditions is suspected, as in this patient.

This patient's troponin level and electrocardiogram findings suggest the presence of myocardial ischemia. Myocardial ischemia occurs in roughly one third of patients with carbon monoxide poisoning, often independent of any known history of, or risk factors for, coronary artery disease. Vascular occlusive coronary artery disease is also less likely in this patient without clear cardiovascular risk factors. Therefore, cardiac catheterization would not be an appropriate next diagnostic step in this patient with possible myocardial ischemia due to carbon monoxide poisoning.

Electroencephalography is also not appropriate for this patient. Although he may have developed a seizure or acute coronary syndrome after pulling his car into the garage, neither possibility fully accounts for the multiple signs of end-organ damage seen with carbon monoxide poisoning. This patient has a history of seizures and could have postictal encephalopathy with an accompanying lactic acidosis, but this would not explain his myocardial ischemia. There are no corroborating signs of seizure such as a tongue laceration. Given the absence of hemodynamic instability, acute coronary syndrome is unlikely to present with encephalopathy.

This patient's clinical scenario is highly consistent with carbon monoxide poisoning, and the combination of obtundation, preserved respiratory drive, low blood pressure, and normal pupil findings are not typical of sedating or sympathomimetic drug ingestions.

KEY POINT

- Patients with carbon monoxide poisoning may have normal oxygen saturation measured by pulse oximetry; therefore, co-oximetry of an arterial blood gas sample should be used to measure the carboxyhemoglobin level and confirm the diagnosis.

Bibliography

Hampson NB, Piantadosi CA, Thom SR, Weaver LK. Practice recommendations in the diagnosis, management, and prevention of carbon monoxide poisoning. Am J Respir Crit Care Med. 2012 Dec 1;186(11):1095-101. [PMID: 23087025]

Item 84   Answer: B

Educational Objective: Treat sympathomimetic overdose with lorazepam.

The most appropriate next step in treatment is to start lorazepam on an as-needed basis. The combination of hypertension, tachycardia, fever, diaphoresis, mydriasis, and rhabdomyolysis is most consistent with sympathomimetic intoxication. Common causes of sympathomimetic intoxication include cocaine, amphetamines, ephedrine, and caffeine. Benzodiazepines are first-line therapy for sympathomimetic intoxication.

Activated charcoal can be used to reduce drug levels in patients with therapeutic drug overdose but generally should not be administered if the patient is at risk of aspirating or more than 1 to 2 hours have elapsed since the time of ingestion. The potential harms of activated charcoal outweigh the benefits for this patient.

Physostigmine is an antidote for anticholinergic toxicity, which also presents with agitation, mydriasis, fever, and tachycardia. However, this degree of hypertension and the presence of diaphoresis rather than anhidrosis make anticholinergic toxicity less likely in this patient.

Experience in patients with cocaine-induced hypertension suggests use of β-blockers can paradoxically worsen hypertension due to loss of β-mediated vascular smooth muscle relaxation. Given these concerns with cocaine, it is reasonable to avoid β-blockers, such as propranolol, in sympathomimetic intoxication in general. Furthermore, this patient has no clear evidence of end-organ damage (for example, stroke, acute coronary syndrome, aortic dissection) that would mandate rapid, tightly controlled blood pressure reduction.

> **KEY POINT**
>
> • The combination of hypertension, tachycardia, fever, diaphoresis, mydriasis, and rhabdomyolysis is most consistent with sympathomimetic intoxication; benzodiazepines are first-line therapy for sympathomimetic toxicity.

Bibliography
Holstege CP, Borek HA. Toxidromes. Crit Care Clin. 2012 Oct;28(4):479-98. [PMID: 22998986]

Item 85   Answer: C

Educational Objective: Treat localized non-small cell lung cancer.

The most appropriate treatment is resection. The transthoracic needle biopsy obtained in this patient was consistent with a diagnosis of adenocarcinoma of the lung. After non–small cell lung cancer (NSCLC) is diagnosed based on biopsy findings of a suspicious lung mass, staging studies are obtained to develop an appropriate treatment plan. Because the cancer may spread systemically, studies are also done to detect common sites of involvement, typically liver, bone, adrenal glands, or brain. Imaging studies include CT of the chest and abdomen plus a bone scan or PET/CT plus contrast-enhanced MRI of the brain. In this patient, the PET/CT showed only localized disease and his MRI of the brain did not show evidence of metastatic disease. If the mediastinum and distant sites are disease-free, surgical resection is considered feasible. The next steps are determining the extent of the surgical procedure to remove all known disease and deciding whether postoperative residual lung function will be adequate. Because most patients with lung cancer have damage to the lungs from tobacco use, pulmonary function studies should be obtained to evaluate total lung capacity, forced expiratory volumes, and D$_{LCO}$. Values below a certain level may preclude surgery. In this patient with localized NSCLC who can tolerate surgery, complete resection should be attempted. The 5-year survival rate in patients diagnosed

with resectable disease ranges from 30% to 75%. If surgery is not possible, radiation therapy is recommended as an alternative.

Airway stent placement can be performed in instances of airway obstruction, including those caused by endobronchial involvement of a primary lung cancer. However, this patient has no evidence of airway obstruction on chest imaging and is currently asymptomatic.

In more advanced NSCLC that includes mediastinal, hilar, or contralateral lymph node involvement, outcomes have not been shown to be improved with surgical resection; therefore, chemotherapy in combination with radiation therapy is considered first-line therapy. This patient has no evidence of advanced disease. Patients with distant metastasis are generally treated with chemotherapy alone, but this patient has no evidence of metastatic disease. Adjuvant chemotherapy could be considered in some patients with resectable disease.

> **KEY POINT**
>
> • In patients with localized non–small cell lung cancer who can tolerate surgery, complete resection should be attempted.

Bibliography
Collins LG, Haines C, Perkel R, Enck RE. Lung cancer: diagnosis and management. Am Fam Physician. 2007 Jan 1;75(1):56-63. [PMID: 17225705]

Item 86   Answer: A

Educational Objective: Diagnose pulmonary sarcoidosis with bronchoscopic biopsy.

The most appropriate next step in management is to perform a bronchoscopic biopsy of the mediastinal lymph nodes and lung. The diagnosis is most likely sarcoidosis. Sarcoidosis is a multiorgan inflammatory disease characterized by tissue infiltration by mononuclear phagocytes, lymphocytes, and noncaseating granulomas. The cause remains unknown, but there is increasing evidence to suggest it is the end result of interactions among a persistent antigen, HLA class II molecules, and T-cell receptors. Ninety percent of patients with sarcoidosis have pulmonary involvement; however, diagnosis is often difficult because symptoms can be nonspecific. Pulmonary function tests often show restriction, but obstruction can be seen as well; these findings are not specific to sarcoidosis. Sarcoidosis is a diagnosis of exclusion based on multisystem involvement and histologic evidence of noncaseating granulomas when all other causes are ruled out. Bronchoscopy with transbronchial biopsies combined with endobronchial biopsies has been shown to have sensitivities as high as 90% for diagnosing sarcoidosis. Most patients require a tissue diagnosis, but there are some exceptions that do not warrant histologic confirmation. These include classic clinical presentations of known sarcoid syndromes such as Löfgren syndrome (hilar lymphadenopathy, acute oligoarthritis, and erythema nodosum) and Heerfordt syndrome (uveitis, parotid gland enlargement, and fever).

Sarcoidosis often spontaneously resolves and the decision to treat is based on symptoms. Glucocorticoids are the treatment of choice, but in this patient the decision to treat should be made only after confirming a diagnosis and then assessing the risks and benefits of treatment.

The Centers for Disease Control and Prevention endorses the use of interferon-γ release assays (IGRAs) in all clinical settings in which the tuberculin skin test (TST) is recommended. IGRAs are as sensitive as but more specific than the TST in diagnosing tuberculosis. Testing for tuberculosis with both an IGRA and TST is generally not recommended, and this patient's recent negative TST makes a diagnosis of tuberculosis an unlikely cause of his clinical findings.

Although serum angiotensin-converting enzyme levels are elevated in 75% of patients with chronic sarcoidosis, the test lacks specificity and is therefore of limited use diagnostically.

KEY POINT

- Sarcoidosis is a diagnosis of exclusion based on multisystem involvement and histologic evidence of noncaseating granulomas when all other causes are ruled out.

Bibliography

Sun J, Yang H, Teng J, et al. Determining factors in diagnosing pulmonary sarcoidosis by endobronchial ultrasound-guided transbronchial needle aspiration. Ann Thorac Surg. 2015 Feb;99(2):441-5. [PMID: 25497069]

Item 87   Answer: B

Educational Objective: Manage hypoxic and hypercapnic respiratory failure in a patient with a contraindication to noninvasive ventilation.

The most appropriate next step in management is intubation and mechanical ventilation. This patient is experiencing an exacerbation of his COPD with hypercapnic respiratory failure with hypoxia and mental status changes. Although the majority of patients with acute exacerbation of COPD should undergo a trial of noninvasive ventilation (NIV) and reevaluation prior to intubation and mechanical ventilation, encephalopathy that impairs the ability to cooperate with NIV or manage secretions is a contraindication to NIV. Other contraindications to NIV include conditions that make airway protection difficult (for example, bulbar dysfunction or ineffective gag or cough reflexes), medical instability (such as hemodynamic instability, severe acidosis, arrhythmias, or active upper gastrointestinal bleeding), and mechanical issues associated with NIV (including upper airway obstruction, recent facial trauma or surgery, or esophageal or transsphenoidal surgery). Because this patient would likely not be able to adhere with NIV because of confusion and may not be able to protect his airway, intubation and mechanical ventilation are indicated.

Although increasing the level of inspired oxygen to maintain an oxygen saturation of greater than 90% in acute COPD exacerbations has been shown to be beneficial, doing so would not address this patient's hypercapnia and associated mental status changes, which need to be treated with ventilatory support.

The use of NIV in eligible patients is effective and can avoid intubation in several disease states, particularly with COPD exacerbations or decompensated heart failure. In COPD, NIV has been shown to decrease the need for intubation, decrease mortality, and reduce length of hospital stay and complication rates. Compared with invasive mechanical ventilation, NIV uses pressure instead of volume to assist ventilation, and multiple different modes are available for use with limited data regarding the effectiveness of one mode of ventilation relative to another. However, none of the NIV modes would be appropriate in this patient with a contraindication to this therapy.

KEY POINT

- Contraindications to noninvasive ventilation (NIV) include conditions that make airway protection difficult (for example, encephalopathy or bulbar dysfunction), medical instability (such as hemodynamic instability, severe acidosis, arrhythmias, or active upper gastrointestinal bleeding), and mechanical issues associated with NIV (including upper airway obstruction, recent facial trauma or surgery, or esophageal or transsphenoidal surgery).

Bibliography

Keenan SP, Sinuff T, Burns KE, et al; Canadian Critical Care Trials Group/Canadian Critical Care Society Noninvasive Ventilation Guidelines Group. Clinical practice guidelines for the use of noninvasive positive-pressure ventilation and noninvasive continuous positive airway pressure in the acute care setting. CMAJ. 2011 Feb 22;183(3):E195-214. [PMID: 21324867]

Item 88   Answer: C

Educational Objective: Manage a pulmonary nodule with a high pretest probability of primary lung cancer.

The most appropriate management is to refer for thoracic surgery. One year ago this patient had a 3-mm pulmonary nodule. As a cigarette smoker, she is at high risk for lung cancer and was managed appropriately with repeat imaging in 12 months. On repeat imaging, the nodule has enlarged. The pretest probability that this nodule represents a primary lung cancer is high. Not only is this patient an active and long-time smoker, but her nodule has more than doubled in size over the previous year. Therefore, tissue diagnosis is warranted. An enlarging pulmonary nodule warrants more aggressive evaluation with tissue diagnosis or excision depending on the nodule's pretest probability of malignancy. Provided she is an appropriate candidate, surgical resection may be the best management. It would confirm the suspected diagnosis of primary lung cancer and would also be curative in this patient with likely stage I non–small cell lung cancer (based on the small size and absence of lymphadenopathy or other evidence of metastatic disease).

Although bronchoscopy could potentially provide a diagnosis, resection is the treatment of choice in a patient with stage IA lung cancer. Since she has no evidence of lymphadenopathy or other nodules, surgical resection may provide both diagnosis and cure. If the bronchoscopy is negative, the pretest probability of a primary lung cancer is high enough that the patient would still require further tissue diagnosis as well.

Similarly, a negative transthoracic needle aspiration would not be reassuring since it only obtains a small number of cells; therefore, if the needle aspiration were negative for malignancy the patient would still require a second diagnostic procedure. If the transthoracic needle aspiration confirmed malignancy, surgical resection would be indicated in the absence of any evidence of additional foci of malignancy.

This patient's pulmonary nodule has already significantly increased in size. Therefore, further surveillance imaging, even if obtained sooner, is not indicated at this time. At this point, the clinician should focus on the diagnosis, staging, and treatment.

KEY POINT

- An enlarging pulmonary nodule warrants more aggressive evaluation with tissue diagnosis or excision depending on the nodule's pretest probability of malignancy.

Bibliography

Gould MK, Fletcher J, Iannettoni MD, et al; American College of Chest Physicians. Evaluation of patients with pulmonary nodules: when is it lung cancer?: ACCP evidence-based clinical practice guidelines (2nd edition). Chest. 2007 Sep;132(3 Suppl):108S-130S. [PMID: 17873164]

Item 89   Answer: A

Educational Objective: Understand the role of the rapid response team in managing deteriorating clinical status in hospitalized patients.

Activation of a rapid response team would be expected to decrease the chance of cardiopulmonary arrest in a patient such as this. Unrecognized deterioration of a patient's clinical status in general medical settings allows patients to progress to cardiopulmonary arrest, which carries a very poor prognosis for hospital outcome and survival. It has been found that the signs and symptoms of deterioration are usually present several hours before arrest (with a median time of 6 hours). A strategy to improve the recognition and response to deteriorating patients has been developed in the form of rapid response systems. These systems seek to alter management in deteriorating patients who are at risk of cardiopulmonary collapse by intervening before irreversible instability occurs.

Although there are no standard structures of rapid response teams, they are frequently composed of intensivists and others with experience in identifying and managing patients with worsening clinical parameters who may be helpful in guiding further treatment interventions and assist

in determining the appropriate setting of care for a specific patient. Unfortunately, clear criteria do not exist for activating rapid response teams. However, a number of indicators have been identified that are associated with increased risk of decompensation; when these indicators are present, rapid response intervention may be effective. These indicators include changes in vital signs (heart rate of <30/min or ≥139/min; systolic blood pressure <70 mm Hg or ≥200 mm Hg; respiration rate <9/min or >35/min, temperature <34.0 °C [93.2 °F] or ≥39.0 °C [102.2 °F]), oxygen saturation less than 85%, and development of altered mental status or coma. This patient's persistent tachycardia indicates possible vital sign instability warranting further evaluation as a potential early indicator of deterioration. Studies of rapid response teams have shown reduced rates of cardiopulmonary arrest outside of the ICU and reduced mortality.

Implementation of rapid response teams has not been consistently shown to reduce rates of intubation, ICU utilization, or length of hospital stay.

KEY POINT

- Indicators for activating rapid response teams may include changes in vital signs (heart rate of <30/min or ≥139/min; systolic blood pressure <70 mm Hg or ≥200 mm Hg; respiration rate <9/min or >35/min, temperature <34.0 °C [93.2 °F] or ≥39.0 °C [102.2 °F]), oxygen saturation less than 85%, and development of altered mental status or coma

Bibliography

Winters BD, Weaver SJ, Pfoh ER, Yang T, Pham JC, Dy SM. Rapid-response systems as a patient safety strategy: a systematic review. Ann Intern Med. 2013 Mar 5;158(5 Pt 2):417-25. [PMID: 23460099]

Item 90   Answer: D

Educational Objective: Treat shift work sleep disorder.

The most appropriate management is sleep hygiene counseling. This patient has symptoms of shift work sleep disorder, in which sleepiness and fatigue occur during the nighttime work shift and insomnia occurs during the daytime sleep period. The first step in management is to address sleep-related behaviors and the sleep environment, referred to as sleep hygiene. Strategies that may be useful include caffeinated beverages and bright light exposure during the evening work shift; avoiding direct sunlight in the early morning (by using sunglasses and darkening the bedroom); avoiding exertion, eating, and alcohol prior to the morning sleep period; and, if feasible, considering a short (30-minute) nap overnight, perhaps during a meal break.

Modafinil, a novel stimulant, is approved for use in shift work sleep disorder. However, it should be considered only after conservative measures such as sleep hygiene counseling are tried. Modafinil is limited by cost and side effects, which include headache, anxiety, and (rarely) serious skin reactions.

Multiple sleep latency testing (MSLT) is a laboratory-based sleep test that objectively measures sleepiness and is used primarily as a diagnostic aid in testing for narcolepsy or idiopathic hypersomnia. MSLT should not be performed in sleep-deprived patients. There is no indication for MSLT in this patient.

Polysomnography is indicated when there is strong pretest evidence of a primary sleep disorder, such as sleep-disordered breathing. Because of this patient's lack of previous symptoms and association of her symptoms with her work schedule, there is low suspicion for an underlying sleep problem requiring diagnosis by polysomnography. However, if her symptoms persist following conservative therapy, in-laboratory polysomnography could be considered for a more comprehensive evaluation.

Hypnotic medications such as zolpidem have been used empirically to aid sleep initiation following a night shift, but their efficacy is not well known. Furthermore, there is increasing concern about side effects and complex behaviors (sleep driving and sleep eating) associated with hypnotics in patients who may be sleep-deprived. A short course of hypnotics could be considered, but only after conservative measures, such as sleep hygiene counseling, are attempted.

KEY POINT

- The first step in management of shift work sleep disorder is to address sleep-related behaviors and the sleep environment, referred to as sleep hygiene.

Bibliography

Morgenthaler TI, Lee-Chion T, Alessi C, et al; Standards of Practice Committee of the American Academy of Sleep Medicine. Practice parameters for the clinical evaluation and treatment of circadian rhythm sleep disorders. An American Academy of Sleep Medicine Report. Sleep. 2007 Nov;30(11):1445-59. Erratum in: Sleep. 2008 Jul 1;31(7):table of contents. [PMID: 18041479]

Item 91   Answer: A

Educational Objective: Diagnose hypersensitivity pneumonitis.

The most likely diagnosis is acute hypersensitivity pneumonitis (HP). HP is the result of an immunologic response to repetitive inhalation of antigens. Acute HP presents within 48 hours of a high-level exposure and is often associated with fever, flulike symptoms, cough, and shortness of breath. Radiographic imaging can demonstrate bilateral hazy opacities, and high-resolution CT imaging of the chest shows findings of ground-glass opacities and centrilobular micronodules that are upper- and mid-lobe predominant. Symptoms typically wane within 24 to 48 hours after removal from the exposure. Recurrence of symptoms with exposure to the respiratory antigen is the hallmark of this disorder, and careful attention to the history helps identify the cause. This patient presents with a known or likely exposure to a possible antigen related to his work as a timber trimmer (exposure to agricultural dusts that can readily become colonized with mold), symptoms occurring shortly after possible exposure, a history of similar symptoms, and inspiratory crackles on examination. This constellation of signs and symptoms in conjunction with the radiographic appearance makes HP the most likely diagnosis.

Acute interstitial pneumonia (AIP) is an uncommon form of diffuse lung injury that develops in response to an often unknown insult over a short period of time (days to weeks). Clinically, AIP presents with findings similar to the acute respiratory distress syndrome (ARDS), with severe and progressive hypoxia and imaging showing diffuse bilateral air space opacification. Although the time course of this patient's presentation might be consistent with this diagnosis, his other clinical findings do not support a diagnosis of AIP.

Idiopathic pulmonary fibrosis typically presents in older individuals, and its presentation is more chronic, usually with symptom duration greater than 6 months at the time of presentation. It is therefore not a likely diagnosis in this patient.

Although nonspecific interstitial pneumonia presents in younger patients such as this one, it typically presents as a chronic, rather than acute, process.

KEY POINT

- Acute hypersensitivity pneumonitis presents within 48 hours of a high-level exposure to respiratory antigens and often is associated with fever, flulike symptoms, cough, and shortness of breath; high-resolution CT imaging of the chest shows findings of ground-glass opacities and centrilobular micronodules that are upper- and mid-lobe predominant.

Bibliography

Lacasse Y, Girard M, Cormier Y. Recent advances in hypersensitivity pneumonitis. Chest. 2012 Jul;142(1):208-17. [PMID: 22796841]

Item 92   Answer: D

Educational Objective: Treat a patient with a recent COPD exacerbation with pulmonary rehabilitation.

The most appropriate treatment is to start pulmonary rehabilitation. Pulmonary rehabilitation is recommended for all symptomatic patients with COPD and an FEV_1 less than 50% of predicted and specifically for those hospitalized with an acute exacerbation of COPD. Pulmonary rehabilitation may also be considered in symptomatic or exercise-limited patients with an FEV_1 greater than or equal to 50% of predicted, such as this patient. This patient has had a recent acute exacerbation, has diminished exercise capacity, and is on maximal medical treatment; therefore, she would benefit from pulmonary rehabilitation.

Roflumilast is indicated only in patients with severe or very severe COPD with recurrent exacerbations. This is this patient's first exacerbation, and this treatment is therefore not indicated.

Long-term glucocorticoid therapy is not indicated in patients with COPD owing to serious side effects; however, short-term use is helpful during an acute exacerbation. A recent study showed that, in addition to optimizing COPD therapy, a 5-day course of an oral glucocorticoid is adequate for most patients with COPD exacerbation. Increasing the duration of therapy by an additional 5 days would not likely be of benefit because this patient is completing a 5-day course of glucocorticoids, her symptoms have already improved, and the anti-inflammatory effect of glucocorticoids extends beyond completion of the course of medication.

Long-term oxygen therapy is indicated in patients with an arterial P_{O_2} at or below 55 mm Hg (7.3 kPa) or oxygen saturation breathing ambient air at or below 88% (confirmed twice over a 3-week period), with or without hypercapnia. Other indications are evidence of pulmonary hypertension, peripheral edema suggesting right-sided heart failure, or polycythemia, in combination with an arterial P_{O_2} less than 60 mm Hg (8.0 kPa), or oxygen saturation less than 88% breathing ambient air. This patient's oxygen saturation is 92% breathing ambient air; therefore, oxygen supplementation is not currently indicated.

KEY POINT

- Pulmonary rehabilitation is recommended for all symptomatic patients with COPD who have an FEV_1 less than 50% of predicted and specifically for those hospitalized with an acute COPD exacerbation; it may also be considered for symptomatic or exercise-limited patients with an FEV_1 greater than or equal to 50% of predicted.

Bibliography

Spruit MA, Singh SJ, Garvey C, et al; ATS/ERS Task Force on Pulmonary Rehabilitation. An official American Thoracic Society/European Respiratory Society statement: key concepts and advances in pulmonary rehabilitation. Am J Respir Crit Care Med. 2013 Oct 15;188(8):e13-64. Erratum in: Am J Respir Crit Care Med. 2014 Jun 15;189(12):1570. [PMID: 24127811]

Item 93   Answer: D

Educational Objective: Manage anemia in the ICU setting.

The most appropriate management of this patient's anemia is to not transfuse. This patient is hemodynamically stable with no evidence of active bleeding. The decision to transfuse erythrocytes should be based on hemodynamic parameters, the acuity of anemia, coexisting medical problems, and ongoing blood loss. In patients with critical illness, restricting blood transfusions for a hemoglobin of less than 7 g/dL (70 g/L) significantly reduces cardiac events, rebleeding, bacterial infections, and total mortality as compared with a less restrictive strategy allowing transfusion at higher hemoglobin levels. Four critical care organizations (the American College of Chest Physicians, the American Thoracic Society, the Society of Critical Care Medicine, and the Association of Critical Care Nurses) recommend avoiding transfusion of erythrocytes in nonbleeding, hemodynamically stable

patients with a hemoglobin concentration greater than 7 g/dL (70 g/L). Because this patient's hemoglobin is above the recommended threshold and he is hemodynamically stable with no clinical findings suggesting the need for increased oxygen-carrying capacity, transfusion is not indicated.

The recommendation to avoid transfusion in nonbleeding, hemodynamically stable patients has been included in the Choosing Wisely Campaign, an initiative of the American Board of Internal Medicine Foundation to encourage physicians, patients, and other health care agencies to consider the risks and benefits of medical tests and procedures, noting that all tests may not be necessary and some, in fact, may cause harm. Part of the initiative is to help physicians be better stewards of finite health care resources.

The erythropoiesis-stimulating agents (ESAs) should be considered for patients with chronic kidney disease (CKD) and symptomatic anemia attributable to erythropoietin deficiency when the hemoglobin level is less than 10 g/dL (100 g/L). Before attributing anemia to CKD, it is important to exclude other causes. Iron deficiency is common in patients with CKD. ESAs are associated with an increased risk of thrombotic and cardiovascular events as well as increased blood pressure and are generally not an appropriate intervention for a critically ill patient.

KEY POINT

- Do not routinely transfuse erythrocytes in nonbleeding, hemodynamically stable patients in the ICU with a hemoglobin concentration greater than 7 g/dL (70 g/L).

Bibliography

Salpeter SR, Buckley JS, Chatterjee S. Impact of more restrictive blood transfusion strategies on clinical outcomes: a meta-analysis and systematic review. Am J Med. 2014 Feb;127(2):124-131.[PMID: 24331453]

Item 94   Answer: B

Educational Objective: Diagnose obstructive sleep apnea complicating anesthesia.

The most appropriate next step in management is polysomnography in this patient with likely undiagnosed obstructive sleep apnea (OSA). OSA may first come to clinical recognition immediately following a surgical procedure involving general anesthesia and/or narcotic analgesia that exacerbates the underlying pathophysiologic processes that contribute to OSA, and it may present with repeated episodes of postoperative hypoxia or as frank respiratory failure. The increased risk of postoperative complications associated with OSA highlights the importance of identifying the presence of the disorder preoperatively in high-risk patients. This patient has multiple risk factors for OSA, including age, male gender, obesity, hypertension, and a thick neck. His need for reintubation in the postanesthesia period suggests the possible presence of a sleep-related breathing disorder. Therefore, testing with polysomnography is indicated for further evaluation.

Overnight pulse oximetry has not been validated as a method for evaluating for OSA, primarily because of a high rate of false-positive and false-negative results. It would therefore not be an appropriate next study in this patient with a high pretest probability of OSA.

Multiple screening instruments are available that use clinical parameters to assess for the possible presence of OSA; these include the STOP-Bang questionnaire, Sleep Apnea Clinical Score, and the Berlin questionnaire. They are most commonly used to assess risk in patients with symptoms possibly attributable to OSA or as part of preoperative pulmonary assessment. This patient, however, already has a high probability of disease given his known risk factors for OSA along with his postoperative respiratory complications. A low score on a screening instrument would not alter the need for further evaluation.

Not pursuing further diagnostic information in this patient with multiple risk factors accompanied by postoperative pulmonary complications would be inappropriate.

KEY POINT

- Polysomnography is indicated in patients at high risk for obstructive sleep apnea due to the increased risk of postoperative complications, which may manifest as repeated episodes of postoperative hypoxia or frank respiratory failure.

Bibliography

American Society of Anesthesiologists Task Force on Perioperative Management of patients with obstructive sleep apnea. Practice guidelines for the perioperative management of patients with obstructive sleep apnea: an updated report by the American Society of Anesthesiologists Task Force on Perioperative Management of patients with obstructive sleep apnea. Anesthesiology. 2014 Feb;120(2):268-86. [PMID: 24346178]

Item 95   Answer: D

Educational Objective: Diagnose postintensive care syndrome.

The most likely diagnosis is postintensive care syndrome. The patient was severely ill and in an ICU for several days where she was treated for severe sepsis and shock. Postintensive care syndrome is a term used to describe new or worsening function in one or more physical, cognitive, or mental domains that persists after hospital discharge following a critical illness, as in this patient. Examples of clinical findings include cognitive deficits resembling traumatic brain injury or mild cognitive impairment; psychiatric symptoms such as depression, anxiety, and posttraumatic stress disorder (PTSD); and physical deficits such as weakness and fatigue. Although the cause of this syndrome is not understood, possible mechanisms include hypoxia, hypotension, inflammation, the catabolic state, hypoglycemia, other nutritional disorders, immobility, and agents used for sedation. This syndrome may also be applied to symptoms experienced by family members of post-ICU patients who may experience sleep disturbances, anxiety, depression, a complicated grief reaction, and PTSD. The efficacy of preventive measures and

treatment interventions is not known, but efforts to maintain light sedation and avoid glycemic extremes and hypoxia may be of benefit. Treatment otherwise focuses on the specific symptoms experienced by the patient or family.

Critical illness neuromyopathy is a generalized axonal sensorineural polyneuropathy associated with severe illness and treatment in an ICU setting. Although it could explain this patient's physical limitations, it is not associated with psychiatric symptoms such as anxiety or cognitive deficits such as difficulty multitasking.

Similarly, prolonged bed rest in patients in the ICU may result in significant deconditioning and physical limitations following recovery from acute illness; however, it would not be expected to cause problems with psychiatric or cognitive function.

Patients treated in the ICU for severe illness are at increased risk for depression, anxiety, and PTSD, which may result in the psychiatric and cognitive symptoms seen in this patient. Generalized anxiety disorder develops over time and is characterized by excessive worrying about many things of little or no need for concern. Sleep disturbances along with anxiety are reasons patients seek help from their physicians. However, this diagnosis would not explain this patient's overall symptom complex, which includes cognitive limitations and physical symptoms such as weakness.

KEY POINT

- Postintensive care syndrome is a term used to describe new or worsening function in one or more physical, cognitive, or mental domains that persists after hospital discharge following a critical illness.

Bibliography

Needham DM, Davidson J, Cohen H, et al. Improving long-term outcomes after discharge from intensive care unit: report from a stakeholders' conference. Crit Care Med. 2012 Feb;40(2):502-9. [PMID: 21946660]

Item 96   Answer: A   [H]

Educational Objective: Diagnose acute mesenteric ischemia.

The most likely diagnosis is acute mesenteric ischemia. Acute mesenteric ischemia is caused by inadequate blood flow to all or part of the small bowel. Causes include superior mesenteric artery (SMA) embolism, SMA thrombosis, nonocclusive mesenteric ischemia (usually due to splanchnic vasoconstriction), mesenteric venous thrombosis, and focal segmental ischemia. SMA embolism from the left atrium or ventricular mural thrombi is the most common cause. The classic presentation is acute onset of severe abdominal pain; the abdomen is typically soft and less tender than expected based on the patient's symptoms (pain out of proportion to the examination). This patient has many findings that should heighten the suspicion for acute mesenteric ischemia including chronic atrial fibrillation, onset of periumbilical abdominal pain, emesis, hypotension, abdominal pain that is out of proportion to the abdominal examination, and

CONT.

a forceful bowel evacuation. An elevated leukocyte count, metabolic acidosis, and elevated plasma lactate level are common, but their absence should not exclude the diagnosis. Plain abdominal films may be normal early in the course of disease. A high degree of clinical suspicion is necessary to diagnose mesenteric ischemia in time for potentially life-saving interventions to be effective. Immediate surgical consultation and angiography are appropriate for this patient.

Acute pancreatitis is almost always associated with the sudden onset of pain. The pain is generally located in the epigastrium and radiates to the back. Pain is often accompanied by fever, nausea, and repeated vomiting. Although an elevated serum amylase level is usually from a pancreatic source, hyperamylasemia can be seen in a variety of other conditions including intestinal ischemia. This patient's presentation is not typical for acute pancreatitis.

Campylobacter enteritis could account for this patient's abdominal pain, elevated leukocyte count, and hypotension; however, this patient's absence of bloody stools and diarrhea, along with the presence of persistent hypotension, make this diagnosis less likely.

Colonic ischemia comprises 75% of all cases of intestinal ischemia. Typical symptoms are the acute onset of mild, crampy abdominal pain with tenderness on examination over the affected region of colon. Bleeding often occurs within a few days of pain onset. The location of this patient's pain and early vomiting are not compatible with colonic ischemia.

KEY POINT

- The abrupt onset of central abdominal pain, emesis, forceful bowel evacuation, and severe hypotension along with an unremarkable abdominal examination in the setting of atrial fibrillation is highly suggestive of acute embolic mesenteric ischemia.

Bibliography

Wyers MC. Acute mesenteric ischemia: diagnostic approach and surgical treatment. Semin Vasc Surg. 2010 Mar;23(1):9-20. [PMID: 20298945]

 ### Item 97   Answer: C

Educational Objective: Manage acute respiratory distress syndrome using positive end-expiratory pressure.

The most appropriate management is to increase the positive end-expiratory pressure (PEEP). This patient is hypoxic due to acute respiratory distress syndrome (ARDS). Her gas exchange has worsened to the point of an arterial Po_2/FiO_2 ratio of 54 mm Hg (7.2 kPa), which indicates very severe ARDS. PEEP improves lung compliance, ventilation-perfusion (V/Q) matching, and oxygenation. A 2013 systematic review found no difference in survival using higher PEEP (approximately 15 cm H_2O) versus lower PEEP (approximately 8 cm H_2O); however, the patients with the most severe ARDS did show improvement in oxygenation when treated with

higher PEEP, but there was no improvement in the number of ventilator-free days. Current recommendations are to use a PEEP level that achieves adequate oxygenation with an FiO_2 of less than 0.6 and does not cause hypotension.

Decreasing the tidal volume could be considered a lung-protective measure, but this patient's tidal volume is already at the target of 6 mL/kg of ideal body weight. Reducing the tidal volume further will likely result in greater alveolar hypoventilation and increasing hypoxemia.

Prone positioning is a maneuver for improving oxygenation, and may be helpful in patients with ARDS in whom it is difficult to maintain adequate levels of oxygenation. However, its effect on oxygenation is slow, and it would not be the best next step toward improving this patient's gas exchange.

Increasing the set respiration rate on the ventilator probably would not improve this patient's oxygenation unless it induced auto-PEEP, which would raise the effective PEEP level indirectly. This would not be the best way to recruit alveoli, however, because the auto-PEEP in this situation is impossible to regulate as lung mechanics change over time. It is safer and more reliable to raise the set level of PEEP.

KEY POINT

- In patients with severe acute respiratory distress syndrome, current recommendations are to use a positive end-expiratory pressure level that achieves adequate oxygenation with an FiO_2 of less than 0.6 and does not cause hypotension.

Bibliography

Santa Cruz R, Rojas JI, Nervi R, Heredia R, Ciapponi A. High versus low positive end-expiratory pressure (PEEP) levels for mechanically ventilated adult patients with acute lung injury and acute respiratory distress syndrome. Cochrane Database Syst Rev. 2013 Jun 6;6:CD009098. [PMID: 23740697]

Item 98   Answer: B

Educational Objective: Recommend appropriate influenza and pneumococcal vaccinations in a patient with COPD.

This patient should receive inactivated influenza vaccine and 23-valent polysaccharide pneumococcal vaccine (PPSV23). Influenza vaccination has been shown to reduce serious illness (such as lower respiratory tract infections that require hospitalization) and death in patients with COPD. These vaccines should be administered annually in all patients with COPD. Pneumococcal vaccination with PPSV23 should be given to all patients aged 19 to 64 years with COPD, with revaccination at age 65 years if 5 years have elapsed since the previous pneumococcal immunization. All patients (with or without COPD) should also receive the 13-valent pneumococcal conjugate vaccine (PCV13) at age 65 years, although the polysaccharide and conjugate vaccines should be given sequentially rather than together for optimal effect. Ideally, PCV13 should be administered at least 1 year following PPSV23. PPSV23 and PCV13 are also indicated in patients with functional or anatomic asplenia, cochlear implants, persistent cerebrospinal fluid leak, and significant immuno-compromising conditions. Preferably, these patients should receive PCV13 first followed by PPSV23 at least 8 weeks later. This patient will require another dose of PPSV23 at the age of 65 years. Patients with COPD who received their first PPSV23 dose at age 65 years or older do not require revaccination.

Because this patient is younger than 65 years, she does not require the PCV13 vaccination at this time.

The live attenuated influenza vaccination is recommended for healthy persons between the ages of 2 and 49 years. Because this patient has COPD and because she is older than 49 years, live attenuated influenza vaccination should not be administered.

KEY POINT

- Patients with COPD should receive inactivated influenza vaccination annually, and the 23-valent polysaccharide pneumococcal vaccine (PPSV23) should be given to all patients aged 19 to 64 years with COPD, with revaccination at age 65 years or older if 5 years have elapsed since the previous pneumococcal immunization; the 13-valent pneumococcal conjugate vaccine should also be administered at age 65 years or older if 1 year has elapsed since the last PPSV23 immunization.

Bibliography

Bridges CB, Coyne-Beasley T; Advisory Committee on Immunization Practices. Advisory committee on immunization practices recommended immunization schedule for adults aged 19 years or older: United States, 2014. Ann Intern Med. 2014 Feb 4;160(3):190. [PMID: 24658695]

Item 99   Answer: E

Educational Objective: Manage auto-positive end-expiratory pressure.

The most appropriate immediate next step in management is to disconnect the endotracheal tube from the ventilator circuit and reconnect it after a few seconds. This patient has developed severe auto-positive end-expiratory pressure (auto-PEEP) as a result of breath stacking on the ventilator due to her obstructive lung disease. The intrathoracic pressure has risen to the point of impairing her central venous return, so her cardiac output is falling because of inadequate preload. Her oxygenation has worsened, owing to both her low cardiac output and to ventilation-perfusion mismatch in the lungs resulting from hyperinflation. The most immediate need is to release the pressure by disconnecting the ventilator circuit and allowing her to passively exhale for several seconds. The ventilator should then be reconnected and the settings changed to allow for more expiratory time.

Slowing the respiration rate, decreasing the tidal volume, and increasing the inspiratory flow rate while tolerating respiratory acidosis are strategies to increase the exhaled volume with each cycle. However, these interventions are

not appropriate until after the increased intrathoracic pressure is released by temporarily disconnecting the ventilator circuit. This patient's unstable condition must be addressed before changes to the ventilator settings will be helpful.

Similarly, increased sedation and preparation for therapeutic paralysis may be useful for this patient, but her increased intrathoracic pressure must be released before other interventions are pursued.

KEY POINT

- If auto-positive end-expiratory pressure (auto-PEEP) is observed in a patient on mechanical ventilation, the most appropriate initial intervention is to disconnect the ventilator circuit from the patient's endotracheal tube for a few seconds to allow for a prolonged exhalation to release the increased intrathoracic pressure.

Bibliography

Brochard L. Intrinsic (or auto-) positive end-expiratory pressure during spontaneous or assisted ventilation. Intensive Care Med. 2002 Nov;28(11):1552-4. [PMID: 12583374]

Item 100   Answer: B

Educational Objective: Treat acute respiratory distress syndrome using a lung-protective ventilator strategy.

The intervention most likely to improve this patient's chance of survival is maintaining the tidal volume at 360 mL. This patient has acute respiratory distress syndrome (ARDS); he meets the criteria for ARDS with bilateral lung opacities and very poor oxygenation with an arterial P_{O_2}/F_{IO_2} ratio of 101 mm Hg (13.4 kPa). Very few interventions have evidence supporting a survival benefit in ARDS, but the mainstay of management is a lung-protective ventilator strategy, with low tidal volume (6 mL/kg of ideal body weight [IBW]) and low plateau pressure (<30 cm H_2O). Other interventions with supporting evidence include a conservative fluid strategy to keep the lungs as dry as possible, prone positioning, and early therapeutic paralysis (for the first 48 hours) if severely hypoxemic.

The physiologic result of reducing the tidal volume would be a lower minute ventilation, and the P_{CO_2} would likely rise further above its current elevated level, resulting in an additional decrease in arterial pH. Allowing hypercapnia to achieve lung-protective ventilation goals in ARDS (termed permissive hypercapnia) is acceptable and even desirable if it means ventilating at lower tidal volumes and plateau pressures despite causing a reduction in arterial pH. In general, a pH as low as 7.25 is considered acceptable in this situation; however, decreasing the minute ventilation would likely lower the pH below this level. Some evidence exists that hypercapnia may also be protective in ARDS independent of the low tidal volume strategy that causes it, but this is controversial.

Raising the tidal volume would improve the abnormal P_{CO_2}, but might cause greater injury to the lung tissue, leading to higher risk of mortality.

- The mainstay of management for acute respiratory distress syndrome is a lung-protective ventilator strategy, with low tidal volume (6 mL/kg of ideal body weight) and low plateau pressure (<30 cm H_2O), even if this results in hypercapnia.

Bibliography

Laffey JG, O'Croinin D, McLoughlin P, Kavanagh BP. Permissive hypercapnia-role in protective lung ventilatory strategies. Intensive Care Med. 2004 Mar;30(3):347-56. [PMID: 14722644]

Item 101   Answer: C

Educational Objective: Diagnose idiopathic pulmonary fibrosis.

The most likely diagnosis is idiopathic pulmonary fibrosis (IPF). This patient's presentation of progressively worsening cough and dyspnea is typical for this rare disease. He has multiple risk factors, including smoking history, organic dust exposure from his previous work as a carpenter, and current age; the prevalence of IPF increases significantly with each decade of life, and the disease essentially only affects individuals who are older than 50 years. This is important because an individual younger than 40 years who presents with similar symptoms has a significantly higher likelihood of an alternative cause, such as connective tissue disease-related pulmonary disease. Therefore, in younger patients with a similar presentation, more intensive screening for autoimmune disorders may be appropriate. In addition, this patient's high-resolution CT (HRCT) findings are classic for usual interstitial pneumonia (UIP), which is the typical pathologic correlate of IPF. A definite UIP pattern on CT imaging in a patient whose clinical history does not suggest an underlying alternative disorder is consistent with a diagnosis of IPF.

Although this patient is at risk for COPD because of his smoking history, his pulmonary function tests show a normal FEV_1/FVC ratio. Clubbing is also noted on physical examination. Although the etiology of clubbing remains unclear, this is more commonly reported in patients with diffuse parenchymal lung disease rather than COPD. Most importantly, CT imaging is not consistent with the findings usually seen with COPD.

Hypersensitivity pneumonitis presents in acute and chronic forms. This patient's presentation is not consistent with acute disease given the lack of flulike symptoms. The chronic form of the disease can present similarly to IPF, but this patient lacks a history of a clear ongoing exposure to a likely offending agent associated with hypersensitivity pneumonitis (such as organic antigens from domestic birds), and his CT findings are basal predominant. Hypersensitivity pneumonitis typically affects the upper and mid-lung zones, and micronodules are often present.

Respiratory bronchiolitis–associated interstitial lung disease is strongly associated with smoking exposure. However, the CT imaging demonstrates mid to upper lung–predomi-

nant centrilobular micronodules. Although advanced cases can be associated with septal line thickening and scarring, the distribution on the CT scan is not consistent with this.

- Idiopathic pulmonary fibrosis is characterized by progressive dyspnea and cough, with high-resolution CT findings of peripheral- and basal-predominant septal line thickening and honeycomb change; risk factors include smoking history, organic dust exposure, and older age.

Bibliography

Raghu G, Collard HR, Egan JJ, et al; ATS/ERS/JRS/ALAT Committee on Idiopathic Pulmonary Fibrosis. An official ATS/ERS/JRS/ALAT statement: idiopathic pulmonary fibrosis: evidence-based guidelines for diagnosis and management. Am J Respir Crit Care Med. 2011 Mar 15;183(6):788-824. [PMID: 21471066]

Item 102   Answer: D

Educational Objective: Diagnose and stage lung cancer.

The most appropriate diagnostic test to perform next is needle aspiration of the left supraclavicular lymph nodes. Given this patient's significant smoking history and his imaging findings consistent with a pulmonary mass and associated lymphadenopathy, he has a high pretest probability of primary lung cancer. The most appropriate diagnostic test is the one that not only confirms the diagnosis but also provides adequate staging to help plan treatment options. Needle aspiration of the left supraclavicular lymph nodes is the least invasive procedure, and it would also stage the likely malignancy by documenting metastatic disease to these lymph nodes.

Bronchoscopy with needle aspiration of the mediastinal lymph nodes would both diagnose and provide some information about staging. However, it is more invasive than aspiration of the palpable supraclavicular lymph nodes.

Bronchoscopy with transbronchial biopsy of the left apical mass may be technically difficult given the apical position of the mass. However, more importantly, it would not provide any information about possible metastases to the lymph nodes.

CT-guided needle biopsy could potentially diagnose the patient with lung cancer. However, the needle would need to pass through normal lung tissue, which carries a risk of inducing pneumothorax. In addition, similar to bronchoscopy with transbronchial biopsy of the left apical mass, it would not provide information on staging because it would not assess whether there is involvement of the mediastinal or supraclavicular lymph nodes.

- The most appropriate diagnostic test for lung cancer is the one that not only confirms the diagnosis in the least invasive fashion but also provides adequate staging to help plan treatment options.

Bibliography

Alberts WM; American College of Chest Physicians. Diagnosis and management of lung cancer executive summary: ACCP evidence-based clinical practice guidelines (2nd Edition). Chest. 2007 Sep;132(3 Suppl):1S-19S. [PMID: 17873156]

Item 103   Answer: D

Educational Objective: Treat high-altitude pulmonary edema.

The most appropriate adjunctive treatment is nifedipine. This patient is exhibiting signs of high-altitude pulmonary edema (HAPE). The mechanism of HAPE is believed to be a noncardiogenic exaggerated hypoxic vasoconstriction of the pulmonary vasculature. HAPE usually occurs at altitudes in excess of 2500 meters (8200 feet). Typical symptoms consist of cough, dyspnea, and exertional intolerance; symptoms are usually insidious in onset but may occasionally occur abruptly and awaken a patient from sleep. Other features, such as headache, fatigue, nausea, vomiting, and disturbed sleep, may or may not be present. Dyspnea at rest is a key feature of HAPE. On physical examination, tachypnea and tachycardia are typical, and crackles or wheezing can be auscultated. Pink frothy sputum or frank hemoptysis may occur, followed by worsening gas exchange and possibly respiratory failure. Treatment is with supplemental oxygen and rest, both of which will acutely reduce pulmonary artery pressures. Descent from altitude should be considered, particularly if oxygen is not available. Adjunctive therapies include vasodilators such as nifedipine or phosphodiesterase-5 inhibitors (sildenafil or tadalafil). Nifedipine may act by relaxing vascular smooth muscle and can be used as a treatment as well as a preventive agent in patients who have previously experienced HAPE.

Acetazolamide is the preferred drug for preventing acute mountain sickness and high-altitude cerebral edema, but it is not useful in preventing HAPE.

Dexamethasone is the preferred drug (in addition to supplemental oxygen) for the treatment of severe acute mountain sickness and high-altitude cerebral edema. It is not effective in the treatment of HAPE.

Ibuprofen is a reasonable first choice for symptoms of mild acute mountain sickness such as headache and nausea; however, it is not useful in treating HAPE.

KEY POINT

- Treatment of high-altitude pulmonary edema is with supplemental oxygen, rest, and consideration of descent from altitude; vasodilators such as nifedipine can be used as adjunctive treatment.

Bibliography

Bärtsch P, Swenson ER. Clinical practice: Acute high-altitude illnesses. N Engl J Med. 2013 Jun 13;368(24):2294-302. [PMID: 23758234]

Index

A

NAME AND ADDRESS (Please complete.)

Last Name   First Name   Middle Initial

Address

Address cont.

City   State   ZIP Code

Country

Email address

ACP®

American College of Physicians
Leading Internal Medicine, Improving Lives

Medical Knowledge Self-Assessment Program® 17

TO EARN *AMA PRA CATEGORY 1 CREDITS*™ YOU MUST:

1. Answer all questions.
2. Score a minimum of 50% correct.

==

TO EARN *FREE* INSTANTANEOUS *AMA PRA CATEGORY 1 CREDITS*™ ONLINE:

1. Answer all of your questions.
2. Go to **mksap.acponline.org** and enter your ACP Online username and password to access an online answer sheet.
3. Enter your answers.
4. You can also enter your answers directly at **mksap.acponline.org** without first using this answer sheet.

To Submit Your Answer Sheet by Mail or FAX for a $15 Administrative Fee per Answer Sheet:

1. Answer all of your questions and calculate your score.
2. Complete boxes A–F.
3. Complete payment information.
4. Send the answer sheet and payment information to ACP, using the FAX number/address listed below.

B

Order Number

(Use the Order Number on your MKSAP materials packing slip.)

C

ACP ID Number

(Refer to packing slip in your MKSAP materials for your ACP ID Number.)

COMPLETE FORM BELOW ONLY IF YOU SUBMIT BY MAIL OR FAX

Last Name   First Name   MI

Payment Information. Must remit in US funds, drawn on a US bank.

The processing fee for each paper answer sheet is $15.

☐ Check, made payable to ACP, enclosed

Charge to   ☐ **VISA**   ☐ **MasterCard**   ☐ **American Express**   ☐ **DISCOVER**

Card Number _____

Expiration Date _____ / _____   Security code (3 or 4 digit #s) _____
              MM   YY

Signature _____

Fax to: 215-351-2799

Mail to:
Member and Customer Service
American College of Physicians
190 N. Independence Mall West
Philadelphia, PA 19106-1572

1 Ⓐ Ⓑ Ⓒ Ⓓ Ⓔ
2 Ⓐ Ⓑ Ⓒ Ⓓ Ⓔ
3 Ⓐ Ⓑ Ⓒ Ⓓ Ⓔ
4 Ⓐ Ⓑ Ⓒ Ⓓ Ⓔ
5 Ⓐ Ⓑ Ⓒ Ⓓ Ⓔ

6 Ⓐ Ⓑ Ⓒ Ⓓ Ⓔ
7 Ⓐ Ⓑ Ⓒ Ⓓ Ⓔ
8 Ⓐ Ⓑ Ⓒ Ⓓ Ⓔ
9 Ⓐ Ⓑ Ⓒ Ⓓ Ⓔ
10 Ⓐ Ⓑ Ⓒ Ⓓ Ⓔ

11 Ⓐ Ⓑ Ⓒ Ⓓ Ⓔ
12 Ⓐ Ⓑ Ⓒ Ⓓ Ⓔ
13 Ⓐ Ⓑ Ⓒ Ⓓ Ⓔ
14 Ⓐ Ⓑ Ⓒ Ⓓ Ⓔ
15 Ⓐ Ⓑ Ⓒ Ⓓ Ⓔ

16 Ⓐ Ⓑ Ⓒ Ⓓ Ⓔ
17 Ⓐ Ⓑ Ⓒ Ⓓ Ⓔ
18 Ⓐ Ⓑ Ⓒ Ⓓ Ⓔ
19 Ⓐ Ⓑ Ⓒ Ⓓ Ⓔ
20 Ⓐ Ⓑ Ⓒ Ⓓ Ⓔ

21 Ⓐ Ⓑ Ⓒ Ⓓ Ⓔ
22 Ⓐ Ⓑ Ⓒ Ⓓ Ⓔ
23 Ⓐ Ⓑ Ⓒ Ⓓ Ⓔ
24 Ⓐ Ⓑ Ⓒ Ⓓ Ⓔ
25 Ⓐ Ⓑ Ⓒ Ⓓ Ⓔ

26 Ⓐ Ⓑ Ⓒ Ⓓ Ⓔ
27 Ⓐ Ⓑ Ⓒ Ⓓ Ⓔ
28 Ⓐ Ⓑ Ⓒ Ⓓ Ⓔ
29 Ⓐ Ⓑ Ⓒ Ⓓ Ⓔ
30 Ⓐ Ⓑ Ⓒ Ⓓ Ⓔ

31 Ⓐ Ⓑ Ⓒ Ⓓ Ⓔ
32 Ⓐ Ⓑ Ⓒ Ⓓ Ⓔ
33 Ⓐ Ⓑ Ⓒ Ⓓ Ⓔ
34 Ⓐ Ⓑ Ⓒ Ⓓ Ⓔ
35 Ⓐ Ⓑ Ⓒ Ⓓ Ⓔ

36 Ⓐ Ⓑ Ⓒ Ⓓ Ⓔ
37 Ⓐ Ⓑ Ⓒ Ⓓ Ⓔ
38 Ⓐ Ⓑ Ⓒ Ⓓ Ⓔ
39 Ⓐ Ⓑ Ⓒ Ⓓ Ⓔ
40 Ⓐ Ⓑ Ⓒ Ⓓ Ⓔ

41 Ⓐ Ⓑ Ⓒ Ⓓ Ⓔ
42 Ⓐ Ⓑ Ⓒ Ⓓ Ⓔ
43 Ⓐ Ⓑ Ⓒ Ⓓ Ⓔ
44 Ⓐ Ⓑ Ⓒ Ⓓ Ⓔ
45 Ⓐ Ⓑ Ⓒ Ⓓ Ⓔ

46 Ⓐ Ⓑ Ⓒ Ⓓ Ⓔ
47 Ⓐ Ⓑ Ⓒ Ⓓ Ⓔ
48 Ⓐ Ⓑ Ⓒ Ⓓ Ⓔ
49 Ⓐ Ⓑ Ⓒ Ⓓ Ⓔ
50 Ⓐ Ⓑ Ⓒ Ⓓ Ⓔ

51 Ⓐ Ⓑ Ⓒ Ⓓ Ⓔ
52 Ⓐ Ⓑ Ⓒ Ⓓ Ⓔ
53 Ⓐ Ⓑ Ⓒ Ⓓ Ⓔ
54 Ⓐ Ⓑ Ⓒ Ⓓ Ⓔ
55 Ⓐ Ⓑ Ⓒ Ⓓ Ⓔ

56 Ⓐ Ⓑ Ⓒ Ⓓ Ⓔ
57 Ⓐ Ⓑ Ⓒ Ⓓ Ⓔ
58 Ⓐ Ⓑ Ⓒ Ⓓ Ⓔ
59 Ⓐ Ⓑ Ⓒ Ⓓ Ⓔ
60 Ⓐ Ⓑ Ⓒ Ⓓ Ⓔ

61 Ⓐ Ⓑ Ⓒ Ⓓ Ⓔ
62 Ⓐ Ⓑ Ⓒ Ⓓ Ⓔ
63 Ⓐ Ⓑ Ⓒ Ⓓ Ⓔ
64 Ⓐ Ⓑ Ⓒ Ⓓ Ⓔ
65 Ⓐ Ⓑ Ⓒ Ⓓ Ⓔ

66 Ⓐ Ⓑ Ⓒ Ⓓ Ⓔ
67 Ⓐ Ⓑ Ⓒ Ⓓ Ⓔ
68 Ⓐ Ⓑ Ⓒ Ⓓ Ⓔ
69 Ⓐ Ⓑ Ⓒ Ⓓ Ⓔ
70 Ⓐ Ⓑ Ⓒ Ⓓ Ⓔ

71 Ⓐ Ⓑ Ⓒ Ⓓ Ⓔ
72 Ⓐ Ⓑ Ⓒ Ⓓ Ⓔ
73 Ⓐ Ⓑ Ⓒ Ⓓ Ⓔ
74 Ⓐ Ⓑ Ⓒ Ⓓ Ⓔ
75 Ⓐ Ⓑ Ⓒ Ⓓ Ⓔ

76 Ⓐ Ⓑ Ⓒ Ⓓ Ⓔ
77 Ⓐ Ⓑ Ⓒ Ⓓ Ⓔ
78 Ⓐ Ⓑ Ⓒ Ⓓ Ⓔ
79 Ⓐ Ⓑ Ⓒ Ⓓ Ⓔ
80 Ⓐ Ⓑ Ⓒ Ⓓ Ⓔ

81 Ⓐ Ⓑ Ⓒ Ⓓ Ⓔ
82 Ⓐ Ⓑ Ⓒ Ⓓ Ⓔ
83 Ⓐ Ⓑ Ⓒ Ⓓ Ⓔ
84 Ⓐ Ⓑ Ⓒ Ⓓ Ⓔ
85 Ⓐ Ⓑ Ⓒ Ⓓ Ⓔ

86 Ⓐ Ⓑ Ⓒ Ⓓ Ⓔ
87 Ⓐ Ⓑ Ⓒ Ⓓ Ⓔ
88 Ⓐ Ⓑ Ⓒ Ⓓ Ⓔ
89 Ⓐ Ⓑ Ⓒ Ⓓ Ⓔ
90 Ⓐ Ⓑ Ⓒ Ⓓ Ⓔ

91 Ⓐ Ⓑ Ⓒ Ⓓ Ⓔ
92 Ⓐ Ⓑ Ⓒ Ⓓ Ⓔ
93 Ⓐ Ⓑ Ⓒ Ⓓ Ⓔ
94 Ⓐ Ⓑ Ⓒ Ⓓ Ⓔ
95 Ⓐ Ⓑ Ⓒ Ⓓ Ⓔ

96 Ⓐ Ⓑ Ⓒ Ⓓ Ⓔ
97 Ⓐ Ⓑ Ⓒ Ⓓ Ⓔ
98 Ⓐ Ⓑ Ⓒ Ⓓ Ⓔ
99 Ⓐ Ⓑ Ⓒ Ⓓ Ⓔ
100 Ⓐ Ⓑ Ⓒ Ⓓ Ⓔ

101 Ⓐ Ⓑ Ⓒ Ⓓ Ⓔ
102 Ⓐ Ⓑ Ⓒ Ⓓ Ⓔ
103 Ⓐ Ⓑ Ⓒ Ⓓ Ⓔ
104 Ⓐ Ⓑ Ⓒ Ⓓ Ⓔ
105 Ⓐ Ⓑ Ⓒ Ⓓ Ⓔ

106 Ⓐ Ⓑ Ⓒ Ⓓ Ⓔ
107 Ⓐ Ⓑ Ⓒ Ⓓ Ⓔ
108 Ⓐ Ⓑ Ⓒ Ⓓ Ⓔ
109 Ⓐ Ⓑ Ⓒ Ⓓ Ⓔ
110 Ⓐ Ⓑ Ⓒ Ⓓ Ⓔ

111 Ⓐ Ⓑ Ⓒ Ⓓ Ⓔ
112 Ⓐ Ⓑ Ⓒ Ⓓ Ⓔ
113 Ⓐ Ⓑ Ⓒ Ⓓ Ⓔ
114 Ⓐ Ⓑ Ⓒ Ⓓ Ⓔ
115 Ⓐ Ⓑ Ⓒ Ⓓ Ⓔ

116 Ⓐ Ⓑ Ⓒ Ⓓ Ⓔ
117 Ⓐ Ⓑ Ⓒ Ⓓ Ⓔ
118 Ⓐ Ⓑ Ⓒ Ⓓ Ⓔ
119 Ⓐ Ⓑ Ⓒ Ⓓ Ⓔ
120 Ⓐ Ⓑ Ⓒ Ⓓ Ⓔ

121 Ⓐ Ⓑ Ⓒ Ⓓ Ⓔ
122 Ⓐ Ⓑ Ⓒ Ⓓ Ⓔ
123 Ⓐ Ⓑ Ⓒ Ⓓ Ⓔ
124 Ⓐ Ⓑ Ⓒ Ⓓ Ⓔ
125 Ⓐ Ⓑ Ⓒ Ⓓ Ⓔ

126 Ⓐ Ⓑ Ⓒ Ⓓ Ⓔ
127 Ⓐ Ⓑ Ⓒ Ⓓ Ⓔ
128 Ⓐ Ⓑ Ⓒ Ⓓ Ⓔ
129 Ⓐ Ⓑ Ⓒ Ⓓ Ⓔ
130 Ⓐ Ⓑ Ⓒ Ⓓ Ⓔ

131 Ⓐ Ⓑ Ⓒ Ⓓ Ⓔ
132 Ⓐ Ⓑ Ⓒ Ⓓ Ⓔ
133 Ⓐ Ⓑ Ⓒ Ⓓ Ⓔ
134 Ⓐ Ⓑ Ⓒ Ⓓ Ⓔ
135 Ⓐ Ⓑ Ⓒ Ⓓ Ⓔ

136 Ⓐ Ⓑ Ⓒ Ⓓ Ⓔ
137 Ⓐ Ⓑ Ⓒ Ⓓ Ⓔ
138 Ⓐ Ⓑ Ⓒ Ⓓ Ⓔ
139 Ⓐ Ⓑ Ⓒ Ⓓ Ⓔ
140 Ⓐ Ⓑ Ⓒ Ⓓ Ⓔ

141 Ⓐ Ⓑ Ⓒ Ⓓ Ⓔ
142 Ⓐ Ⓑ Ⓒ Ⓓ Ⓔ
143 Ⓐ Ⓑ Ⓒ Ⓓ Ⓔ
144 Ⓐ Ⓑ Ⓒ Ⓓ Ⓔ
145 Ⓐ Ⓑ Ⓒ Ⓓ Ⓔ

146 Ⓐ Ⓑ Ⓒ Ⓓ Ⓔ
147 Ⓐ Ⓑ Ⓒ Ⓓ Ⓔ
148 Ⓐ Ⓑ Ⓒ Ⓓ Ⓔ
149 Ⓐ Ⓑ Ⓒ Ⓓ Ⓔ
150 Ⓐ Ⓑ Ⓒ Ⓓ Ⓔ

151 Ⓐ Ⓑ Ⓒ Ⓓ Ⓔ
152 Ⓐ Ⓑ Ⓒ Ⓓ Ⓔ
153 Ⓐ Ⓑ Ⓒ Ⓓ Ⓔ
154 Ⓐ Ⓑ Ⓒ Ⓓ Ⓔ
155 Ⓐ Ⓑ Ⓒ Ⓓ Ⓔ

156 Ⓐ Ⓑ Ⓒ Ⓓ Ⓔ
157 Ⓐ Ⓑ Ⓒ Ⓓ Ⓔ
158 Ⓐ Ⓑ Ⓒ Ⓓ Ⓔ
159 Ⓐ Ⓑ Ⓒ Ⓓ Ⓔ
160 Ⓐ Ⓑ Ⓒ Ⓓ Ⓔ

161 Ⓐ Ⓑ Ⓒ Ⓓ Ⓔ
162 Ⓐ Ⓑ Ⓒ Ⓓ Ⓔ
163 Ⓐ Ⓑ Ⓒ Ⓓ Ⓔ
164 Ⓐ Ⓑ Ⓒ Ⓓ Ⓔ
165 Ⓐ Ⓑ Ⓒ Ⓓ Ⓔ

166 Ⓐ Ⓑ Ⓒ Ⓓ Ⓔ
167 Ⓐ Ⓑ Ⓒ Ⓓ Ⓔ
168 Ⓐ Ⓑ Ⓒ Ⓓ Ⓔ
169 Ⓐ Ⓑ Ⓒ Ⓓ Ⓔ
170 Ⓐ Ⓑ Ⓒ Ⓓ Ⓔ

171 Ⓐ Ⓑ Ⓒ Ⓓ Ⓔ
172 Ⓐ Ⓑ Ⓒ Ⓓ Ⓔ
173 Ⓐ Ⓑ Ⓒ Ⓓ Ⓔ
174 Ⓐ Ⓑ Ⓒ Ⓓ Ⓔ
175 Ⓐ Ⓑ Ⓒ Ⓓ Ⓔ

176 Ⓐ Ⓑ Ⓒ Ⓓ Ⓔ
177 Ⓐ Ⓑ Ⓒ Ⓓ Ⓔ
178 Ⓐ Ⓑ Ⓒ Ⓓ Ⓔ
179 Ⓐ Ⓑ Ⓒ Ⓓ Ⓔ
180 Ⓐ Ⓑ Ⓒ Ⓓ Ⓔ

MK4001